SATISFACTION IN CLOSE RELATIONSHIPS

SATISFACTION IN CLOSE RELATIONSHIPS

Edited by
Robert J. Sternberg
Mahzad Hojjat

THE GUILFORD PRESS
New York   London

©1997 The Guilford Press
A Division of Guilford Publications, Inc.
72 Spring Street, New York, NY 10012

Printed in the United States of America

This book is printed on acid-free paper.

Last digit is print number: 9   8   7   6   5   4   3   2   1

Library of Congress Cataloging-in-Publication Data

Satisfaction in close relationships / edited by Robert J. Sternberg
and Mahzad Hojjat.
    p.   cm.
Includes bibliographical references and index.
ISBN 1-57230-217-8
    1. Interpersonal relations.   2. Marriage.   3. Couples.
4. Satisfaction.   I. Sternberg, Robert J.   II. Hojjat, Mahzad.
HM132.S3454   1997
158.2—dc21   97-13530
                                                                  CIP

Contributors

Robert J. Sternberg, PhD, is an IBM Professor of Psychology and Education in the Department of Psychology at Yale University. He is the author of two forthcoming books on love.

Mahzad Hojjat, MS, MPhil., is a doctoral student in the Department of Psychology at Yale University. She specializes in the study of close relationships.

Michael L. Barnes, PhD, Department of Psychology, Yale University, New Haven, Connecticut

Steven R. H. Beach, PhD, Department of Psychology, University of Georgia, Athens, Georgia

Ellen Berscheid, PhD, Department of Psychology, University of Minnesota, Minneapolis, Minnesota

David M. Buss, PhD, Department of Psychology, The University of Texas at Austin, Austin, Texas

Andrew Christensen, PhD, Department of Psychology, University of California at Los Angeles, Los Angeles, California

Mari L. Clements, PhD, Department of Psychology, Pennsylvania State University, University Park, Pennsylvania

Allan D. Cordova, MA, Center for Marital and Family Studies, Department of Psychology, University of Denver, Denver, Colorado

James V. Cordova, PhD, Department of Psychology, University of Illinois, Champaign, Illinois

Steve W. Duck, PhD, Department of Communication Studies, University of Iowa, Iowa City, Iowa

Larry A. Erbert, PhD, Department of Speech and Corporate Communication, Baruch College, New York, New York

Judith A. Feeney, PhD, Department of Psychology, University of Queensland, Queensland, Australia

Frank D. Fincham, PhD, Department of Psychology, University of Wales, Cardiff, Wales, United Kingdom

Vicki Gluhoski, PhD, Sociomedical Research Unit, Memorial Sloan-Kettering Cancer Center, New York, New York

Clyde Hendrick, PhD, Department of Psychology, Texas Tech University, Lubbock, Texas

Susan S. Hendrick, PhD, Department of Psychology, Texas Tech University, Lubbock, Texas

Neil S. Jacobson, PhD, Department of Psychology, University of Washington, Seattle, Washington

Susan I. Kemp-Fincham, MA, Department of Psychology, University of Wales, Cardiff, Wales, United Kingdom

Lilah Raynor Koski, MA, Director of Research, Kingsley & Associates, San Francisco, California

Samuel L. Lashley, MA, Department of Psychology, Catholic University of America, Washington, DC

Jean-Philippe Laurenceau, MS, Department of Psychology, Pennsylvania State University, University Park, Pennsylvania

George Levinger, PhD, Department of Psychology, University of Massachusetts at Amherst, Amherst, Massachusetts

Jason Lopes, BA, Department of Psychology, University of Minnesota, Minneapolis, Minnesota

Howard J. Markman, PhD, Center for Marital and Family Studies, Department of Psychology, University of Denver, Denver, Colorado

Patricia Noller, PhD, Department of Psychology, University of Queensland, Queensland, Australia

Clifford I. Notarius, PhD, Department of Psychology, The Catholic University of America, Washington, DC

Todd K. Shackelford, MA, Department of Psychology, The University of Texas at Austin, Austin, Texas

Phillip R. Shaver, PhD, Department of Psychology, University of California at Davis, Davis, California

Debra J. Sullivan, PhD, Clinical Psychologist, Washington, DC

Pamela T. Walczynski, MA, Department of Psychology, University of California at Los Angeles, Los Angeles, California

Carla Ward, BA, Department of Psychology, University of Queensland, Queensland, Australia

Mark A. Whisman, PhD, Department of Psychology, Yale University, New Haven, Connecticut

Jeffrey Young, PhD, Department of Psychiatry, Columbia University and Cognitive Therapy Center of New York, New York, New York

Preface

Why are some people satisfied in their close relationships, and others not? This is the question that has motivated the present volume. Our goal is to provide a psychologically sound compendium on the factors that lead people to be either satisfied or dissatisfied with their close relationships.

The chapters in this volume are written for academicians and clinicians with an interest in close relationships. Research psychologists will find an overview of the latest theory and research findings pertaining to satisfaction in close relationships. Psychotherapists from all kinds of backgrounds will find the volume a valuable source of concrete suggestions for dealing with clients who are experiencing distress in their relationships.

The volume is divided into five main parts plus a prologue. In his prologue, George Levinger discusses the field of satisfaction in close relationships, and sets the stage for what is to come.

In Part I, "Models of Love and Satisfaction in Close Relationships," authors show how models of love can be applied to understanding satisfaction in close relationships. The models are of diverse kinds: Todd K. Shackelford and David M. Buss use an evolutionary model, Lilah Raynor Koski and Phillip R. Shaver a model of attachment, Susan S. Hendrick and Clyde Hendrick a model of love styles, Michael L. Barnes and Robert J. Sternberg a hierarchical model of love, and Mahzad Hojjat a model of philosophy of life to show how satisfaction can be understood in terms of elements of love that are or are not present in relationships. Many of the authors also discuss how these elements come to appear in or disappear from relationships.

In Part II, "Satisfaction over the Course of Close Relationships," authors discuss the time course of relationships and its relation to satisfaction. Ellen Berscheid and Jason Lopes show how the individual, couple, and relationship change over time. Judith A. Feeney, Patricia Noller, and Carla Ward consider stages of the life cycle and marital quality. And Larry A. Erbert and Steve W. Duck view the time course of satisfaction in close relationships from a dialectical perspective.

In Part III, "Conflict and Satisfaction in Close Relationships," authors look in particular at the role of conflict in marital satisfaction as well as dissatisfaction. Clifford I. Notarius, Samuel L. Lashley, and Debra J. Sullivan discuss the role of anger and the ways it can destroy relationships. Andrew Christensen and Pamela T. Walczynski discuss various relations between conflict and satisfaction. And Frank D. Fincham, Steven R. H. Beach, and Susan I. Kemp-Fincham look at how positive and negative factors interact to produce varying levels of marital quality.

In Part IV, "Psychotherapy and Satisfaction in Close Relationships," authors discuss the role of therapy in understanding as well as treating problems related to clients' satisfaction with their close relationships. James V. Cordova and Neil S. Jacobson discuss the role of acceptance in couple therapy, and the implications of acceptance for treating depression. Mari L. Clements, Allan D. Cordova, Howard J. Markman, and Jean-Philippe Laurenceau show how marital satisfaction can erode over time, and they suggest steps to prevent this pattern of erosion. Jeffrey Young and Vicki Gluhoski present a schema-focused perspective on satisfaction in close relationships.

In Part V, Mark A. Whisman masterfully integrates the chapters that have come before; he provides a unifying model that encompasses the diverse points of view presented in the varied chapters.

We are grateful to Seymour Weingarten for contracting this book and for making various suggestions along the way for its improvement.

ROBERT J. STERNBERG
MAHZAD HOJJAT

Contents

Prologue   1
George Levinger

PART 1.
MODELS OF LOVE AND SATISFACTION
IN CLOSE RELATIONSHIPS

1. Marital Satisfaction in Evolutionary   7
   Psychological Perspective
   Todd K. Shackelford and David M. Buss

2. Attachment and Relationship Satisfaction   26
   across the Lifespan
   Lilah Raynor Koski and Phillip R. Shaver

3. Love and Satisfaction   56
   Susan S. Hendrick and Clyde Hendrick

4. A Hierarchical Model of Love and Its Prediction 79
   of Satisfaction in Close Relationships
   Michael L. Barnes and Robert J. Sternberg

5. Philosophy of Life as a Model   102
   of Relationship Satisfaction
   Mahzad Hojjat

xi

PART 2.
SATISFACTION OVER THE COURSE
OF CLOSE RELATIONSHIPS

6. A Temporal Model of Relationship Satisfaction   129
    and Stability
    Ellen Berscheid and Jason Lopes

7. Marital Satisfaction and Spousal Interaction   160
    Judith A. Feeney, Patricia Noller, and Carla Ward

8. Rethinking Satisfaction in Personal Relationships   190
    from a Dialectical Perspective
    Larry A. Erbert and Steve W. Duck

PART 3.
CONFLICT AND SATISFACTION
IN CLOSE RELATIONSHIPS

9. Angry at Your Partner?: Think Again   219
    Clifford I. Notarius, Samuel L. Lashley,
    and Debra J. Sullivan

10. Conflict and Satisfaction in Couples   249
    Andrew Christensen and Pamela T. Walczynski

11. Marital Quality: A New Theoretical Perspective   275
    Frank D. Fincham, Steven R. H. Beach, and
    Susan I. Kemp-Fincham

PART 4.
PSYCHOTHERAPY AND SATISFACTION
IN CLOSE RELATIONSHIPS

12. Acceptance in Couple Therapy and Its Implications   307
    for the Treatment of Depression
    James V. Cordova and Neil S. Jacobson

13. The Erosion of Marital Satisfaction over Time   335
    and How to Prevent It
    Mari L. Clements, Allan D. Cordova,
    Howard J. Markman, and Jean-Philippe Laurenceau

14. A Schema-Focused Perspective on Satisfaction   356
    in Close Relationships
    Jeffrey Young and Vicki Gluhoski

PART 5.
CONCLUSION

15. Satisfaction in Close Relationships: 385
    Challenges for the 21st Century
    Mark A. Whisman

    Author Index   411

    Subject Index   421

SATISFACTION IN CLOSE RELATIONSHIPS

Prologue

GEORGE LEVINGER

Several years ago a cartoon in *The New Yorker*, captioned "Critics in Love," showed a man sitting next to a woman on a couch with his arm around her shoulders and her hand on his knee. Above the man's head was a balloon with four stars in it, indicating his extreme attraction to her; a similar balloon above the woman's head contained only two and a half stars. Both of these partners were carefully monitoring their ongoing satisfaction with their relationship. In a parallel vein, it is common practice today for married individuals to ask themselves periodically how well their marriage is going and how much they are getting out of it.

Contrast these practices with those typical in past centuries. For example, in 17th-century England it was usual among propertied parents to select a possible spouse for their offspring and—if prospects looked good—to negotiate a preliminary financial settlement before the couple were brought together "to discover whether or not they found each other personally obnoxious. If no strong [negative] feelings were aroused, the couple normally consented . . . and the arrangements for a formal church wedding went forward" (Stone, 1992, p. 7).

Why do people today show such a high need to monitor their "satisfaction in close relationships"? What is there in present-day Western culture that virtually requires laypeople—as well as psychological experts, such as the eminent contributors to this volume—to worry about the assessing, building, eroding, and repairing of couple satisfaction?

1

To address such questions, I want to look back briefly through history and across cultures. Looking backward, we see that people once spent far less effort on analyzing the quality of their personal relationships. In earlier eras, interpersonal relationships, family, and community were relatively fixed; it was taken for granted that spouses would stay together until death parted them, that families would govern an individual's choice of mate, and that these choices would be made from a rather confined field of eligible partners. Looking cross-culturally, we find that in more collectivistic cultures the success of couple relationships is far less tied to personal rewards and far more to family and communal interdependence than in Western society (Dion & Dion, 1996; Markus & Kitayama, 1991). For instance, a study of Japanese marriages found that, overall, the more that parents had given approval to a marriage, the greater was the spouses' subsequent marital satisfaction (Blood, 1967).

I think that today's preoccupation with close relationships in Western society can be traced to several converging historical trends. First, in past centuries there was much less emphasis on each person's individuality and a greater homogeneity in people's life experience; it seemed to matter less whom one might choose to marry within one's field of eligible mates. The alternatives were relatively limited.

Second, until the 18th or 19th century in Protestant countries, and until even more recently in Catholic countries, two persons who had entered into a formal union could not legitimately separate from each other. These societies insisted that marriage must last forever (granted, "forever" often used to mean a much shorter lifetime). Having little opportunity for exit, partners had little motivation for monitoring their ongoing marital satisfaction. A better strategy for sustaining personal well-being was to tolerate one's situation and to perform one's daily duties cheerfully—or, in some circles, to find ways of mitigating one's tedium in extramarital liaisons.

Third, modern Western society is characterized not only by a wider range of alternatives and a greater opportunity for exit from unsatisfactory bonds, but also by a greater fuzziness about what sorts of relationships are approved. Until recently, normative couple ties were either marital or premarital; today there is far more toleration of unmarried cohabitation, of long-term same-sex unions, and of various forms of "reconstituted" families. I might add that the term "close relationship" was coined only about 20 years ago, for an interdisciplinary conference addressing diverse perspectives on human intimacy (Levinger & Raush, 1977), to provide a broadly inclusive label for all sorts of highly interdependent relationships—not merely to refer to marriage or intended marriage.

Amid today's greatly increased alternatives, decreased social con-
straints, and heightened pair instability, therefore, it matters far more
how well two partners are pleased with the quality of their relationship. Today's relational continuance depends less on duty or obligation
and much more on satisfaction; if one or both partners are dissatisfied,
they must either strive to improve their connection or risk its likely
collapse. And, as Berscheid and Lopes (Chapter 6, this volume) and
others have pointed out, increased opportunities for breakup—and
projected marital divorce rates of up to 67%—put additional pressures
on existing ties.

"To satisfy" means "to fulfill a need or desire" or "to free from doubt
or question" (*American Heritage Dictionary*, 1992, p. 1604). It derives
from the Latin roots of *facere* ("to do") and *satis* ("enough"). But how indeed can one "do enough" to fulfill ever-rising needs and expectations for
happiness in one's closest relationship, in a society where breaking up has
become more normal than staying together for life? If "dissatisfaction results from an excess of wants over abilities" (Levinger, 1966, p. 803), how
can partners free each other from doubting that their mutual resources
and skills will continue to meet their needs for the indefinite future?

The contributors to this volume make important advances in clarify-
ing both the bases of such questions and their consequences. Rather
than delving into matters of history or cultural context, they focus mainly
on the psychology of satisfaction or dissatisfaction. Some chapters address general issues about the nature of love, the foundations of satisfaction, and the dynamics of its maintenance and deterioration across
a broad spectrum of close relationships. Adult satisfaction or intimacy
is linked to childhood attachment (Koski & Shaver, Chapter 2), to the
partners' value similarity (Hojjat, Chapter 5), to relational dialectics
(Erbert & Duck, Chapter 8), and to diverse conceptions of love (Barnes
& Sternberg, Chapter 4; Hendrick & Hendrick, Chapter 3). There is
also a theoretical analysis of how temporal changes in relational satisfaction are affected by a couple's social or physical environment (Berscheid & Lopes, Chapter 6).

Other chapters provide conceptual and empirical analyses of spouses'
beliefs about the quality of their marriage. Differences between wives'
and husbands' marital satisfaction are discussed from the viewpoint of
evolutionary psychology (Shackelford & Buss, Chapter 1). The rewards
of marital interaction are analyzed empirically, and explained by means
of five factors that especially emphasize a couple's consensus and communication (Feeney, Noller, & Ward, Chapter 7). And the entire concept of "marital quality" is reconceptualized in terms of both its positive
and negative dimensions, and their accessibility to the spouses' own
awareness (Fincham, Beach, & Kemp-Fincham, Chapter 11).

The remaining contributions focus on the problems, conflicts, and deterioration of relationships; they address ways of helping partners cope with difficulties in their own relationship. One chapter reinterprets decreasing marital satisfaction in terms of an active "erosion" of positive interactions, and discusses a tested program for helping young couples inoculate their relationships to prevent such deterioration (Clements, Cordova, Markman, & Laurenceau, Chapter 13). Another describes how "integrative behavioral couple therapy" aims to help couples deal with existing conflicts; it highlights building "acceptance" of weaknesses, as well as making positive changes in a relationship (Christensen & Walczynski, Chapter 10). Still another piece shows how such an integrative therapy can help a couple build acceptance and maintain relationship satisfaction when one member is deeply depressed (Cordova & Jacobson, Chapter 12). There is also a developmental analysis of anger in relationships, which discusses how couples can deal with anger constructively (Notarius, Lashley, & Sullivan, Chapter 9). Yet another chapter introduces "schema-focused therapy" as an approach to rebuilding relationship satisfaction (Young & Gluhoski, Chapter 14).

Together, these 14 chapters convey much of the best current knowledge about how to define, assess, and maintain or improve love and satisfaction in close relationships. Rather than commenting any further, I invite readers to examine these chapters for themselves. I believe that they contribute substantially to an understanding of this significant contemporary topic.

REFERENCES

American heritage dictionary (3rd ed.). (1992). Boston: Houghton Mifflin.

Blood, R. O. (1967). *Love match and arranged marriage.* New York: Free Press.

Dion, K. K., & Dion, K. L. (1996). Cultural perspectives on romantic love. *Personal Relationships, 3,* 5–17.

Levinger, G. (1966). Sources of marital dissatisfaction among applicants for divorce. *American Journal of Orthopsychiatry, 36,* 803–807.

Levinger, G., & Raush, H. L. (1977). *Close relationships: Perspectives on the meaning of intimacy.* Amherst: University of Massachusetts Press.

Markus, H. R., & Kitayama, S. (1991). Culture and the self: Implications for cognition, emotion, and motivation. *Psychological Review, 98,* 224–253.

Stone, L. (1992). *Uncertain unions: Marriage in England 1660–1753.* Oxford: Oxford University Press.

PART 1

MODELS OF LOVE
AND SATISFACTION
IN CLOSE RELATIONSHIPS

CHAPTER 1

Marital Satisfaction in Evolutionary Psychological Perspective

TODD K. SHACKELFORD
DAVID M. BUSS

Formal marriage arrangements between men and women exist in every known culture around the world (Brown, 1991; Buss, 1985; Buss & Schmitt, 1993; Epstein & Guttman, 1984; Vandenberg, 1972). Moreover, more than 90% of the world's population will marry at least once during their lifetime (Buss, 1985; Buss & Schmitt, 1993; Epstein & Guttman, 1984; Vandenberg, 1972). Equally revealing, however, is that the vast majority of human societies also have instituted formal procedures for marital divorce (Betzig, 1989). Fewer than one in two marriages in the Western world lasts a lifetime; indeed, the majority end within the first 4 years of marriage (Fisher, 1992). This astonishing rate of conjugal dissolution is not peculiar to Western culture (Betzig, 1989; Fisher, 1992).

The cross-cultural ubiquity of marriage and divorce suggest the potential utility of, and insight that can be provided by, an evolutionary psychological perspective (Buss, 1995; Daly & Wilson, 1988; Kenrick, Sadalla, Groth, & Trost, 1990; Symons, 1992; Tooby & Cosmides, 1992). In this chapter, we present a conceptual overview of marital satisfaction and discontent as seen through the lens of evolutionary psychology. We begin by reconceptualizing marital satisfaction from the framework offered by this perspective. Next, we discuss the notion of "mate value," and examine the reasons why a discrepancy in relative spousal mate value is likely to translate into marital dissatisfaction. We then offer an evolutionary psychological personality profile of spouses who evoke in their partners dissatisfaction with their relationships. We then consider the use of "mate-guarding" tactics among married couples, and discuss which of these tactics are likely to promote marital happiness and which are likely to lead to marital decay. Next, we provide an evolutionary psychological prescription for how to guarantee an unhappy marriage, focusing on sources of marital anger, upset, and irritation. We close with a summary of spousal and relationship qualities that promote marital satisfaction, as gleaned from an evolutionary psychological perspective.

Our aim in this chapter is primarily to elucidate the *conceptual* utility of adopting an evolutionary psychological framework for understanding marital satisfaction. Throughout the chapter, however, we provide supportive data, where available, collected from an intensive study of 107 married couples (see Buss, 1991a, 1992).

RECONCEPTUALIZING MARITAL SATISFACTION WITHIN AN EVOLUTIONARY PSYCHOLOGICAL FRAMEWORK

The marital relationship is in many ways unique among human relationships. Marriage entails processes and expectations not present in other intimate relationships. Rarely is there an expectation of sexual fidelity or romantic/emotional exclusivity, for example, among even the closest of friends (Shackelford & Buss, 1996; Shackelford, 1997). Romantic exclusivity and sexual fidelity are, however, among the expected benefits of participation in a presumably monogamous marriage in all cultures that prescribe this mating arrangement (Betzig, 1989; Brown, 1991; Buss, 1994; Daly & Wilson, 1988). Marriage is a universal human institution; no fewer than 9 of every 10 humans worldwide marry (Brown, 1991; Buss, 1985; Buss & Schmitt, 1993; Epstein & Guttman, 1984; Vandenberg, 1972). Given its cross-cultural prevalence, marriage is likely to have posed a recurrent set of adaptive problems for ancestral men and women throughout human evolutionary history (Buss, 1994; Buss & Schmitt, 1993; Daly & Wilson, 1988).

Many of these adaptive challenges would have been equally confronted by ancestral men and women. Marriage is fundamentally a reproductive union (Betzig, 1989; Buss & Schmitt, 1993; Daly & Wilson, 1988), and in this regard ancestral men and women alike would have confronted the basic adaptive challenge of identifying potential marriage partners capable of producing offspring. Those early humans who were less adept at discriminating the reproductively fertile from the less fertile among the pool of potential spouses are less likely to be our ancestors, for they would have been outreproduced by their more perceptive conspecifics. The marital choices and underlying psychological mechanisms of the more reproductively successful among early humans have become instantiated in the human mind over the hundreds of thousands of generations of our evolutionary history. The marital choices we make today are in this respect the marital choices that our ancestors made millennia ago.

Various authors have expanded on the multiplicity of adaptive challenges that men and women confront in the context of marriage (see, e.g., Buss, 1991b, 1994; Daly & Wilson, 1988). These adaptive challenges include the following, in addition to identifying a reproductively fertile spouse: achieving successful conception, or engaging in the necessary sexual and social activities to fertilize or be fertilized by one's spouse; mate retention, or preventing the defection or desertion of one's spouse, as well as preventing encroachment by intrasexual competitors; and parental care and socialization, or acting to ensure the successful survival and reproduction of offspring produced within the marriage.

Other adaptive challenges of marriage are sex-specific and, as a consequence, have selected for sex-differentiated mating psychologies. Ancestral men, but not women, faced the adaptive problem of being certain that the offspring produced by their spouses were indeed their own. Because fertilization occurs within women, men can never be 100% certain that the children their mates bear are their own. Ancestral men, of course, did not have access to DNA-fingerprinting technology, or even to the much less accurate blood-grouping techniques that are now employed today. Women's sexual infidelity placed ancestral men at risk of investing in offspring to whom they were genetically unrelated. Those males who were indifferent to the sexual fidelity of their spouses are less likely to be our evolutionary ancestors, for they would have been outreproduced by males who invested effort in retaining exclusive sexual access to their spouses. A man's sensitivity to and concern about the sexual infidelity of his spouse can be understood as a solution to the adaptive problem of threatened cuckoldry (Buss, Larsen, Westen, & Semmelroth, 1992; Buss & Schmitt, 1993; Daly, Wilson, & Weghorst, 1982; Wilson & Daly, 1992).

Although women have not faced the adaptive problem of parental certainty, the sexual infidelity of their spouses probably provided a cue to the potential loss of other reproductively valuable resources garnered from the marital relationship (Buss et al., 1992; Daly, Wilson, & Weghorst, 1982). A woman may fear that the time, attention, investment, commitment, and resources her spouse contributes will be diverted to another woman and her children (Buss et al., 1992; Buss & Schmitt, 1993; Daly & Wilson, 1988). A woman's sensitivity to the sexual infidelity of her spouse can thus be understood as a solution to the adaptive problem of threatened loss of reproductively valuable resources (Buss et al., 1992; Buss & Schmitt, 1993).

From an evolutionary psychological perspective, marital satisfaction or dissatisfaction can be viewed as psychological states that track the overall benefits and costs associated with a particular marital union. The costs and benefits are gauged psychologically, but our evolved psychological mechanisms for gauging them have been forged over the vast expanse of evolutionary time. At an ultimate level, therefore, the psychological mechanisms track what would have been costs and benefits in ancestral times. A marriage partner who is unfaithful, for example, inflicts a probabilistic cost of lowered paternity certainty or the diversion of resources and commitment to another. Infidelity, therefore, can be expected to lower the partner's marital satisfaction because it is tracking costs of this sort. Thus, marital satisfaction can be regarded as a psychological device that tracks the overall costs and benefits of a marriage. Marital dissatisfaction can serve the adaptive function of motivating the individual to attempt to change the existing relationship, or to seek another one that may be more propitious.

In summary, the marital alliance is a reproductive union forged by nearly every man and woman the world over. It is very likely to have been a recurrent feature of the human "adaptive landscape" (Buss, 1991b) over our evolutionary history. Marriage entails many and varied adaptive challenges, some of which are sex-specific, but many of which are confronted by men and women alike. The adaptive problems of marriage are not static, but change with the fluctuating context of the enduring marriage. It is the *continuously* successful solving of the adaptive problems posed by the marital alliance that produces a state of relative marital satisfaction, happiness, and contentment.

WHEN ONE SPOUSE IS WORTH MORE THAN THE OTHER: "MATE VALUE" DISCREPANCY AND MARITAL DISSATISFACTION

People differ in their ability to attract, acquire, and retain marriage partners. That is, people differ in their "mate value," or their overall attractiveness (physical and otherwise) as potential spouses, relative to other potential spouses on the current "mating market" (Buss, 1994; Symons, 1979). In a study of over 10,000 people across 37 cultures, Buss (1989a) identified the primary constituents of men's and women's mate value. Cross-culturally, women more than men were found to value cues to resource acquisition (e.g., ambition, industriousness, earning capacity) in a potential spouse. Men more than women were found to value cues to reproductive capacity (e.g., youth, physical attractiveness) in a potential spouse. Because women and not men bear the time- and energy-intensive burden of gestation, parturition, and lactation, more of their value as potential spouses is tied up in their reproductive capacity. Two of the most reliable cues to reproductive value in women are physical attractiveness and age (Buss, 1989a; Symons, 1979). Those early human males who selected as spouses relatively more physically attractive and youthful females would probably have outreproduced those males who did not attend to these cues to reproductive capacity.

Because human offspring can garner tremendous benefits from the additional investment provided by an adult male (Buss, 1989a, 1994), ancestral women who selected as marriage partners men with relatively greater ability and willingness to invest their current and future resources in the women and their offspring would probably have produced a greater number of healthy offspring. Thus, relative to women, more of men's mate value is tied up in their ability and willingness to invest acquired resources in their spouses and children.

Mate value is, of course, much more than the reproductive capacity of women and the resource acquisition potential of men. In his cross-cultural study, Buss (1989a) found that members of both sexes valued intelligence, kindness, and dependability more than any other attributes in a potential spouse. Nonetheless, sex differences in spouse preferences exist.

The mate value of spouses is positively correlated. In general, men with greater resources or resource acquisition potential tend to marry younger and more physically attractive women (Buss, 1994; Elder, 1969; Taylor & Glenn, 1976; Udry & Eckland, 1984). People with a good sense of humor tend to have spouses with a good sense of humor (Buss, 1994); intelligent people tend to marry those of approximately equal intelligence (Buss, 1994); and so on, for a vast array of personality and demographic variables (Buss, 1984, 1994). In our sample of 107 married couples, the spousal cross-correlation of mate value as assessed by two independent interviewers (one male and one female) was .63 ($p < .001$).

Working within an evolutionary framework, we predicted that a discrepancy in mate value within a couple would be associated with marital dissatisfaction in both spouses, regardless of which spouse was judged to be the more valuable mate. A discrepancy in mate value is likely to produce anxiety in the less valuable partner concerning his or her spouse's possible defection from the relationship or extramarital liaison, in search of someone of more comparable value. This anxiety may translate into marital dissatisfaction. The spouse of higher relative mate value also may express dissatisfaction with an arrangement where the benefits received may be less than the costs of remaining in the relationship to the exclusion of other possible relationships. In our sample of married couples, this prediction was supported, at least in part: The greater the mate value discrepancy, the less satisfied men, but not women, were with their marriages. It is not clear why this prediction held for men but not their wives.

SPOUSAL PERSONALITY ATTRIBUTES
THAT SIGNAL TROUBLE FOR A MARRIAGE

In this section of the chapter, we offer predictions regarding spousal personality traits as conceptualized within the five-factor model of personality and the partner's marital satisfaction. The five-factor model of personality (Norman, 1963; Goldberg, 1981) proposes that five major dimensions capture the bulk of significant individual differences in personality. These bipolar factors are Surgency (dominant, extraverted vs. submissive, introverted), Agreeableness (warm, trusting vs. cold, suspicious), Conscientiousness (reliable, well-organized vs. undependable, disorganized), Emotional Stability (secure, even-tempered vs. nervous, temperamental), and Openness/Intellect (perceptive, curious vs. imperceptive, uncurious).

Some research has been conducted on the covariation of marital dissatisfaction with spousal markers of the "Big Five." The most consistent predictor of marital unhappiness for both men and women is a spouse's low standing on Emotional Stability, emerging in nearly every study that has included a marker of this dimension (Buss, 1991a). A spouse exhibiting low Conscientiousness evokes marital dissatisfaction in his or her partner (Bentler & Newcomb, 1978; Kelly & Conley, 1987), as does a spouse manifesting low Agreeableness (Burgess & Wallen, 1953; Kelly & Conley, 1987). A spouse who exhibits low Emotional Stability, low Conscientiousness, and low Agreeableness is likely to inflict substantial costs on his or her partner, rendering the relationship a much less beneficial and therefore much less satisfying arrangement.

Buss (1991a) found that women married to men who displayed low Agreeableness tended to complain that their husbands were condescending toward them, neglecting, rejecting, unreliable, physically and verbally abusive, unfaithful, inconsiderate, moody, abusive of alcohol, emotionally constricted, insulting of their appearance, and self-centered. Women married to men who exhibited low Conscientiousness complained that their husbands were unfaithful, and those married to emotionally unstable men complained that their husbands were condescending, possessive, dependent, jealous, physically and verbally abusive, unfaithful, inconsiderate, physically self-absorbed, moody, abusive of alcohol, emotionally constricted, and self-centered. Buss (1991a) also found that women married to men who scored low on Openness/Intellect tended to complain that their husbands were neglecting, rejecting, unreliable, abusive, inconsiderate, physically self-absorbed, moody, sexually withholding and rejecting, abusive of alcohol, and emotionally constricted.

Men's complaints about their wives also covaried with their wives' personalities, but less so than was the case for women's complaints about their husbands. Men married to women who scored low on Agreeableness complained that their wives were condescending, unfaithful, and self-centered. Men married to women who exhibited low Conscientiousness complained that their wives were abusive of alcohol and emotionally constricted. Men married to emotionally unstable women complained that their wives were possessive, dependent, jealous, and self-centered. Finally, men married to women scoring low on Openness/Intellect complained that their spouses tended to sexualize other men, abused alcohol, and were emotionally constricted.

Thus, men and women whose spouses exhibit low levels of Agreeableness, Conscientiousness, Emotional Stability, and Openness/Intellect are exposed to a variety of significant costs. Early males and females who remained in relationships with spouses imposing such costs are less likely to be our ancestors, for they would have been outreproduced by men and women who either refrained from involvement with people exhibiting these undesirable personality characteristics, or defected from the relationships once they were involved. One facet of the psychological and emotional machinery that may have been selected for over human evolutionary history is the triggering of feelings of dissatisfaction, unhappiness, and discontent with marriage to a spouse exhibiting disagreeableness, undependability, emotional instability, and stupidity or closed-mindedness. These developing feelings of marital dissatisfaction might then have prompted the beguiled spouse to defect from the reproductively costly relationship in search of a more beneficial arrangement. In the sample of 107 married couples, this prediction was supported: Disagreeableness, undependability, emotional instability, and stupidity or closed-mindedness of a spouse were impressively associated with a partner's marital dissatisfaction.

From an evolutionary psychological perspective, one of the most serious transgressions of the presumably monogamous marital alliance is a partner's infidelity. Such unfaithfulness is likely to have imposed serious reproductive costs on ancestral men and women alike (see above). Because of the asymmetry in parental certainty, however, a wife's infidelity is potentially much more costly to her husband than is a husband's infidelity to his wife. The wife of a philandering man stands to lose some portion of his investment to another woman and her children. Even if she loses the bulk of his investment, any children she bears are unquestionably her genetic progeny. The husband of an unfaithful wife stands to lose the entire reproductive capacity of his spouse, for at least one childbearing cycle. Moreover, the unsuspecting cuckold risks investing years, even decades, of precious tangible and intangible resources in a rival's offspring.

Elsewhere (Buss & Shackelford, in press), we examined the relationship between a spouse's susceptibility to varying degrees of infidelity and his or her standings on the Big Five. We found that wives who exhibited a low level of Conscientiousness were more likely to flirt with another man, passionately kiss another man, go on a romantic date with another man, have a one-night stand with another man, have a brief affair with another man, and have a serious affair with another man. No clear relationship emerged between husbands' standings on the five factors and their susceptibility to infidelity. On the basis of these findings, and in conjunction with the asymmetry in parental certainty, we expected to find the strongest marital unhappiness–spousal personality correlation for men married to women scoring low on Conscientiousness. This was precisely what we found: With regard to his wife's personality, the best predictor of a husband's marital satisfaction was his spouse's Conscientiousness.

A powerful selective pressure that would have been differentially confronted by ancestral men and women is damaging physical abuse at the hands of a spouse. Although men and women may be equally likely to engage in physical abuse (as distinct from legal "battering"; e.g., Dobash, Dobash, Wilson, & Daly, 1992) of their spouse (Buss, 1991a; de Weerth & Kalma, 1993; Dobash et al., 1992), a history of intense sexual selection for intersexual physical competitive ability among men but not women has produced men that today are, on average, substantially larger and stronger than women (Daly & Wilson, 1983; Trivers, 1985). The result is that the physical abuse of a woman by her husband is more damaging than is the physical abuse of a man by his wife (Daly & Wilson, 1988; Daly et al., 1982; Dobash et al., 1992). Physical abuse is one of the greatest costs that men can inflict on their wives (Daly & Wilson, 1988; Daly et al., 1982; Dobash et al., 1992). Buss (1991a) reported substantial negative correlations between a wife's complaints that her husband abused her and his Agreeableness and Emotional Stability. We would expect, therefore, to find the strongest marital unhappiness–spousal personality correlations between women's unhappiness and their partners' standing on Agreeableness and Emotional Stability. We would expect these results to the extent that modern women are descended from ancestral women who defected from reproductively costly relationships with abusive—that is, disagreeable and emotionally unstable—husbands. This was just what we found upon examining the married couples' data: With regard to her husband's personality, the best predictors of a woman's marital satisfaction were her spouse's Agreeableness and Emotional Stability.

SPOUSAL TACTICS OF MATE GUARDING AND THEIR IMPACT ON MARITAL SATISFACTION

In this section of the chapter, we provide an evolutionary psychological analysis of the impact of various mate-guarding tactics employed by one spouse and the impact of these tactics on the marital satisfaction of his or her partner. We open with a brief discussion of several mate-guarding tactics that evoke marital dissatisfaction in the recipient of these tactics. Next we consider two mate-guarding tactics husbands employ that appear to be successful, insofar as the use of these tactics covaries positively with their spouses' marital satisfaction.

"To Have and to Hold from This Day Forward . . .": Spousal Mate-Guarding Tactics That Evoke Marital Dissatisfaction

Once the initial adaptive problems of locating, attracting, and wedding a suitable marriage partner have been successfully solved, many adaptive challenges follow, not the least of which is guarding one's spouse from encroachment by intrasexual competitors. Those early human men and women who successfully guarded their spouses from would-be poachers probably would have been more reproductively prosperous than were those men and women who did not guard their spouses as successfully. The mate-guarding tactics that men and women enact today are produced by the psychological mechanisms that encouraged successful mate guarding by our ancestors (Buss & Shackelford, 1997).

Remarkably little research has investigated human mate-guarding tactics. What little work has been done has focused almost exclusively on wife guarding by husbands (e.g., Daly et al., 1982; Ghiselin, 1974;

Wilson, 1975). The most comprehensive taxonomy of mate guarding was developed in a series of studies by Buss (1988). Importantly, Buss's (1988) taxonomy includes tactics used by men *and* women in an effort to guard or retain their partners.

From an evolutionary psychological perspective, mate guarding is a tricky business indeed. Excessive mate guarding runs the risk of being interpreted by the object of the guarding as evidence that he or she is of exceptionally greater mate value than is the guarder. Total abstention from mate guarding, however, may send one of two messages to the unguarded spouse:

1. The unguarded spouse is so much *more* valuable a mate than his or her partner that the partner is unwilling to spend limited energy guarding a spouse who is likely to defect from the marriage in search of a more beneficial arrangement. Moreover, the partner who perceives his or her spouse to be of exceptionally greater relative mate value may well decide to cut his or her losses and go in search of a spouse of more nearly equal value.

2. The unguarded spouse is so much *less* valuable a mate than his or her partner that the partner is unwilling to spend limited energy guarding a mate that he or she plans to abandon in search of a mate of greater value. In this case, the unguarded spouse may act to preempt the inevitable rather than squander limited time and resources, and defect from the marriage to seek out a spouse of more nearly equal value.

If excessive mate guarding and total abstention from mate guarding are both likely to prove detrimental to a marriage, this suggests that some level of mate guarding is optimal, from the guarder's perspective. Up to this point, we have discussed mate guarding as if it were a single behavior or collection of behaviors. On the contrary, Buss (1988) identified 19 tactics subsuming 104 acts that men and women employ to guard their partners from intrasexual encroachment. These 19 tactics represent an impressively diverse array of guarding strategies. Each of the tactics has one of three goals: (1) to make the current relationship more attractive or beneficial to the guarded spouse, thereby reducing the likelihood that the guarded spouse will defect; (2) to impose or threaten to impose severe costs on the guarded partner if he or she attempts to defect from the relationship, reducing the likelihood that the guarded spouse will defect; or (3) to dissuade intrasexual competitors from poaching. We would predict that tactics consisting of threatening to impose or actually imposing severe costs on a defecting spouse will evoke feelings of marital dissatisfaction in the guarded spouse. Tactics consisting of bestowing benefits on the guarded spouse to make the current marriage more attractive, on the other hand, are likely to evoke feelings of marital happiness.

Four tactics, in particular, appear to represent an imposition or threatened imposition of costs in the event of spousal defection: (1) monopolization of the mate's time (e.g., He spent all of his free time with her so that she could not meet anyone else; She would not let him go out without her; He insisted that she spend all of her free time with him); (2) threatening infidelity (e.g., He talked to another woman at the party to make her jealous; She went out with other men to make him jealous; He showed interest in other women to make her angry); (3) punishing or threatening to punish the mate's infidelity (e.g., He hit her when he caught her flirting with someone else; She threatened to break up if he ever cheated on her; He said that he would never talk to her again if he ever saw her with someone else); and (4) emotional manipulation (e.g., He told her he would "die" if she ever left; She threatened to harm herself if he ever left; He pleaded that he could not live without her). Insofar as each of these four tactics represents an imposition or threatened imposition of costs for spousal defection, the recipient of these tactics should experience less marital satisfaction. This prediction was generally supported in our sample of married couples, regardless of the sex of the guarded spouse. Men and women whose spouses monopolized their time, threatened infidelity, punished or threatened to punish their infidelity, and manipulated them emotionally were less satisfied with their marriages than were men and women whose spouses did not employ these mate-guarding tactics.

"To Love, Honor, and Cherish . . . ": Mate-Guarding Tactics That Evoke Marital Satisfaction

In his cross-cultural study of characteristics desired in a spouse, Buss (1989a) found that women more than men desired spouses who were willing and able to invest resources in the women and their children. Women more than men also value spouses who are willing and able to invest emotional resources, time, effort, and energy in the women and their children (Buss et al., 1992; Shackelford, 1997; Shackelford & Buss, 1996, in press; Wiederman & Algeier, 1993). We would predict, therefore, that women married to men who invest more tangible resources, emotional resources, time, energy, and effort in them will report greater marital satisfaction than will women whose husbands invest less in them. A woman's channeling of tangible and intangible resources to her husband is predicted to be uncorrelated with his marital satisfaction.

Two of the mate-guarding tactics identified by Buss (1988) are relevant to these predictions: resource provisioning (e.g., He spent a lot

of money on her; She bought him an expensive gift; He took her out
to a nice restaurant) and expressing love and caring (e.g., He told her
that he loved her; She went out of her way to be kind, nice, and caring; He displayed greater affection for her). What do we find in the
married couples' data? Consistent with our predictions, women's—but
not men's—marital satisfaction was positively correlated with their
spouses' resource provisioning and expression of love.

SOURCES OF ANGER, IRRITATION, AND UPSET: HOW TO GUARANTEE AN UNHAPPY MARRIAGE

No marriage is perfect. Conflict between spouses is an inevitable consequence of the many and varied compromises that a man and a woman must make in their efforts to initiate and maintain an effective and
efficient reproductive partnership. In an effort to identify the themes
and topics that generate the most conflict, Buss (1989b) empirically developed a taxonomy of the sources of anger, upset, and irritation between long-term partners. Buss (1989b) identified 15 categories subsuming
147 acts that a man or woman might commit that would elicit irritation, anger, or upset in his or her partner. Our aim in this section of
the chapter is to provide an evolutionary psychological account of which
sources of anger, upset, and irritation are likely to be most distressing
for husbands and for wives. Some of the relationships we report here
have been described in Buss (1989b).

The most costly action a wife can impose on her husband is sexual
infidelity. A woman's sexual infidelity places her husband at risk of investing tremendous resources in offspring to whom he is genetically
unrelated—an irrevocable catastrophe in reproductive currency, from
the husband's perspective. Modern men are descended from an unbroken
chain of ancestral men who invested substantial time and effort in en-
suring the sexual fidelity of their partners. Ancestral men whose partners were sexually unfaithful probably would have imposed substantial
retributive costs on them (including damaging physical abuse), and would
have cut their losses and defected from the relationships rather than
risk the reproductive tragedy of cuckoldry. Cross-culturally, suspicion
of a wife's infidelity is today the leading cause of wife battery and wife
killing (Daly & Wilson, 1988; Daly et al., 1982), and the reason most
frequently given for a man's decision to divorce his wife (Betzig, 1989).
We would therefore predict that among the variety of means by which
a woman might upset, anger, or irritate her husband, the best predictor
of a man's marital dissatisfaction will be his wife's infidelity.

One of the most costly actions a man can impose on his wife is
physical abuse. The minimum obligatory parental investment of women

in their offspring is far greater than the minimum obligatory parental investment of men. In evolutionary psychological terms, women are the limiting reproductive resource (Trivers, 1972). One consequence of this sex difference in minimum obligatory parental investment is that competition among men for sexual access to reproductively valuable women tends to be more intense than is competition among women for access to reproductively valuable men. As noted earlier, greater male than female intrasexual competition for mates has selected over evolutionary history for a significant size and strength differential between men and women. Men, on average, and across a variety of measures, tend to be larger and stronger than women (Daly & Wilson, 1983; Trivers, 1985). Although the sexes do not appear to differ in the frequency with which they inflict physical abuse on their spouses (Buss, 1991a; de Weerth & Kalma, 1993; but see Dobash et al., 1992, for important qualifications), men's abuse of their wives tends to be much more physically damaging than women's abuse of their husbands (Daly & Wilson, 1988; Daly et al., 1982; Dobash et al., 1992). We would therefore predict that among the variety of means by which a husband might upset, anger, or irritate his wife, the best predictor of a woman's marital dissatisfaction will be abuse at the hands of her husband.

Of all the things a wife might do that distress her husband, which is the best predictor of his marital dissatisfaction? We predicted that a wife's infidelity would fit this bill. Looking at the married couples' data, we found that a wife's infidelity was *not* the best predictor of her husband's marital unhappiness; it was, however, the second best predictor. The best predictor of a husband's marital dissatisfaction was his wife's level of moodiness or emotional instability. Interestingly, an excellent predictor of a man's estimate that his wife will commit a variety of infidelities is her level of moodiness (Buss & Shackelford, in press).

Of the hundreds of things a husband might do that evoke anger, upset, and irritation in his wife, which of these actions best predicts his wife's marital discontent? We predicted that a woman's marital satisfaction would be most negatively affected by her husband's abuse of her. This was just what we found in our sample of married couples. It appears, therefore, that abusive husbands and unfaithful, emotionally unstable wives all but guarantee their spouses miserable marriages.

CONCLUSIONS: TAKING STOCK
OF THE HAPPY MARRIAGE
IN EVOLUTIONARY PSYCHOLOGICAL PERSPECTIVE

In this final section of the chapter, we take stock of the ins and outs, the dos and don'ts of a rewarding, satisfying, and generally happy marriage. Each of the insights we present was harvested only after a careful tilling of an evolutionary psychological perspective on human nature in general, and on the marital alliance in particular. Throughout this chapter, we have speculated that feelings of marital dissatisfaction may function as a psychological and emotional trigger of sorts, inducing or encouraging the dissatisfied spouse to take action to render the marriage more satisfying, or to begin considering alternative marital arrangements, or both. In this section we summarize those aspects of the conjugal relationship, spousal personality characteristics, spousal mate-guarding tactics, and spousal sources of anger, irritation, and upset that evoke marital dissatisfaction. The absence of these events, actions, or characteristics define the relatively happy marriage. Tables 1.1 and 1.2 present the predictors of a husband's and a wife's marital satisfaction, respectively, that we have discussed in this chapter.

TABLE 1.1. Predictors of a Husband's Marital Satisfaction as Gleaned from an Evolutionary Psychological Perspective

Mate value discrepancy

Little or no mate value discrepancy between husband and wife

Wife's personality

High Agreeableness
High Conscientiousness
High Emotional Stability
High Openness/Intellect

Mate-guarding tactics employed by wife

Less monopolization of spouse's time
Less threatening to be unfaithful
Less punishing or threatening to punish spouse's infidelity
Less emotional manipulation

Spousal sources of anger, upset, and irritation

Absence of wife's infidelity[a]
Less condescension toward husband
Less self-centeredness exhibited by wife
Less alcohol abuse by wife
Less emotional constriction exhibited by wife
Less possessiveness exhibited by wife
Less jealousy exhibited by wife
Less dependency exhibited by wife
Less sexualizing of others exhibited by wife

[a]Appears to be the best predictor of a husband's marital satisfaction.

TABLE 1.2. Predictors of a Wife's Marital Satisfaction as Gleaned from an Evolutionary Psychological Perspective

Husband's personality

High Agreeableness
High Conscientiousness
High Emotional Stability
High Openness/Intellect

Mate-guarding tactics employed by husband

Less monopolization of spouse's time
Less threatening to be unfaithful
Less punishing or threatening to punish spouse's infidelity
Less emotional manipulation
More resource provisioning
More expression of love and caring

Spousal sources of anger, upset, and irritation

Less physical and verbal abuse exhibited by husband[a]
Less condescension toward wife
Less neglect exhibited by husband
Less rejection exhibited by husband
Less unreliability exhibited by husband
Absence of husband's infidelity
Less inconsiderateness exhibited by husband
Less moodiness exhibited by husband
Less alcohol abuse by husband
Less emotional constriction exhibited by husband
Less insulting by husband of wife's physical appearance
Less possessiveness exhibited by husband
Less jealousy exhibited by husband
Less dependency exhibited by husband
Less physical self-absorption exhibited by husband
Less sexual withholding and rejection exhibited by husband

[a]Appears to be the best predictor of a wife's marital satisfaction.

The spouses in a mutually satisfying, mutually beneficial marriage are likely to be of relatively equal mate value. From our limited research on married couples, the relationship between mate value discrepancy and marital satisfaction appears to be especially true for husbands. When either spouse is much more valuable or much less valuable than the other as a potential mate on the current "spouse market," a husband is likely to report feelings of marital dissatisfaction. It is not clear to us at this time why husbands' but not wives' marital satisfaction is predictable from the mate value discrepancy between the spouses. Future research is needed to clarify this finding.

Men and women married to agreeable, conscientious, emotionally stable, and open spouses are happier with their marriages. Because of the substantial reproductive costs involved, we have predicted and found that, in terms of spousal personality characteristics, the greatest predictor of a man's marital satisfaction is his wife's level of Conscientiousness. Women low in Conscientiousness are more likely than women high on this personality dimension to be sexually unfaithful to their husbands. Less conscientious women are thus more likely than more conscientious women to place their husbands at risk of investing substantial resources in another man's progeny. The greatest predictors of a woman's marital satisfaction are her husband's levels of Agreeableness and Emotional Stability. Disagreeable, emotionally unstable men are more likely than agreeable, emotionally stable men to inflict physical abuse on their wives.

From an evolutionary psychological perspective, guarding a spouse from intrasexual poaching is a tremendously important adaptive problem recurrently faced by men and women over human evolutionary history. Mate guarding is a tricky enterprise. We have speculated that either excessive mate guarding or total abstention from mate guarding may evoke feelings of marital dissatisfaction in one's spouse. There may be some optimal level of mate guarding that effectively thwarts intrasexual poachers while maintaining or even increasing the guarded spouse's marital happiness.

Mate guarding is not a single behavior, nor is it even a collection of related behaviors. Mate guarding represents a wide range of strategies; some of these increase a spouse's marital happiness, whereas others decrease a spouse's satisfaction with the marriage. Monopolizing a spouse's time, threatening infidelity, punishing or threatening to punish a spouse's infidelity, and emotionally manipulating a spouse are mate-guarding tactics that impose or threaten the imposition of costs for spousal defection. Men and women whose spouses employ these tactics are less satisfied with their marriages than are men and women whose spouses do not employ these mate-guarding tactics.

Women around the world desire husbands who are willing and able to invest their limited time, energy, love, affection, and tangible resources in the women and their children (Buss, 1989a). Not surprisingly, then, women married to men who employ the mate-guarding tactics of resource provisioning and expressing love and caring are more satisfied with their marriages than are women married to men who do not employ these tactics.

The single best predictor of a woman's marital dissatisfaction is the extent to which her spouse abuses her. Although we had predicted that the best predictor of a man's marital happiness would be his partner's infidelity, in fact a wife's unfaithfulness ranked second to her level of moodiness or emotional instability. As we discuss elsewhere (Buss & Shackelford, in press), however, a wife's moodiness or emotional instability is one of the most impressive predictors of a husband's estimate that his wife will cheat on him.

The vast majority of men and women around the world will marry at least once in their lifetimes (Brown, 1991; Buss, 1985; Buss & Schmitt, 1993; Epstein & Guttman, 1984; Vandenberg, 1972). In no culture, however, is marital satisfaction a given. Divorce, whether formal or informal, appears to be a cross-culturally ubiquitous phenomenon (Betzig, 1989). An evolutionary psychological perspective on marriage brings into clear focus the many roads that lead to conjugal distress between husbands and wives. Careful consideration of the many and varied adaptive challenges that our ancestors successfully negotiated helps us to pinpoint the greatest sources of conflict among modern married couples. Although wedded bliss may be a romantic fantasy of young lovers, some marriages do bring lifelong joy and happiness. An evolutionary psychological framework affords a profitable conceptual backdrop for identifying the constituents of these happy marriages, and provides direction for reducing the sources of conflict that lead to marital dissatisfaction.

ACKNOWLEDGMENT

This chapter was prepared while Todd K. Shackelford was a Jacob K. Javits Graduate Fellow.

REFERENCES

Bentler, P. M., & Newcomb, M. D. (1978). Longitudinal study of marital success and failure. *Journal of Consulting and Clinical Psychology, 46,* 1053–1070.

Betzig, L. (1989). Causes of conjugal dissolution: A cross-cultural study. *Current Anthropology, 30,* 654–676.

Brown, D. (1991). *Human universals.* New York: McGraw-Hill.

Burgess, E. W., & Wallen, P. (1953). *Engagement and marriage.* Philadelphia: Lippincott.

Buss, D. M. (1984). Marital assortment for personality dispositions: Assessment with three different data sources. *Behavior Genetics, 14,* 111–123.

Buss, D. M. (1985). Human mate selection. *American Scientist, 73,* 47–51.

Buss, D. M. (1988). From vigilance to violence: Tactics of mate-retention in American undergraduates. *Ethology and Sociobiology, 9,* 219–317.

Buss, D. M. (1989a). Sex differences in human mate preferences: Evolutionary hypotheses tested in 37 cultures. *Behavioral and Brain Sciences, 12,* 1–49.
Buss, D. M. (1989b). Conflict between the sexes: Strategic interference and the evocation of anger and upset. *Journal of Personality and Social Psychology, 56,* 735–747.
Buss, D. M. (1991a). Conflict in married couples: Personality predictors of anger and upset. *Journal of Personality, 59,* 663–688.
Buss, D. M. (1991b). Evolutionary personality psychology. *Annual Review of Psychology, 42,* 459–491.
Buss, D. M. (1992). Manipulation in close relationships: The five factor model of personality in interactional context. *Journal of Personality, 60,* 477–499.
Buss, D. M. (1994). *The evolution of desire.* New York: Basic Books.
Buss, D. M. (1995). Evolutionary psychology: A new paradigm for psychological science. *Psychological Inquiry, 6,* 1–30.
Buss, D. M., Larsen, R. J., Westen, D., & Semmelroth, J. (1992). Sex differences in jealousy: Evolution, physiology, and psychology. *Psychological Science, 3,* 251–255.
Buss, D. M., & Schmitt, D. P. (1993). Sexual strategies theory: An evolutionary perspective on human mating. *Psychological Review, 100,* 204–232.
Buss, D. M., & Shackelford, T. K. (1997). From vigilance to violence: Mate retention tactics in married couples. *Journal of Personality and Social Psychology, 72,* 346–361.
Buss, D. M., & Shackelford, T. K. (in press). Susceptibility to infidelity in the first year of marriage. *Journal of Research in Personality.*
Daly, M., & Wilson, M. (1983). *Sex, evolution, and behavior* (2nd ed.). Boston: Willard Grant.
Daly, M., & Wilson, M. (1988). *Homicide.* Hawthorne, NY: Aldine de Gruyter.
Daly, M., Wilson, M., & Weghorst, S. J. (1982). Male sexual jealousy. *Ethology and Sociobiology, 3,* 11–27.
de Weerth, C., & Kalma, A. P. (1993). Female aggression as a response to sexual jealousy: A sex-role reversal? *Aggressive Behavior, 19,* 265–279.
Dobash, R. P., Dobash, R. E., Wilson, M., & Daly, M. (1992). The myth of sexual symmetry in marital violence. *Social Problems, 39,* 71–91.
Elder, G. H., Jr. (1969). Appearance and education in marriage mobility. *American Sociological Review, 34,* 519–533.
Epstein, E., & Guttman, R. (1984). Mate selection in man: Evidence, theory, and outcome. *Social Biology, 31,* 243–278.
Fisher, H. E. (1992). *Anatomy of love.* New York: Norton.
Ghiselin, M. T. (1974). *The economy of nature and the evolution of sex.* Berkeley: University of California Press.
Goldberg, L. (1981). Language and individual differences: The search for universals in personality lexicons. In L. Wheeler (Ed.), *Review of personality and social psychology* (Vol. 2, pp. 141–165). Beverly Hills, CA: Sage.
Kelly, E. L., & Conley, J. J. (1987). Personality and compatibility: A prospective analysis of marital stability and marital satisfaction. *Journal of Personality and Social Psychology, 52,* 27–40.
Kenrick, D. T., Sadalla, E. K., Groth, G., & Trost, M. R. (1990). Evolution,

traits, and the stages of humans courtship: Qualifying the parental invest-ment model. *Journal of Personality, 58,* 97–116.

Norman, W. T. (1963). Toward an adequate taxonomy of personality attrib-utes: Replicated factor structure in peer nomination personality ratings. *Journal of Personality and Social Psychology, 66,* 574–583.

Shackelford, T. K. (1997). Perceptions of betrayal and the design of the mind. In J. A. Simpson & D. T. Kenrick (Eds.), *Evolutionary social psychology* (pp. 73–107). Mahwah, NJ: Erlbaum.

Shackelford, T. K., & Buss, D. M. (1996). Betrayal in mateships, friendships, and coalitions. *Personality and Social Psychology Bulletin, 22,* 1151–1164.

Shackelford, T. K., & Buss, D. M. (in press). Cues to infidelity. *Personality and Social Psychology Bulletin.*

Symons, D. (1979). *The evolution of human sexuality.* New York: Oxford Univer-sity Press.

Symons, D. (1992). On the use and misuse of Darwinism in the study of hu-man behavior. In J. Barkow, L. Cosmides, & J. Tooby (Eds.), *The adapted mind* (pp. 137–159). New York: Oxford University Press.

Taylor, P. A., & Glenn, N. D. (1976). The utility of education and attractive-ness for females' status attainment through marriage. *American Sociologi-cal Review, 41,* 484–498.

Tooby, J., & Cosmides, L. (1992). Psychological foundations of culture. In J. Barkow, L. Cosmides, & J. Tooby (Eds.), *The adapted mind* (pp. 19–136). New York: Oxford University Press.

Trivers, R. (1972). Parental investment and sexual selection. In B. Campbell (Ed.), *Sexual selection and the descent of man* (pp. 136–179). Chicago: Aldine.

Trivers, R. (1985). *Social evolution.* Menlo Park, CA: Benjamin/Cummings.

Udry, J. R., & Eckland, B. K. (1984). Benefits of being attractive: Differential payoffs for men and women. *Psychological Reports, 54,* 47–56.

Vandenberg, S. (1972). Assortative mating, or who married whom? *Behavior Genetics, 2,* 127–158.

Wiederman, M. W., & Algeier, E. R. (1993). Gender differences in sexual jealousy: Adaptationist or social learning explanation? *Ethology and Socio-biology, 14,* 115–140.

Wilson, E. O. (1975). *Sociobiology.* Cambridge, MA: Harvard University Press.

Wilson, M., & Daly, M. (1992). The man who mistook his wife for chattel. In J. Barkow, L. Cosmides, & J. Tooby (Eds.), *The adapted mind* (pp. 289–322). New York: Oxford University Press.

CHAPTER 2

Attachment and Relationship Satisfaction across the Lifespan

LILAH RAYNOR KOSKI
PHILLIP R. SHAVER

The original aim of attachment theory (Bowlby, 1982, 1988) was to explain the development of personality and psychopathology in the context of close relationships, especially the parent–child relationship. The theory deals mainly with the benefits accrued by a child whose primary caregivers are available, caring, attentive, and responsive, and with the problems encountered by a child whose primary caregivers are neglectful, abusive, or (as a result of death or separation) absent. Despite the theory's not being a theory of relationship satisfaction per se, attachment researchers have gradually been led to map some of the features of psychologically healthy and unhealthy relationships, including relationships between romantic partners. In such relationships, unlike the relationships of the young children initially studied by Bowlby and his followers, it is possible to ask both partners whether or not they are satisfied, and to establish conceptual parallels between adult satisfaction or dissatisfaction and the kinds of emotions evident in the attachment behavior of infants and young children. In some cases, looking carefully at early relationships reveals issues and processes not immediately evident in studies of adult satisfaction.

The purpose of this chapter is to explore potential contributions of lifespan attachment research to an understanding of relationship satisfaction. The chapter begins with a discussion of the concepts "attachment" and "satisfaction," including a brief summary of the key elements of Bowlby and Ainsworth's attachment theory (Ainsworth & Bowlby, 1991). This is followed by a review of discoveries concerning parent–infant attachment relationships, with an emphasis on discoveries related to the processes underlying "satisfaction." The next three sections review studies of attachment and relationship quality in childhood, adolescence and adulthood, and old age. The chapter ends with implications for enhancing satisfaction in close relationships across the lifespan.

WHAT ARE ATTACHMENT AND SATISFACTION?

Attachment

At the center of attachment theory is Bowlby's (1982) assumption that human beings, like other primates, have been equipped by evolution with an "attachment behavioral system." This system causes a human infant to "bond" emotionally with an "attachment figure," and then to scan the environment intermittently to assess the availability and responsiveness of that person (usually a parent or designated caregiver). As long as such a figure is present, the attachment behavioral system remains relatively quiescent, but under certain conditions—for example, when no attachment figure is available or when the environment seems dangerous or unpredictable—the attachment behavioral system is activated. The infant then forgets what he or she was doing a moment before, looks more insistently for the attachment figure, and begins to cry and crawl toward the likely location of that person. Under typical circumstances, these searching, proximity-seeking behaviors increase in intensity until the attachment figure comes to the infant's rescue.

According to Bowlby and Ainsworth, an infant can be viewed as an assembly of behavioral systems, only one of which has to do with attachment. There are also, for example, exploration, affiliation, and sexual systems. At least during infancy, the attachment system takes precedence, so that an infant engaged in exploratory play will suddenly abandon that activity upon noticing that his or her attachment figure is leaving or is unavailable. Once comforting contact with the attachment figure has been reestablished, the infant can return to play or engage in some other activity. Attachment researchers, following Ainsworth (1967), refer to the attachment figure as a "safe haven" in times of distress and a "secure base" from which to explore the environment. Later researchers, beginning with Sroufe and Waters (1977), have postulated that the presence of a responsive caregiver who effectively serves as a safe haven and secure base causes an infant to experience a positive emotional state, "felt security." More generally, the theory portrays positive and negative emotions, such as joy, love, anger, anxiety, sadness, and grief, as consequences of attachment figures' supportive or unsupportive actions. And it characterizes defenses, such as denial, repression, and hypervigilance, as modes of regulating attachment-related emotions. (See Shaver, Collins, & Clark, 1996, for a detailed discussion of attachment and emotion regulation.)

Attachment theory focuses on the gradual development of individual differences in relationship styles as a function of the behavior of primary caregivers. If a child comes, in the context of attachment relationships, to feel largely secure, he or she develops what Bowlby (1982) called secure "internal working models" of self and relationship partners. If a child has reason to feel rejected or coolly received by one or more attachment figures, he or she may develop an insecure sense of self and a distrust of others. A somewhat different set of working models evolves if a child finds key attachment figures to be unpredictable or unreliable in their responsiveness—sometimes available, warm, and interested; sometimes self-preoccupied, anxious, and unavailable. Also important are a child's experiences with losses and separations. According to attachment theory, such experiences strongly activate the attachment behavioral system and initiate a series of stages labeled "protest," "despair," and "detachment" (Bowlby, 1973, 1980). The outcome of major losses depends in part on the support given a child following the loss, and on the willingness of substitute attachment figures to tolerate grief and discuss the child's feelings openly.

Much of attachment research has been designed to identify patterns of infant–parent attachment and to assess their sequelae later in childhood—for example, in the context of peer relationships or student–teacher relationships. In recent years, the patterns first identified in infancy and childhood have been assessed in studies of adolescent and adult friendships and romantic relationships, where the topics of interest include the effects of relationship patterns, or "attachment styles" (Levy & Davis, 1988; Shaver, Hazan, & Bradshaw, 1988), on relationship satisfaction (e.g., Brennan & Shaver, 1995; Collins & Read, 1990).

Relationship Satisfaction

The word "satisfaction" implies that a need or debt has been satisfied or fulfilled. In the literature on close relationships, "satisfaction" has been used to label evaluative scales that assess how a relationship is faring according to participants' self-reports. In the literature on romantic and marital relationships, satisfactory relationships are often labeled "nondistressed," to distinguish them from relationships that are troubled, "distressed," and perhaps headed for divorce or breakup.

Attachment theory provides a particular perspective on the relationship-related needs that must be met in order for relationship partners to describe themselves as satisfied. These needs have to do, at their root, with the desirability of feeling protected, loved, and secure. Secondarily, they concern the ability to engage in exciting, rewarding exploratory activities that depend on a foundation of attachment-related felt security. Moreover, the theory suggests that certain personal needs and preferences—for example, for an unusual degree of certainty about a partner's affection and commitment, or for a partner's willingness to allow a certain degree of autonomy and privacy—result from a person's previous history of relationships with attachment figures. In order for an adult relationship to be viewed as satisfying, the partners in the relationship presumably have to have their attachment-related needs largely met, including needs for a lack of interference with favorite affect-regulating strategies and defenses.

This approach to relationship satisfaction applies across the lifespan because, according to Bowlby (1982), the need for attachment figures persists "from the cradle to the grave" (p. 208). Of course, the nature of attachment relationships changes with development (Main, Kaplan, & Cassidy, 1985; Shaver et al., 1988). As a child develops, attachment relationships depend more extensively on linguistic expressions of needs and feelings. "Availability" becomes more abstract and no longer requires constant, immediate physical presence. "Responsiveness" changes, depending on the needs to which an attachment figure is expected to respond.

ATTACHMENT AND RELATIONSHIP SATISFACTION IN INFANCY

According to Bowlby (1982), emotional responses reflect the short-term status and long-term quality of the attachment between a child and his or her primary caregivers. For example, infants and children display a predictable set of reactions (protest) when they are about to be separated from an attachment figure. Some of the first research on infant–caregiver attachment consisted of case studies and filmed observations of small samples of children who were forced to endure extended separations from their parents (e.g., Robertson, 1952; Robertson & Robertson, 1967). Findings from those studies revealed, as expected, that children exhibited certain patterns of distress (anxiety, anger, withdrawal from others) in response to separations.

These case studies led Ainsworth (1967) to conduct a systematic study of infants and mothers in Uganda, and eventually to create a laboratory situation, the "Strange Situation," that reliably elicited attachment behaviors in the United States (Ainsworth, Blehar, Waters, & Wall, 1978). In the Strange Situation, 12-month-old infants are observed during a series of separations and reunions from their primary caregivers. Based on the infants' behavior during the separation and reunion episodes, the infants are classified into one of three attachment categories: "secure," "anxious–ambivalent," or "avoidant." Recently, a fourth category, "disorganized/disoriented," has been added (Main et al., 1985). (For the sake of brevity, the second, third, and fourth categories are referred to from here on as "anxious," "avoidant," and "disorganized.")

The four types of infants differ markedly in their behavior and in the positivity and negativity of their interactions with caregivers. In the Strange Situation, infants classified as secure tend to show distress during separations, but they recover quickly upon reunion and continue to explore their environment with interest. When secure infants are reunited with their caregivers, they greet them with joy and affection. At home, secure infants cry less than insecure infants, respond more positively to being held, and initiate more contact with their mothers (Ainsworth et al., 1978). Mothers of secure infants are responsive to their babies' cries, hold them affectionately, have relatively harmonious and cooperative interactions with them, and are emotionally expressive (Ainsworth et al., 1978; Belsky, Rovine, & Taylor, 1984; Isabella & Belsky, 1991; Isabella, Belsky, & von Eye, 1989). It seems reasonable, in the context of the present chapter, to characterize these relationships as mutually satisfying.

Avoidant infants appear to have much less satisfying interactions with their caregivers. In the Strange Situation, they show little distress when separated from their mothers, engage in little creative, fluid exploratory behavior, and avoid their mothers when reunited with them. At home, avoidant infants cry more and are more angry than secure infants. The mothers of avoidant infants tend to be emotionally rigid, as well as angry at and rejecting of their young children. They tend to withdraw support precisely when their infants most need it, during periods of distress. Some of these mothers say explicitly that they do not enjoy physical contact (touching, cuddling, nursing) with their infants. Anxious infants and their mothers, on the other hand, appear to have conflicted and ambivalent interactions. In the Strange Situation, anxious infants are extremely distressed upon separation from their mothers, explore relatively little, and exhibit conflicted responses toward their mothers at reunion (e.g., these infants may cling one moment and angrily resist comforting the next moment). At home, anxious infants cry more and are angrier and less compliant than secure infants. Interactions between anxious infants and their mothers are characterized by a lack of harmony and especially by chronic anxiety on the infants' part, perhaps because the infants cannot rely on the caregivers' consistent responsiveness (Ainsworth et al., 1978; Isabella et al., 1989). Mothers of anxious infants tend to be insensitive to their infants' emotional signals, perhaps because they are somewhat anxious and preoccupied with their own feelings (Main et al., 1985).

The fourth group, disorganized infants, are characterized by odd, awkward behaviors during the Strange Situation. For example, when reunited with their mothers, disorganized infants may begin to approach but then suddenly stop and avert their gaze or physically "freeze" (see Main & Solomon, 1990, for a summary of disorganized attachment behaviors). Disorganized infants are much more common in maltreated and high-risk samples than in the usual samples that volunteer for university studies of child development (Carlson, Cicchetti, Barnett, & Braunwald, 1989; van IJzendoorn, Goldberg, Kroonenberg, & Frenkel, 1992). Their odd behavior is thought to be a result of their attachment figure's helpless, frightened, or frightening behavior (Main & Hesse, 1990).

To summarize, research on infant–caregiver attachment suggests that relationship satisfaction is higher in secure than in insecure infant–caregiver dyads. Satisfaction is indicated behaviorally by the secure infants' greater positivity: greater physical affection, emotional expressivity, and active exploration of the world. Among their mothers, greater satisfaction is expressed behaviorally by sensitivity and responsiveness to infant signals, positive affect, and maternal affection, and verbally in self-reports of feelings related to the parent–child relationship. Maternal self-reports reveal, for example, that mothers of secure babies are more interested in and satisfied with their children than are mothers of insecure babies (Egeland & Farber, 1984). Attachment behaviors and maternal self-reports in insecure dyads indicate lower levels of satisfaction. Anxious dyads are characterized by relatively frequent inharmonious and uncooperative interactions and by the babies' prevalent negative expressivity (crying and angry aggression), despite some affectionate episodes. Avoidant dyads generally lack signs of warmth, joy, and affection; disorganized dyads are marked by fear and confusion.

ATTACHMENT AND RELATIONSHIP SATISFACTION IN YOUNG CHILDREN

As children develop beyond the first year of life, they acquire cognitive skills that allow them to adopt the perspectives of others and to express themselves verbally (Bretherton & Beeghly, 1982; Bretherton, McNew, & Beeghly-Smith, 1981). These cognitive and communication skills affect the nature of the attachment relationship and the ways in which satisfaction and dissatisfaction are expressed. Secure children can articulate their emotions verbally, and can understand and label other people's emotions (Beeghly & Cicchetti, 1994; Morisset, Barnard, Greenberg, Booth, & Spieker, 1990). For example, Bretherton, Ridgeway, and Cassidy (1990) studied the responses of 29 children aged 3 years to a series of potentially anxiety-provoking situations, and assessed their behavior during separation and reunion episodes. Security of responses during separations and reunions was associated with children's self-described ability to cope with a potential 2-week separation. Secure children talked about feeling angry or upset, but also about doing something constructive about the situation. In contrast, avoidant children said, "I don't know," when asked about how to deal with a potential separation; disorganized children responded in odd, nonsensical, or excessively violent ways. (The authors did not find a consistent pattern of responding among anxious children.) Secure children were also more likely than insecure children to imagine a happy reunion with their parents, saying they would hug their parents or go out for pizza with them.

Secure children's ability to express themselves verbally is evident throughout their development. In a study of 5-year-olds, Slough and Greenberg (1990) found security to be correlated with less avoidant and more emotionally open responses to pictures of potential separations. In a sample of 6-year-olds, Main et al. (1985) found security in infancy to be correlated with the security and reasonableness of later narrative responses to potential separations. Secure children in this study were also more likely to respond positively (smiling and showing interest, making positive comments) to photographs of their families, whereas children who had been classified as insecure in infancy were more likely to respond with discomfort or lack of disinterest.

The open, well-developed, and positive emotional expressions of secure children, in contrast to the constrained and negative emotional expressions of insecure children, affect the relationships children form and the satisfaction experienced in those relationships. Secure children are more nurturing (Troy & Sroufe, 1987), more involved with others (LaFraniere & Sroufe, 1985), and more agentic and independent (Erickson, Sroufe, & Egeland, 1985; Sroufe, 1983) than insecure children. In contrast, anxious children are relatively dependent and helpless, have difficulty interacting with others, and are likely to be victimized by peers (see Cassidy & Berlin, 1994, for a review). Berlin, Cassidy, and Belsky

(1995) found that 5- to 7-year-old children who had been classified as anxious during infancy reported more social loneliness than children who had been classified during infancy as secure or avoidant. Whereas anxious children tend to emphasize their emotional vulnerability in interactions with others (Berlin et al., 1995), avoidant children deemphasize or dismiss their need for attachment figures. In response to potential separations from parents, avoidant children minimize their distress (Cassidy, 1988; Main et al., 1985), are rigid and tense in their representations of attachment relationships (e.g., Kaplan & Main, 1985), and are more likely to pick on other children (Troy & Sroufe, 1987). Disorganized children, who have been studied less extensively to date, exhibit hostile behaviors toward their peers (Lyons-Ruth, Alpern, & Repacholi, 1993) and engage in controlling, role-reversing behaviors with their parents (Main & Solomon, 1990).

Longer-term studies of the sequelae of infant attachment patterns also reveal theoretically predictable effects on close relationships. Children aged 10 and 11 years who were secure with their mothers as infants enjoy close friendships with a small number of children later on (Elicker, Englund, & Sroufe, 1992; Grossmann & Grossmann, 1991) and seek help and comfort from their parents when they need it (Grossmann & Grossmann, 1991). Children who were avoidant or anxious as infants report having either no friends or many friends whose names they cannot remember (Grossmann & Grossmann, 1991). These children also harbor relatively negative impressions of relationships and tend to lack social skills (Elicker et al., 1992; Sroufe, Carlson, & Shulman, 1993).

In short, extensive research suggests that as children develop beyond infancy, early behavioral indicators of satisfying or distressed relationships with attachment figures become transformed into a more complex array of cognitive, linguistic, and empathic tendencies and skills. Secure children establish openly expressive, warm, and generally satisfying interactions with others. Insecure children's interactions are more frequently constrained, dissatisfying, or conflictual. Anxious children's dissatisfaction takes the form of feeling needy and emotionally vulnerable; avoidant children's dissatisfaction includes suppressed anger and a tendency to deny their need for close relationships; and disorganized children's dissatisfaction is evident in their hostility and inappropriate social behavior. Viewed from the perspective of adult relationships, studies of attachment-related behavior in childhood suggest that some people will have an easier time than others applying what they learned in childhood to the formation of a mutually satisfying romantic or marital relationship.

MEASUREMENT OF ATTACHMENT IN ADOLESCENCE AND ADULTHOOD

In order to extend attachment research into adolescence and adulthood, it has been necessary to create new measures of attachment orientations or styles suitable for those age groups. Several different kinds of measures have been developed and validated. All involve the use of interviews and self-report questionnaires that probe attachment-related mental representations and feelings.

The Adult Attachment Interview

George, Kaplan, and Main (1985) devised the Adult Attachment Interview (AAI), in which adolescents or adults answer several open-ended questions about their childhood relationships with attachment figures. The answers are then coded in ways designed to predict how the interviewees' children will score in Ainsworth's Strange Situation. In other words, the validation criterion for the AAI is child behavior, not the interviewees' other characteristics or the quality of their adult relationships. On the basis of the interview, a person can be placed into one of three attachment categories: "secure" (or, free and autonomous with respect to attachment), "dismissing" (of attachment), or "preoccupied" (with attachment).

Secure adults are at ease discussing attachment experiences and can describe them fluently and coherently. In Ainsworth's Strange Situation, their children tend to behave securely. Dismissing adults often describe their parents in vaguely idealistic terms, have difficulty backing up these generalizations with specific memories, and deny the influence of attachment experiences on their development. Their children often turn out to be avoidant in the Strange Situation. Preoccupied adults seem to be entangled in still-intense negative or conflicted feelings about their parents; they can easily retrieve specific attachment-related memories but have trouble discussing them coherently. Their children are generally anxious in the Strange Situation. Each interviewee also receives a score on "lack of resolution" of attachment-related losses or traumas (e.g., losing a parent, being abused as a child). People classified as "unresolved" exhibit unusual lapses in reasoning during the AAI—for example, speaking of a deceased attachment figure as if he or she were still alive, or taking undue responsibility for losses or traumatic events. Such people's children are likely to be classified as disorganized in the Strange Situation (Main & Hesse, 1990).

In a 20-year longitudinal study by Waters and his colleagues (Waters, Merrick, Albersheim, & Treboux, 1995) 70% of infants classified at age 1 in the Strange Situation had the same secure versus insecure attachment status when assessed with the AAI at age 21; 64% had exactly the same specific classification (out of Ainsworth's three). And the degree of stability was related to important life events between ages 1 and 21. Those with no major attachment-related negative life events (e.g., loss of a parent, parental divorce, or physical or sexual abuse) had a stability rate of 72%, whereas those who *had* experienced such life events attained a stability rate of only 44%. Thus, attachment patterns tend to be stable, but they are not unchangeable.

A Questionnaire Measure of Romantic Attachment Style

Hazan and Shaver (1987, 1990) developed a self-report measure of *romantic* attachment style. In its original form, this measure consisted of three brief, written descriptions of behavior in romantic relationships — descriptions that were intended to parallel Ainsworth's three types of infants. Respondents were asked which of these three descriptions (Hazan & Shaver, 1990, p. 272) best characterized them:

> *Avoidant:* "I am somewhat uncomfortable being close to others; I find it difficult to trust them completely, difficult to allow myself to depend on them. I am nervous when anyone gets too close, and often, love partners want to be more intimate than I feel comfortable being."
>
> *Anxious:* "I find that others are reluctant to get as close as I would like. I often worry that my partner doesn't really love me or won't want to stay with me. I want to get very close to my partner, and this sometimes scares people away."
>
> *Secure:* "I find it relatively easy to get close to others and am comfortable depending on them. I don't often worry about being abandoned or about someone getting too close to me."

In most studies using this measure, the proportions of the three styles (approximately 25% avoidant, 20% anxious, and 55% secure) are similar to the proportions of the three kinds of infants in studies based on the Strange Situation. The measure has been validated by establishing a network of associations with theoretically related personality and relationship constructs (see Shaver & Clark, 1994, and Shaver & Hazan, 1993, for reviews). Many investigators ask respondents to rate how self-descriptive each style is, rather than simply asking for the most self-descriptive type.

Bartholomew's Four-Category Measures

Bartholomew (1990; Bartholomew & Horowitz, 1991) created a set of attachment measures that combine some of the features of the AAI and the Hazan and Shaver questionnaire. Bartholomew (1990) argued that there are two kinds of avoidance in adolescent and adult relationships, "dismissing" (as captured by the AAI) and "fearful" (as assessed by Hazan and Shaver). When both are included in a self-report measure or coded from interviews about attachment relationships with parents or peers (including romantic partners), the result is a four-category typology that is defined by two bipolar dimensions: (1) positive versus negative internal working model of self, and (2) positive versus negative internal working model of others.

According to this scheme, the four attachment styles are as follows: "secure" (positive model of self, positive model of others), "preoccupied" (negative model of self, positive model of others), "fearful" (negative model of self, negative model of others), and "dismissing" (positive model of self, negative model of others). The description of each style in the self-report version of Bartholomew's measure (Bartholomew & Horowitz, 1991, p. 244) is as follows:

> *Secure:* "It is easy for me to become emotionally close to others. I am comfortable depending on others and having others depend on me. I don't worry about being alone or having others not accept me."
>
> *Fearful:* "I am uncomfortable getting close to others. I want emotionally close relationships, but I find it difficult to trust others completely, or to depend on them. I worry that I will be hurt if I allow myself to become too close to others."
>
> *Preoccupied:* "I want to be completely emotionally intimate with others, but I often find that others are reluctant to get as close as I would like. I am uncomfortable being without close relationships, but I sometimes worry that others don't value me as much as I value them."
>
> *Dismissing:* "I am comfortable without close emotional relationships. It is very important to me to feel independent and self-sufficient, and I prefer not to depend on others or have others depend on me."

Most recent studies of attachment in adolescence and adulthood are based either on the AAI or on one of the self-report measures just described (or a multi-item extension of them). The AAI has been used primarily in studies of infant–parent attachment; the self-report measures have been used primarily in studies of adult peer and romantic relationships.

ATTACHMENT AND RELATIONSHIP SATISFACTION IN ADOLESCENCE AND YOUNG ADULTHOOD

Continuing Attachments to Parents

Evidence for continuity in the association between attachment and relationship satisfaction is provided by a study of conflict resolution in mother–teen dyads. Kobak, Cole, Ferenz-Gillies, Fleming, and Gamble (1993, Study 2) observed 14- to 18-year-olds and their mothers while each dyad discussed a problematic issue in the relationship. Based on coders' *Q*-sort summaries of AAI interviews with the adolescents, each was assigned scores on two dimensions: security–anxiety (i.e., security vs. insecurity) and deactivation–hyperactivation (i.e., diverting attention away from attachment-related information vs. being preoccupied with attachment). These two dimensions are 45-degree rotations of Bartholomew's two dimensions; they run from secure to fearful and from dismissing to preoccupied in Bartholomew's terms. AAI security was associated with low avoidance, low dysfunctional anger, and relationship balance (i.e., egalitarian give and take between mother and child); deactivation was associated with maternal dominance and dysfunctional anger.

In a slightly older sample of college students, AAI scores also proved to be associated with emotional regulation. Dozier and Kobak (1992) found that use of the deactivating strategy was related to increases in skin conductance when students were asked questions about such childhood experiences as parental rejection and separation from parents. Thus, the deactivating strategy was related to suppression and denial of attachment-related emotions. This avoidance and suppression of attachment-related emotions may help explain some of the communication difficulties encountered by people who use this strategy. Teenagers who are able to discuss problems with their mothers while maintaining balance may have more satisfying relationships partly because they experience relatively little anger and conflict, or are able to articulate rather than suppress negative emotions.

Studies of adolescents making the transition from home to college reveal other aspects of the association between attachment styles and satisfaction. In a study by Hazan and Hutt (1993), for example, secure college freshmen reported being lonely during their first month on campus, but quickly made friends and felt well integrated by the end of their first year of school. They received more calls from their parents than their insecure counterparts received, but felt in control of such contacts, as indicated by their ability to end the conversations when they chose to. Avoidant students were less able to rely on their parents for support during the transition and experienced more psychosomatic symptoms. They had fewer conversations with their parents and had to initiate most of the ones they did have. Anxious (preoccupied) students were initially excited about getting away from home and forming new relationships at college, but were socially dissatisfied and lonely after the first semester. Their conversations with parents were often initiated *and ended* by the parents. Kenny (1987) also studied a group of college freshmen during their adaptation to college. Students' perceived adjustment to the separation from their parents was a significant predictor of the competence they felt in dating situations. (Similar findings have been reported with respect to college students' successful exploration of career possibilities; see Blustein, Prezioso, & Palladino-Schultheiss, 1995.) In sum, relationships with parents foster or inhibit exploratory behaviors in adolescence and early adulthood that are important for identity formation and the creation of satisfying peer and romantic relationships.

Relationships with Peers

As in childhood, college students' attachment patterns are related to the quality of their friendships. Kobak and Sceery (1988) found that secure students were rated higher than insecure students on a measure of ego resilience completed by peers. Preoccupied students were rated by peers as more anxious and less positive in their social behavior than were individuals in the other two attachment categories. Dismissing students were rated as relatively hostile. In another sample of college students, Bartholomew and Horowitz (1991) also found that secure individuals differed from insecure individuals in the quality of their interactions with friends. According to both self-reports and friends' reports, secure students were warm and sociable; dismissing students were somewhat competitive and cold; fearful students were introverted and unassertive; and preoccupied students were sociable and warm, but also overly emotional and dominant. Taken together, these studies reveal distinct patterns of interpersonal behavior associated with different attachment styles.

The findings suggest that secure late adolescents and young adults enjoy more satisfying (warm, open, mutually engaging) relationships with their friends than do their insecure peers. The precise nature of the relatively dissatisfying relationships of insecure young adults depends on attachment style. On the one hand, some avoidant individuals (those who are dismissing, in Bartholomew's terms, or those who use deactivating strategies, in Kobak et al.'s) dismiss the importance of relationships and tend to be somewhat cold and hostile in their interactions with friends. Other avoidant adults (those who are fearful, in Bartholomew's terms) are more likely to want relationships but are unsuccessful at becoming fully engaged with them. Preoccupied adults, on the other hand, exhibit the same kinds of emotional, conflictual interactions characteristic of anxious infants.

Attachment and Romantic Relationships

While in college, many late adolescents and young adults become involved in their first serious romantic relationships. Studies of college dating relationships are important to an understanding of attachment and relationship satisfaction, because they suggest that adult romantic relationships are influenced by a person's attachment history (perhaps beginning in infancy), and that men and women differ in the ways their attachment-related experiences affect the degree of satisfaction they experience. Relationship satisfaction has been measured in these studies by both behavioral indicators and self-reports.

In several studies of college-age dating couples, researchers have found that secure attachment (as assessed with self-report measures) is associated with higher levels of relationship satisfaction than insecure attachment is (e.g., Brennan & Shaver, 1995; Hammond & Fletcher, 1991; Kirkpatrick & Davis, 1994; Pistole, 1989; Simpson, 1990). Researchers have also noted effects of partners' attachment style on relationship satisfaction—effects that frequently differ between men and women. For example, there is growing evidence that women's anxiety (i.e., preoccupation or anxious-ambivalence) influences their male partners' relationship satisfaction, whereas men's security and avoidance influences women's satisfaction.

Collins and Read (1990) reported that women's anxiety and men's security were correlated with couple members' relationship satisfaction. Women's anxiety was negatively correlated with both their own and their partners' relationship satisfaction; men's comfort with closeness (security) was correlated with both their own and their partners' relationship satisfaction. Simpson (1990) also found that men with more anxious partners reported lower levels of relationship satisfaction (as indicated by kindness, loyalty, and similarity of values). For women, however, the more secure their partners were, the higher their relationship satisfaction. Kirkpatrick and Davis (1994) reported that men's relationship satisfaction (e.g., the degree to which their relationships were perceived as successful, met their needs, provided enjoyment, and enhanced their feelings of self-worth) was highest if their partners were secure and lowest if their partners were anxious, but women's relationship satisfaction was unrelated to their partners' attachment style.

There is as yet no widespread agreement about the meaning of this apparently reliable gender difference. One possibility is that men's customary independence is threatened by overly anxious, preoccupied partners, whereas women's well-documented desire for intimacy is thwarted by overly avoidant partners. Another possibility is that relationship dissatisfaction heightens negative emotion, triggering gender-related coping mechanisms (emotional expression on the part of women, emotional suppression and withdrawal on the part of men).

Several studies have found attachment to be related to self-report indices of relationship characteristics other than global self-reports of relationship quality. In Simpson's (1990) previously described study, the less often men and women reported feeling positive emotions (which included intense emotions such as "excited" and "elated," as well as milder positive emotions such as "calm" and "content"), the more anxious or avoidant they or their partners were. For both men and women, security was associated with more self-disclosure and greater feelings of love, dependency, trust, and commitment. Similarly, in a study in which subjects were asked to imagine a relationship with a hypothetical partner who had a particular attachment style, subjects' positive emotions were strongest if they or the hypothetical partner was secure. Subjects also liked the secure partner most and expected the least conflict with that partner (Pietromonaco & Carnelley, 1994). Kirkpatrick and Davis (1994) also found that secure men, and men with secure partners, felt more commitment and intimacy in their relationships than insecure men or men with insecure partners.

Feeney (1995) studied attachment and emotional control in dating couples, and found that couples in which both members were insecure reported a greater frequency of negative emotions and greater control of negative emotions than couples in which at least one partner was secure. Emotional control of negative emotions was significantly greater in these insecure couples even when the frequency of negative emotions was statistically controlled. Couples in which both members were secure exhibited the least emotional control, and couples in which one member was insecure fell in the middle. These findings are compatible with studies reviewed earlier, which indicate that secure children learn to express and articulate their attachment-related feelings in the context of their relationships with parents. Insecure individuals seem to experience frequent negative emotions but are unable to express and discuss them effectively, perhaps because their parents were ineffective in the same ways.

A person's attachment-related internal working models influence the way in which he or she experiences close relationships. There is some evidence, for example, that preoccupied (anxious, hyperactivating) people are both more anxious and more passionate than either secure or avoidant people are (Feeney & Noller, 1990; Hatfield, Brinton, & Cornelius, 1989; Hindy & Schwartz, 1994; Levy & Davis, 1988; Kirkpatrick & Davis, 1994), and that they are more likely to be obsessed with their relationships (Hazan & Shaver, 1987) and to endure frequent or repeated breakups (Kirkpatrick & Davis, 1994; Shaver & Brennan, 1992). Avoidant (dismissing, deactivating) individuals' relationships are characterized by emotional distance (Bartholomew & Horowitz, 1991) and lack of interest (Shaver & Brennan, 1992). Avoidant individuals may withdraw from their romantic partners if they feel pressured or stressed (Simpson, Rholes, & Nelligan, 1992). Secure individuals enjoy stable, friendly relationships with their romantic partners—relationships characterized by trust, commitment, constructive communication, and satisfaction (Brennan & Shaver, 1995; Collins & Read, 1990; Kirkpatrick & Davis, 1994; Pistole, 1989; Scharfe & Bartholomew, 1995; Simpson, 1990).

ATTACHMENT AND RELATIONSHIP SATISFACTION AMONG MARRIED ADULTS

Attachment research on adults who are older than typical college students takes several forms. One line of work focuses on adults' cognitive representations of childhood attachment experiences (assessed with the AAI) and on various correlates of these representations. For example, several studies have documented a correspondence between parents' attachment orientations, as measured by the AAI, and their children's attachment classifications in the Strange Situation (see van IJzendoorn, 1995, for a meta-analysis). These studies suggest that attachment-related experiences and behavior patterns can be transferred from generation to generation. (Benoit & Parker, 1994, have documented this continuity across three generations.) Other AAI studies have shown that adults' early attachment experiences are associated with the nature and quality of marital interactions. In addition, there is self-report research on attachment and relationship satisfaction in married couples.

What accounts for the cross-generational transmission of attachment patterns? One of the most frequently mentioned transmission mechanisms is parents' sensitivity, or responsiveness, to children's needs and emotions. In van IJzendoorn's (1995) meta-analysis of AAI studies, there was considerable evidence for sensitivity and responsiveness as mediators of the association between parents' and children's attachment styles. But the strength of these effects was insufficient to explain the association completely. Another, less well-researched possibility is that secure parents are better able to understand and discuss their children's needs and feelings. This possibility is compatible with the fact that parents classified as secure on the AAI display unusually fluent and coherent discourse when describing attachment-related feelings. In fact, it is possible to conceptualize their secure behavior in the AAI as involving responsiveness to the interviewer, accurate perception of the interviewer's questions, and informative but concise answers to these questions. Dismissing parents come across in the interview as somewhat guarded and hence as uncooperative. Preoccupied parents sometimes lose track of the interviewer's questions and become increasingly entangled in their emotional accounts of their parents' deficiencies.

In a revealing study, Bretherton, Biringen, and Ridgeway (1989) interviewed 37 mothers of 2-year-olds about their experiences as mothers and their perceptions of their children. The interviews were scored for maternal sensitivity to children's needs and communications, and for a mother's ability to reflect on her own and her child's behavior and personality. The more sensitive and insightful the mothers were, the more securely their children had behaved as infants in the Strange Situation, and the more secure these children were as toddlers in responding to an open-ended attachment story.

Of course, it is possible that some of the emotional and behavioral similarity between parents and children can be attributed to shared genes. Perhaps affectively positive parents produce children with affectively positive temperaments. To date it has been difficult to disentangle the effects of parenting from the effects of genes, but intervention experiments (e.g., van den Boom, 1994) indicate that attachment security can be deliberately enhanced, regardless of temperament. Hence, it seems unlikely that temperament research will ever render social-relational explanations unnecessary. (Surprisingly, there is no large-scale behavior-genetic study of identical twins' and same-sex fraternal twins' similarity in attachment style although a relevant study of adults has been completed; see Waller & Shaver, 1994.)

AAI classifications seem to be important predictors of adults' relationships with spouses. Cohn, Silver, Cowan, Cowan, and Pearson (1992) assessed attachment types as well as communication and interaction patterns in a sample of married couples. Couples containing at least one secure partner had more harmonious and less conflicted interactions than insecure couples. Couples in which both members were insecure experienced more conflict, produced less positive interactions, and functioned at a lower level than couples in which one or both members were secure. It seems likely that the presence of one secure partner reduces the frequency of angry, hurtful, destructive interactions.

Researchers who have used measures of attachment other than the AAI have also found that attachment styles are related to the quality of marital interactions and to partners' satisfaction with marital relationships. For example, Kobak and Hazan (1991) assessed attachment, relationship satisfaction, and communication in a sample of 40 married couples. Attachment was measured in terms of two dimensions: reliance on partner and psychological availability. Husbands' and wives' reliance on their partners and their ratings of the psychological availability of their partners were associated with constructive communication during problem solving and with relationship satisfaction.

Quality of communication also helped explain the association between attachment style and relationship satisfaction in a large study of Australian married couples. "Mutual expression and understanding" mediated the negative association between anxiety and relationship satisfaction for husbands. For wives, mutual expression and understanding mediated the positive association between relationship satisfaction and security (Feeney, 1994). In another study of Australian couples, the more anxious the husbands were, the less accurate were their wives' nonverbal messages. Wives' security (comfort with closeness) was positively related to the accuracy of their husbands' nonverbal messages (Noller & Feeney, 1994).

In a 2-year longitudinal study of newlyweds, Feeney, Noller, and Callan (1994) found husbands' security and wives' anxiety to be associated with husbands' perceptions of communication quality. For wives, anxiety and partners' security were associated with perceptions of the quality of their communication. For both husbands and wives, anxiety was correlated with the use of coercion and other destructive strategies during communication, and was negatively correlated with the use of mutual understanding and expression. Studies conducted in the United States and Canada have revealed that security is related to the use of constructive accommodation in response to a partner's potentially destructive behaviors (Rusbult, Verette, Whitney, Slovik, & Lipkus, 1991; Scharfe & Bartholomew, 1995) and to a lack of verbal aggression and withdrawal during problem solving (Senchak & Leonard, 1992).

Taken together, these findings highlight the role played by communication in establishing a link between adult attachment style and relationship satisfaction. In interactions between parents and children, adults influence their children's emotions and emerging beliefs about themselves and others, while also modeling certain kinds of behavior (sensitivity, self-centeredness, suppression of feelings, withdrawal of support during times of distress) that will later be copied by the children. Secure, and security-inducing, parents are probably more accurate in sensing their children's needs and concerns, more able to help their children cope with negative experiences and emotions, more affectively positive, and more encouraging. In relationships between adults, especially in the context of marriage, similar forms of verbal and nonverbal communication are important determinants of satisfaction. Secure adults communicate their feelings more accurately and sensitively than insecure adults, perceptively notice their partners' needs and feelings, respond more empathically, and express more optimism about the relationship. Insecure adults, depending on the details of their attachment history, respond with more anger and defensiveness, misread their partners' feelings more often, become demoralized more easily, and frequently attempt to suppress emotion and withdraw from conflict. These are patterns that marital researchers have identified as important predictors of relationship quality and stability.

ATTACHMENT AND RELATIONSHIP SATISFACTION IN OLD AGE

A few researchers have recognized the applicability of attachment theory to the study of relationships in old age (e.g., Antonucci, 1994; Troll & Smith, 1976), but there are almost no studies of the association between attachment styles and relationship satisfaction in this age group. We will therefore reach beyond the existing attachment literature for hints of what may be found in future studies.

As adults age, their social networks decrease in size because of immobility and the deaths of family members and friends. This is not to say, however, that most elderly adults lack close relationships. On the contrary, research shows that intimate relationships are essential for well-being later in life, just as they are at earlier ages (Lowenthal & Haven, 1968); it also shows that although the configuration of social networks may change with age, the quality of the relationships in the network need not decline (Kahn & Antonucci, 1980). Carstensen (1991) has argued that the salience of emotionally close relationships actually increases as old people selectively maintain relationships with emotionally satisfying friends and family members. Lang and Carstensen (1994) found that very old adults (aged 85–104 years) had smaller social networks than a younger sample of elderly adults (aged 70–84 years), but that the two groups did not differ in the number of very close social partners. Rather, the decline in size of the social network could be attributed to a decrease in distant social partners. Interestingly, older adults whose nuclear family members were still alive felt more "socially embedded" (i.e., more socially satisfied, more involved in tender relationships) than older adults without nuclear family members; however, those without family members who nevertheless had emotionally close relationships with others also felt embedded. Although these studies did not include measures of attachment style, they underscore the importance of attachment relationships for elderly adults.

Other researchers have documented important changes in older adults' close relationships. For example, there is evidence that the dynamics of parent–child relationships change as grown children age. Cicirelli (1983, 1991) has proposed that adult children provide care for their aging parents partly in order to protect them, thereby assuring the continued availability of a central attachment figure. Cicirelli's (1983) research uncovered a complex set of dynamics in such role-reversed relationships. Feelings of attachment were associated with both attachment and helping behaviors; negative, conflicted feelings were related to parents' degree of dependency.

In a study of six adults and their elderly parents, Moss and Moss (1992) found further support for the impact of changing roles on the quality of parent–child relationships in later life. They interviewed children whose elderly parents had just moved close to them. In this small sample, there was a tendency for the primary issues in the relationship to be concerned with interdependency: Children felt responsible for their parents' welfare, but parents did not feel completely comfortable relying on their children.

Research on long-term marriages also reveals changes in the nature of marital relationships over time. Levenson, Carstensen, and Gottman (1994) compared a group of middle-aged married couples (aged 40–50, married at least 15 years) with a group of older married couples (aged 60–70 years, married at least 35 years). Relative to the younger couples, the older ones reported less conflict and greater pleasure in their relationships. Interestingly, the older couples ranked communication as the leading source of conflict, whereas the younger couples ranked children first in this respect. As the authors suggested, this difference may represent the availability of communication opportunities for the older couples. In both age groups, couples in which the partners were dissatisfied with their relationships reported significantly more conflict and less pleasure than satisfied couples. We would expect attachment styles (not measured in this study) to explain some of the variance in communication, conflict, and satisfaction.

Studies of relationship satisfaction and social support provide evidence for connections among attachment, satisfaction, and social well-being in the elderly. Mullins and Dugan (1991) assessed social support (with a measure that included an attachment scale different from the ones discussed here) and satisfaction with social relationships in a large sample of residents of an independent living facility in Florida. Regression analyses revealed that attachment and absence of depression were predicted by the frequency of contact with friends and family members. Barnas, Pollina, and Cummings (1991) assessed attachment to children in a sample of women over 65 years of age. They found that security of attachment to children was correlated with reports of social well-being, and that insecurity was correlated with the use of emotion-focused coping techniques. In a large study of adults aged 62 years or older, social attachments predicted self-reported mental health, but not more objective measures of mental health (Harel & Deimling, 1984).

Overall, the few studies that have assessed security of attachment in old age suggest that the link between relationship satisfaction and attachment is similar across the lifespan. Feelings of emotional closeness and intimacy remain significant correlates of satisfaction in attachment relationships. There are also changes in the nature of attachment relationships. Adult children and their aging parents must often renegotiate their relationships to allow the children to help take care of the parents. Research on long-term marriages also implies that marriages change as couples grow older. Marriage becomes less a source of conflict and more a source of pleasure, as long as the quality of communication is high. Finally, intimate, emotionally close relationships remain important, and may even increase in significance, across the lifespan. Bowlby was correct in asserting that attachments are crucial "from the cradle to the grave."

IMPLICATIONS

What can attachment theory and research tell relationship partners and couple therapists about ways to increase relationship satisfaction? The theory provides several core constructs that are important to understanding relationship functioning and individual well-being. The first is sensitivity and responsiveness to a partner's needs, feelings, and emotional communications. Since, according to attachment theory, a person's search for secure attachments continues to be important across the lifespan, the same kinds of sensitivity and responsiveness that foster security in infancy are likely to foster it at later ages as well. A second core construct is felt security—the feeling that one's partner is a safe haven in times of stress and a secure base from which to undertake exciting, challenging activities. When a relationship partner proves unreliable as a secure base and unencouraging about exploring life's challenges, one's sense of security and vitality is likely to be undermined. A third core construct is that of internal working models. According to attachment theory, experience in close relationships is represented in increasingly elaborated mental models of the self and of relationship partners. The memories, beliefs, and expectations embodied in those models influence feelings of self-esteem, optimism, trust, and fear of violation or abandonment. A fourth key construct is coherence of discourse about attachment-related feelings. Attachment researchers have found that coherent communication between caregivers and young children helps the children identify and constructively manage their emotions, and that adults' coherence of discourse about previous attachment experiences predicts the quality of their relationships with their children.

These core constructs are closely related to discoveries made by behaviorally oriented marital researchers (e.g., Gottman, 1994a, 1994b; Markman, Stanley, & Blumberg, 1994; Notarius & Markman, 1993). In their studies it has been possible to predict long-term satisfaction and stability from a handful of communication patterns evident in videotapes of marital conflicts. Conflicts are the focus of this research because, as Gottman (1994b) explains, "A *lasting marriage results from a couple's ability to resolve the conflicts that are inevitable in any relationship*" (p. 28; emphasis in original). Notarius and Markman (1993) agree: "Relationship success depends on the ability of two people to *manage* the conflicts that inevitably occur in all relationships" (p. 17; emphasis in original). As it turns out, the capacity to manage and resolve marital conflicts relies on the same skills identified by researchers studying parent–child attachment. This is not surprising, given that attachment research began with situations—parental departures and reunions—that generate conflicts in every person's first close relationship.

One such skill is the expression and facilitation of positive emotion. "As long as there is five times as much positive feeling and interaction between husband and wife as there is negative, we found [that] the marriage was likely to be stable" (Gottman, 1994a, p. 57). This "magic" 5:1 ratio is maintained by large doses of what attachment researchers call "availability and responsiveness" and Gottman calls "love and respect:"

> The abundance of love and respect in . . . long-term marriages is evident everywhere. Watching the [video]tapes, I see a great deal of affection exchanged through gestures, eye contact, and facial expression. . . . Many jump at the chance to tell the interviewer about the partner's skills and achievements. They also express genuine interest in the details of each other's lives. When conflicts arise, each gives consideration to the other's point of view. (1994a, p. 62)

These are the same kinds of behaviors evident in security-building parent–child relationships. Giving advice to married couples, Gottman suggests a list of behaviors that could also serve as a guide to parents of young children: Show interest, be affectionate, show you care, be appreciative, show your concern, be empathic, be accepting, joke around, and share your joy.

These positivity-enhancing behaviors are the antitheses of the major destructive behaviors that Gottman calls "the four horsemen of the apocalypse": criticism (especially criticism that attacks a partner's personality or character, threatening the partner's self-esteem), contempt (the opposite of love and respect, and another blow to the partner's self-esteem), defensiveness (refusing to take responsibility), and stonewalling (avoiding communication and expression of feelings). These destructive behaviors are, in the language of attachment theory, likely to arouse insecurity in a partner and to chip away at positive components of the partner's working models of self and others. If the partner begins to feel overwhelmed by negative emotions, he or she is likely either to counterattack or to withdraw, become defensive, and stonewall. If both partners begin to make extremely negative attributions (which is especially likely if their internal working models were negatively biased to begin with), the marriage is on its way to dissolution.

Attachment theory differs from the behavioral theories of Gottman, Notarius, and Markman by placing more emphasis on personality and personal history. Beginning from a foundation in behavioral marital therapy, Gottman and his followers deliberately emphasize contemporary, observable communication behaviors while deemphasizing the personal histories that make those behaviors likely. Attachment theory calls attention to the kinds of parental treatment that help a child feel secure, learn to express and understand emotions, and become sensitive and responsive to others' feelings. It also points to the childhood roots of negative emotions and working models, which contribute later to low self-esteem and negative attributions concerning partners' motives and actions.

Attachment theory may shed light on three kinds of stable marriages discovered by Gottman (1994a, 1994b). He calls them "validating," "avoidant," and "volatile," three terms that seem strikingly similar to Ainsworth's three patterns of attachment—secure, avoidant, and anxious. Perhaps each of the three kinds of stable marriages results from one partner's acceptance of the other's defensive style. The avoidant and volatile types of marriage might be especially workable if a person with a secure attachment style accommodates to a partner with an avoidant or anxious style. It seems less likely that two insecure individuals could create a consistently satisfying marriage, although this remains to be studied further.

To some readers, attachment theory may lead to pessimism about the prospects of a person with an insecure attachment style. Recall, however, that intervention studies have shown that parents' behavior can be therapeutically altered, with a resulting increase in their children's attachment security. Also, the same longitudinal studies that have documented stability in child–parent attachment patterns during infancy (e.g., Waters, 1978), childhood (e.g., Elicker et al., 1992), adolescence (Waters et al., 1995), and adulthood (Kirkpatrick & Hazan, 1994) have also shown that approximately 30% of people change attachment styles, often because of changes in important relationships. The evidence suggests that long-term relationship satisfaction can be increased by deliberate efforts to (1) find a secure relationship partner, (2) foster one's partner's self-esteem and felt security, (3) build one's own self-esteem and felt security, (4) improve one's ability to communicate coherently about one's own and one's partner's emotions, and (5) avoid attributing previous attachment figures' negative characteristics to one's partner. These are among the goals of individual psychotherapy as conceptualized by Bowlby (1988), and of marital therapy as conceptualized by Johnson and Greenberg (1995) and Kobak, Ruckdeschel, and Hazan (1994).

Attachment theory is unique among approaches to relationship satisfaction in suggesting that security-enhancing treatment of children is one of the best contributions we can make to the quality of adult relationships in the future. At a time when the divorce rate is high, and when research has shown tendencies for children of divorce to experience a higher than average divorce rate themselves and for once-divorced adults to have an even higher divorce rate in subsequent marriages, it makes sense to take preventive measures.

REFERENCES

Ainsworth, M. D. S. (1967). *Infancy in Uganda: Infant care and the growth of love.* Baltimore: Johns Hopkins University Press.

Ainsworth, M. D. S., Blehar, M. C., Waters, E., & Wall, S. (1978). *Patterns of attachment: A psychological study of the Strange Situation.* Hillsdale, NJ: Erlbaum.

Ainsworth, M. D. S., & Bowlby, J. (1991). An ethological approach to personality development. *American Psychologist, 46,* 333–341.

Antonucci, T. C. (1994). Attachment in adulthood and aging. In M. B. Sperling & W. H. Berman (Eds.), *Attachment in adults: Clinical and developmental perspectives* (pp. 256–272). New York: Guilford Press.

Barnas, M. V., Pollina, L., & Cummings, E. M. (1991). Life-span attachment: Relationship between attachment and socioemotional functioning in women. *Genetic, Social, and General Psychology Monographs, 117,* 177–202.

Bartholomew, K. (1990). Avoidance of intimacy: An attachment perspective. *Journal of Social and Personal Relationships, 7,* 147–178.

Bartholomew, K., & Horowitz, L. M. (1991). Attachment styles among young adults: A test of a four-category model. *Journal of Personality and Social Psychology, 61,* 226–244.

Beeghly, M., & Cicchetti, D. (1994). Child maltreatment, attachment, and the self system: Emergence of an internal state lexicon in toddlers at high social risk. *Development and Psychopathology*, 6, 5–30.

Belsky, J., Rovine, M., & Taylor, D. G. (1984). The Pennsylvania Infant and Family Development Project: III. The origins of individual differences in infant–mother attachment: Maternal and infant contributions. *Child Development*, 55, 718–722.

Benoit, D., & Parker, K. C. H. (1994). Stability and transmission of attachment across three generations. *Child Development*, 65, 1444–1456.

Berlin, L. J., Cassidy, J., & Belsky, J. (1995). Loneliness in young children and infant–mother attachment: A longitudinal study. *Merrill–Palmer Quarterly*, 41, 91–103.

Blustein, D. L., Prezioso, M. S., & Palladino-Schultheiss, D. (1995). Attachment theory and career development: Current status and future directions. *The Counseling Psychologist*, 23, 416–432.

Bowlby, J. (1973). *Attachment and loss: Vol. 2. Separation: Anxiety and anger.* New York: Basic Books.

Bowlby, J. (1980). *Attachment and loss: Vol. 3. Loss: Sadness and depression.* New York: Basic Books.

Bowlby, J. (1982). *Attachment and loss: Vol. 1. Attachment* (2nd ed.). New York: Basic Books.

Bowlby, J. (1988). *A secure base: Clinical applications of attachment theory.* London: Routledge.

Brennan, K. A., & Shaver, P. R. (1995). Dimensions of adult attachment, affect regulation, and romantic functioning. *Personality and Social Psychology Bulletin*, 21, 267–283.

Bretherton, I., & Beeghly, M. (1982). Talking about internal states: The acquisition of an explicit theory of mind. *Developmental Psychology*, 18, 906–921.

Bretherton, I., Biringen, Z., & Ridgeway, D. (1989). The parental side of attachment. In K. A. Pillemar & K. McCartney (Eds.), *Parent–child relations throughout life* (pp. 1–24). Hillsdale, NJ: Erlbaum.

Bretherton, I., Ridgeway, D., & Cassidy, J. (1990). Assessing internal working models of the attachment relationship. In M. T. Greenberg, D. Cicchetti, & E. M. Cummings (Eds.), *Attachment in the preschool years* (pp. 3–50). Chicago: University of Chicago Press.

Bretherton, I., McNew, S., & Beeghly-Smith, M. (1981). Early person knowledge as expressed in gestural and verbal communication: When do infants acquire a "theory of mind"? In M. E. Lamb & L. R. Sherrod (Eds.), *Infant social cognition: Empirical and theoretical considerations* (pp. 333–374). Hillsdale, NJ: Erlbaum.

Carlson, V., Cicchetti, D., Barnett, D., & Braunwald, K. (1989). Disorganized/disoriented attachment relationships in maltreated infants. *Developmental Psychology*, 25, 525–531.

Carstensen, L. L. (1991). Selectivity theory: Social activity in life-span context. *Annual review of gerontology and geriatrics*, 11, 195–217.

Cassidy, J. (1988). Child–mother attachment and the self in six-year-olds. *Child Development*, 59, 121–134.

Cassidy, J., & Berlin, L. J. (1994). The insecure/ambivalent pattern of attachment: Theory and research. *Child Development, 65,* 971–991.

Cicirelli, V. G. (1983). Adult children's attachment and helping behavior to elderly parents: A path model. *Journal of Marriage and the Family, 45,* 815–825.

Cicirelli, V. G. (1991). Attachment theory in old age: Protection of the attached figure. In K. Pillemar & K. McCartney (Eds.), *Parent–child relations throughout life* (pp. 25–42). Hillsdale, NJ: Erlbaum.

Cohn, D. A., Silver, D. H., Cowan, C. P., Cowan, P. A., & Pearson, J. (1992). Working models of childhood attachment and couple relationships. *Journal of Family Issues, 13,* 432–449.

Collins, N. L., & Read, S. J. (1990). Adult attachment, working models, and relationship quality in dating couples. *Journal of Personality and Social Psychology, 58,* 644–663.

Dozier, M., & Kobak, R. R. (1992). Psychophysiology in attachment interviews: Converging evidence for deactivating strategies. *Child Development, 63,* 1473–1480.

Egeland, B., & Farber, E. (1984). Infant–mother attachment: Factors related to its development and changes over time. *Child Development, 55,* 753–771.

Elicker, J., Egeland, M., & Sroufe, L. A. (1992). Predicting peer competence and peer relationships in childhood from early parent–child relationships. In R. Parke & G. Ladd (Eds.), *Family–peer relations: Modes of linkage* (pp. 77–106). Hillsdale, NJ: Erlbaum.

Erickson, M. R., Sroufe, A. L., & Egeland, B. (1985). Attachment theory: Retrospect and prospect. In I. Bretherton & E. Waters (Eds.), Growing points in attachment theory and research. *Monographs of the Society for Research in Child Development, 50*(1–2, Serial No. 209), 147–166.

Feeney, J. A. (1994). Attachment style, communication patterns, and satisfaction across the life cycle of marriage. *Personal Relationships, 1,* 333–348.

Feeney, J. A. (1995). Adult attachment and emotional control. *Personal Relationships, 2,* 143–159.

Feeney, J. A., & Noller, P. (1990). Attachment style as a predictor of adult romantic relationships. *Journal of Personality and Social Psychology, 58,* 281–291.

Feeney, J. A., Noller, P., & Callan, V. J. (1994). Attachment style, communication and satisfaction in the early years of marriage. In K. Bartholomew & D. Perlman (Eds.), *Advances in personal relationships: Vol. 5. Attachment processes in adulthood* (pp. 269–308). London: Jessica Kingsley.

George, C., Kaplan, N., & Main, M. (1985). *Adult Attachment Interview.* Unpublished manuscript, University of California, Berkeley.

Gottman, J. M. (1994a). *Why marriages succeed or fail and how you make yours last.* New York: Simon & Schuster.

Gottman, J. M. (1994b). *What predicts divorce?: The relationship between marital processes and marital outcomes.* Hillsdale, NJ: Erlbaum.

Grossmann, K. E., & Grossmann, K. (1991). Attachment quality as an organizer of emotional and behavioral responses in a longitudinal perspective. In C. M. Parkes, J. Stevenson-Hind, & P. Marris (Eds.), *Attachment across the life cycle* (pp. 93–114). London: Tavistock/Routledge.

Hammond, J. R., & Fletcher, G. J. O. (1991). Attachment styles and relationship satisfaction in the development of close relationships. *New Zealand Journal of Psychology, 20,* 56–62.

Harel, Z., & Deimling, G. (1984). Social resources and mental health: An empirical refinement. *Journal of Gerontology, 39,* 747–752.

Hatfield, E., Brinton, C., & Cornelius, J. (1989). Passionate love and anxiety in young adolescents. *Motivation and Emotion, 13,* 271–289.

Hazan, C., & Hutt, M. (1993). *Patterns of adaptation: Attachment differences in psychosocial functioning during the first year of college.* Unpublished manuscript, Cornell University.

Hazan, C., & Shaver, P. R. (1987). Romantic love conceptualized as an attachment process. *Journal of Personality and Social Psychology, 52,* 511–524.

Hazan, C., & Shaver, P. R. (1990). Love and work: An attachment-theoretical perspective. *Journal of Personality and Social Psychology, 59,* 270–280.

Hindy, C. G., & Schwartz, J. C. (1994). Anxious romantic attachment in adult relationships. In M. B. Sperling & W. H. Berman (Eds.), *Attachment in adults: Clinical and developmental perspectives* (pp. 179–203). New York: Guilford Press.

Isabella, R. A., & Belsky, J. (1991). Interactional synchrony and the origins of infant–mother attachment: A replication study. *Child Development, 62,* 373–384.

Isabella, R. A., Belsky, J., & von Eye, A. (1989). Origins of infant–mother attachment: An examination of the interactional synchrony during the infant's first year. *Developmental Psychology, 25,* 12–21.

Johnson, S. M., & Greenberg, L. S. (1995). The emotionally focused approach to problems in adult attachment. In N. S. Jacobson & A. S. Gurman (Eds.), *Clinical handbook of couple therapy* (pp. 121–141). New York: Guilford Press.

Kahn, R. L., & Antonucci, T. C. (1980). Convoys over the life course: Attachment, roles and social support. In P. B. Baltes & O. G. Brim (Eds.), *Life-span development and behavior* (pp. 254–283). San Diego: Academic Press.

Kaplan, N., & Main, M. (1985, April). Internal representations of attachment at six years as indicated by family drawings and verbal responses to imagined separations. In M. Main (Chair), *Attachment: A move to the level of representation.* Symposium conducted at the meeting of the Society for Research in Child Development, Toronto.

Kenny, M. E. (1987). The extent and function of parental attachment among first-year college students. *Journal of Youth and Adolescence, 16,* 17–29.

Kirkpatrick, L. A., & Davis, K. E. (1994). Attachment style, gender, and relationship stability: A longitudinal analysis. *Journal of Personality and Social Psychology, 66,* 502–512.

Kobak, R. R., Cole, H. E., Ferenz-Gillies, R., Fleming, W. S., & Gamble, W. (1993). Attachment and emotion regulation during mother–teen problem solving: A control theory analysis. *Child Development, 64,* 231–245.

Kobak, R. R., & Hazan, C. (1991). Attachment in marriage: Effects of security and accuracy of working models. *Journal of Personality and Social Psychology, 60,* 861–869.

Kobak, R. R., Ruckdeschel, K., & Hazan, C. (1994). From symptom to signal: An attachment view of emotion in marital therapy. In S. M. Johnson & L. S. Greenberg (Eds.), *The heart of the matter: Perspectives on emotion in marital therapy* (pp. 46–71). New York: Brunner/Mazel.

Kobak, R. R., & Sceery, A. (1988). Attachment in late adolescence: Working models, affect regulation, and representations of self and others. *Child Development, 59,* 135–146.

LaFraniere, P. J., & Sroufe, A. L. (1985). Profiles of peer competence in the preschool: Interrelations between measures, influence of social ecology, and relation to attachment history. *Developmental Psychology, 21,* 56–69.

Lang, F. R., & Carstensen, L. L. (1994). Close emotional relationships in late life: Further support for proactive aging in the social domain. *Psychology and Aging, 9,* 315–324.

Levenson, R. W., Carstensen, L. L., & Gottman, J. M. (1993). Long–term marriage: Age, gender, and satisfaction. *Psychology and Aging, 8,* 301–313.

Levy, M. B., & Davis, K. E. (1988). Lovestyles and attachment styles compared: Their relations to each other and to various relationship characteristics. *Journal of Personal and Social Relationships, 5,* 439–471.

Lowenthal, M. F., & Haven, C. (1968). Interaction and adaptation: Intimacy as a critical variable. *American Sociological Review, 33,* 20–30.

Lyons-Ruth, K., Alpern, L., & Repacholi, B. (1993). Disorganized infant attachment classification and maternal psychosocial problems as predictors of hostile–aggressive behavior in the preschool classroom. *Child Development, 64,* 572–585.

Main, M., & Hesse, E. (1990). Parents' unresolved traumatic experiences are related to infant disorganized status: Is frightened and/or frightening parental behavior the linking mechanism? In M. T. Greenberg, D. Cicchetti, & E. M. Cummings (Eds.), *Attachment in the preschool years: Theory, research, and intervention* (pp. 161–182). Chicago: University of Chicago Press.

Main, M., & Solomon, J. (1990). Procedures for identifying infants as disorganized/disoriented during the Ainsworth Strange Situation. In M. T. Greenberg, D. Cicchetti, & E. M. Cummings (Eds.), *Attachment in the preschool years: Theory, research, and intervention* (pp. 121–160). Chicago: University of Chicago Press.

Main, M., Kaplan, N., & Cassidy, J. (1985). Security in infancy, childhood, and adulthood: A move to the level of representation. In I. Bretherton & E. Waters (Eds.), Growing points of attachment theory and research. *Monographs of the Society for Research in Child Development, 50*(1–2, Serial No. 209), 66–104.

Markman, H., Stanley, S., & Blumberg, S. L. (1994). *Fighting for your marriage: Positive steps for preventing divorce and preserving lasting love.* San Francisco: Jossey-Bass.

Morisset, C. E., Barnard, K. E., Greenberg, M. T., Booth, C. L., & Spieker, S. J. (1990). Environmental influences on early language development: The context of social risk. *Development and Psychopathology, 2,* 127–149.

Moss, M. S., & Moss, S. Z. (1992). Themes in parent–child relationships when elderly parents move nearby. *Journal of Aging Studies, 6,* 259–271.

Mullins, L. C., & Dugan, E. (1991). Elderly social relationships with adult children and close friends and depression. *Journal of Social Behavior and Personality*, 6, 315–328.

Noller, P., & Feeney, J. A. (1994). Relationship satisfaction, attachment, and nonverbal accuracy in early marriage. *Journal of Nonverbal Behavior*, 18, 199–221.

Notarius, C., & Markman, H. (1993). *We can work it out: Making sense of marital conflict*. New York: Putnam.

Pietromonaco, P. R., & Carnelley, K. B. (1994). Gender and working models of attachment: Consequences for perceptions of self and romantic relationships. *Personal Relationships*, 1, 63–82.

Pistole, M. C. (1989). Attachment in adult romantic relationships: Style of conflict resolution and relationship satisfaction. *Journal of Social and Personal Relationships*, 6, 505–510.

Robertson, J. (1952). *A 2-year-old goes to hospital* [Film]. New York: New York University Library.

Robertson, J., & Robertson, J. (1967). *Young children in brief separation: No. 1: Kate, aged 2 years 5 months, in foster care for 27 days* [Film]. New York: New York University Film Library.

Rusbult, C. E., Verette, J., Whitney, G. A., Slovik, L. F., & Lipkus, I. (1991). Accommodation processes in close relationships: Theory and preliminary empirical evidence. *Journal of Personality and Social Psychology*, 60, 53–78.

Scharfe, E., & Bartholomew, K. (1995). Accommodation and attachment representation in young couples. *Journal of Social and Personal Relationships*, 12, 389–401.

Senchak, M., & Leonard, K. E. (1992). Attachment styles and marital adjustment among newlywed couples. *Journal of Social and Personal Relationships*, 9, 51–64.

Shaver, P. R., & Brennan, K. A. (1992). Attachment styles and the "Big Five" personality traits: Their connection with each other and with romantic relationship outcomes. *Personality and Social Psychology Bulletin*, 18, 536–545.

Shaver, P. R., & Clark, C. L. (1994). The psychodynamics of adult romantic attachment. In J. M. Masling & R. F. Bornstein (Eds.), *Empirical perspectives on object relations theories* (pp. 105–156). Washington, DC: American Psychological Association.

Shaver, P. R., Collins, N., & Clark, C. L. (1996). Attachment styles and internal working models of self and relationship partners. In G. J. O. Fletcher & J. Fitness (Eds.), *Knowledge structures in close relationships: A social psychological approach* (pp. 25–61). Hillsdale, NJ: Erlbaum.

Shaver, P. R., & Hazan, C. (1993). Adult romantic attachment: Theory and evidence. In D. Perlman & W. Jones (Eds.), *Advances in personal relationships* (Vol. 4, pp. 29–70). Greenwich, CT: JAI Press.

Shaver, P. R., Hazan, C., & Bradshaw, D. (1988). Love as attachment: The integration of three behavioral systems. In R. J. Sternberg & M. L. Barnes (Eds.), *The psychology of love* (pp. 68–99). New Haven, CT: Yale University Press.

Slough, N. M., & Greenberg, M. T. (1990). Five-year-olds' representations of separation from parents: Responses from the perspective of self and other. *New Directions for Child Development, 48*, 67–83.

Simpson, J. A. (1990). Influence of attachment styles on romantic relationships. *Journal of Personality and Social Psychology, 59*, 971–980.

Simpson, J. A., Rholes, W. S., & Nelligan, J. S. (1992). Support seeking and support giving within couples in an anxiety-provoking situation: The role of attachment styles. *Journal of Personality and Social Psychology, 62*, 434–446.

Sroufe, L. A. (1983). Infant–caregiver attachment and patterns of adaptation in preschool: The roots of maladaptation and competence. In M. Perlmutter (Ed.), *Minnesota Symposia on Child Psychology* (Vol. 16, pp. 41–81). Hillsdale, NJ: Erlbaum.

Sroufe, L. A., Carlson, E., & Shulman, S. (1993). Individuals in relationships: Development from infancy through adolescence. In D. C. Funder, R. D. Parke, C. Tomlinson-Keasey, & K. Widaman (Eds.), *Studying lives through time* (pp. 315–342). Washington, DC: American Psychological Association.

Sroufe, L. A., & Waters, E. (1977). Attachment as an organizational construct. *Child Development, 48*, 1184–1199.

Troll, L., & Smith, J. (1976). Attachment through the life span: Some questions about dyadic bonds among adults. *Human Development, 19*, 156–170.

Troy, M., & Sroufe, A. L. (1987). Victimization among preschoolers: Role of attachment relationship history. *Journal of the American Academy of Child and Adolescent Psychiatry, 26*, 166–172.

van den Boom, D. C. (1994). The influence of temperament and mothering on attachment and exploration: An experimental manipulation of sensitive responsiveness among lower-class mothers with irritable infants. *Child Development, 65*, 1457–1477.

van IJzendoorn, M. (1995). Adult attachment representations, parental responsiveness, and infant attachment: A meta-analysis on the predictive validity of the Adult Attachment Interview. *Psychological Bulletin, 117*, 387–403.

van IJzendoorn, M. H., Goldberg, S., Kroonenberg, P. M., & Frenkel, O. J. (1992). The relative effects of maternal and child problems on the quality of attachment: A meta-analysis of attachment clinical samples. *Child Development, 63*, 840–858.

Waller, N. G., & Shaver, P. R. (1994). The importance of nongenetic influences on romantic love styles: A twin-family study. *Psychological Science, 5*, 268–274.

Waters, E. (1978). The stability of individual differences in infant–mother attachment. *Child Development, 49*, 483–494.

Waters, E., Merrick, S. K., Albersheim, L. J., & Treboux, D. (1995, April). *Attachment security from infancy to early adulthood: A 20-year longitudinal study.* Poster presented at the biennial meeting of the Society for Research in Child Development, Indianapolis, IN.

CHAPTER 3

Love and Satisfaction

SUSAN S. HENDRICK
CLYDE HENDRICK

Maria and José walked into the rather large room, gaily decorated with streamers and flowers, filling up with well-wishers. Maria was more than a little nervous; she and José had been dating steadily for several months, but his first real introduction to her large extended family was to be today, at this party celebrating her grandparents' 50th wedding anniversary. As they approached her grandparents, who were surrounded by friends congratulating them on their 50 years together, Maria stopped, almost ready to turn around and leave. Quietly but firmly, José took her hand and said, "It's okay—let's talk with them." Suddenly Maria was hugging her grandparents, introducing José to everyone, and generally getting caught up in the emotion of the occasion. A bit later, when they had a few moments to talk more quietly, José asked Maria's grandparents the "secret" of their long and seemingly happy marriage. Her grandfather answered first: "It's been a long road that we've traveled together, and not an easy one at that. But we were always in it together; I never felt that I was struggling by myself." And Maria's grandmother added, "And we always loved each other. Right from the first, we fell in love. And then, whatever else was happening, we always had that love." Leaving the party a few hours later, Maria and José talked about her grandparents' marriage—José marveling at how happy the two seemed together, and Maria picturing all the times she had seen her grandfather put his arm around her grandmother's waist and give her a squeeze, or seen her grandmother walk past her grandfather seated at the kitchen table and touch his hair affectionately. Maria also remembered them fighting once in a while, but mostly she remembered their affection. She smiled when she thought of them, wondering if she could ever have as successful a marriage as theirs.

This vignette provides a sketch of *marital* satisfaction, which we broaden in this chapter to "relationship satisfaction." Whether people are in marital, cohabiting, or serious dating relationships, and whether couples are heterosexual or gay or lesbian, issues of satisfaction are terribly important. Satisfaction may have strong implications for whether partners ultimately stay together or break up (e.g., S. S. Hendrick, Hendrick, & Adler, 1988); thus, satisfaction is a significant construct. However, it is also a much-debated one.

WHAT IS SATISFACTION AND WHY IS IT IMPORTANT?

"Satisfaction" is only one of several terms employed to describe some sort of summative judgment about an intimate relationship. Glenn (1990), in a detailed discussion of general marital quality and some of the relevant issues, differentiated "satisfaction" from "happiness," though he characterized both as individually oriented indices of marital quality. As a relationship-oriented index, he employed the term "adjustment."

Although Glenn (1990) divided the descriptive terms into individual and relational terms, we have elsewhere (S. S. Hendrick, 1995) referred to the satisfaction perspective as encompassing partners' subjective feelings about their relationship (e.g., how does the relationship "feel?"), whereas the adjustment perspective may have more to do with actual relationship behaviors (e.g., conflict) and is more accurately captured by how the relationship "works." For example, a couple may have a well-functioning relationship in behavioral terms: The partners agree on parenting strategies, work well together without conflict, budget their money effectively, and have productive careers. They are well adjusted. Yet the partners are far from emotionally close, and they are unsatisfied. Another couple may disagree frequently about particular parenting approaches, have occasional arguments, budget money erratically, and be only marginally content with their work. Yet the partners make love frequently, feel emotionally connected, and are relatively satisfied with their relationship.

Glenn also mentioned the term "success," which refers to how a relationship endures over time. Yet he acknowledged that success must be measured by more than whether a couple stays together or breaks up, but must rather reflect both durability *and* satisfaction. "A marriage that is intact and satisfactory to both spouses is successful, while one that has ended in divorce or separation or is unsatisfactory to one or both spouses is a failure" (Glenn, 1990, p. 821). Our own approach is from the satisfaction perspective, with our interest fixed on people's subjective, affective experiencing of their own happiness and contentment with their close relationship.

Along with definitional differences have come measurement controversies with some scales measuring global individual satisfaction (e.g., Schumm et al., 1986) and others favoring more relational (and behaviorally grounded) items (e.g., Spanier, 1976). Still other measures are exceedingly long and comprehensive (e.g., Snyder, 1979). Marital satisfaction has been criticized selectively for being confounded with a social desirability bias. In other words, it is thought that people may answer relationship questions on the basis of what they believe is a socially appropriate or socially "desirable" response, rather than on the basis of their real attitudes, beliefs, and emotions. However, more recent research indicates that satisfaction and social desirability are quite separate (e.g., Fowers, Applegate, Olson, & Pomerantz, 1994; Russell & Wells, 1992).

Relationship researchers and clinicians may favor one approach (individual vs. relational, global vs. specific) and one measurement style (brief and global vs. lengthy and specific); however, most agree that disparate approaches should at the very least not be included in the same measure (Glenn, 1990). (For a review of relevant measures, see Sabatelli, 1988.) Given our "satisfaction" perspective and the need for a research-appropriate measure, we have found the Relationship Assessment Scale (S. S. Hendrick, 1981, 1988) quite suitable. This seven-item measure, shown in Table 3.1, correlates highly with the well-established but lengthier Dyadic Adjustment Scale (Spanier, 1976) and has been used in much of our research. Other researchers have also used the measure with some success (e.g., Guldner & Swensen, 1995; Sacher & Fine, 1996).

Questions of defining and measuring marital quality/satisfaction/adjustment pose knotty issues of interest to researchers and occasionally to practicing clinicians, but they have little direct relevance to people like Maria's grandparents, who have "lived out" their satisfaction rather than examining it under a microscope. Most people want to know less about the science of being satisfied than they do about the art of being satisfied. What makes for satisfaction? How do partners stay satisfied?

It is questions such as these that have motivated much of our rela-

TABLE 3.1. Instructions and Items for the Relationship Assessment Scale

Please mark on the answer sheet the letter for each item which best answers that item for you:

1. How well does your partner meet your needs?

A	B	C	D	E
Poorly		Average		Extremely well

2. In general, how satisfied are you with your relationship?

A	B	C	D	E
Unsatisfied		Average		Extremely satisfied

3. How good is your relationship compared to most?

A	B	C	D	E
Poor		Average		Excellent

4. How often do you wish you hadn't gotten in this relationship?

A	B	C	D	E
Never		Average		Very often

5. To what extent has your relationship met your original expectations?

A	B	C	D	E
Hardly at all		Average		Completely

6. How much do you love your partner?

A	B	C	D	E
Not much		Average		Very much

7. How many problems are there in your relationship?

A	B	C	D	E
Very few		Average		Very many

Note. Adapted from Hendrick (1988). Copyright 1988 by the National Council on Family Relations. Adapted by permission. To derive a numerical score, A = 1 and E = 5. The greater the total score, the more satisfied. Items 4 and 7 are reverse-scored.

tionship research over the years, and this research has convinced us that one of the major motivators of relationship satisfaction is "love." Thus the current chapter examines love's role in relationship satisfaction. We overview general theories of love, including the evolutionary perspective. We then present the love styles approach, detailing research showing the most effective love predictors of satisfaction. We discuss the importance of passionate and companionate love, highlighting both cross-cultural and cross-generational findings. Finally, we discuss looking for and finding love, and propose some strategies for keeping love (and satisfaction) alive and well in an intimate relationship. Intimate relationships are endlessly complicated, and we do not presume that love, in and of itself, is all that is needed to keep the partners in a relationship satisfied. But love is a substantial part of the package.

A GENERAL LOOK AT LOVE AND SATISFACTION

Although romantic love was not a prerequisite for marriage until the modern era (Singer, 1984), it has assumed a place of considerable preeminence, with college students in the 1980s more strongly viewing romantic love as desirable for establishing a marriage than students who were asked similar questions in the 1960s viewed it (Simpson, Campbell, & Berscheid, 1986). In fact, although marriage is certainly not everyone's goal, a long-term intimate relationship is the ideal for many if not most people. Attridge and Berscheid (1994), in a discussion of their own and other research indicating the critical role that love plays in people's lives, state "that many single men and women today worry about the prospects of finding a lasting love" (p. 134). One need spend only a few hours perusing the pop psychology shelves at the local bookstore or channel-surfing the daytime TV talk shows to know that love is not seasonal—people's thoughts turn to love in spring, but also in summer, fall, and winter—and that questions about how to find it and how to keep it are everywhere.

Why is love so important? Elsewhere (S. S. Hendrick & Hendrick, 1992b), we have talked about love from both the evolutionary and the sociological perspectives. The latter perspective views love primarily as learned and culturally transmitted. In fact, it is important to recognize that central to the concept of loving another is the concept of the self as one who loves, and our modern notions of "self" have developed only in recent centuries (e.g., Morris, 1972). The sociological perspective would imply that romantic love is a relatively recent cultural invention, and indeed research exploring love orientations in three different cultures and countries (the United States, Russia, and Japan; Sprecher et al., 1994) found a number of cultural differences. However, cultural differences in love do not negate the possibility of certain cultural universals in love, such as passionate love (Hatfield & Rapson, 1987). And a focus on universals is what characterizes the evolutionary approach to love.

The Evolutionary Perspective

As social scientists continue to seek understanding of human relationships, the evolutionary approach (see Shackelford & Buss, Chapter 1, this volume) has offered persuasive explanations for the role love might play. Mellen (1981) speculated at length about men's and women's evolution as hunters and gatherers, with females bearing and caring for the young and concerned with gathering plants close to home, and men, free from constant child care responsibilities, concerned with roaming widely and hunting. Over countless generations, biological evolution as well as probable cultural developments favored those who were most successful in their respective tasks, with nurturing women and men who were good food providers (and protectors as well) most able to rear offspring successfully and thus pass on their genes. Mellen's (1981) thesis was that successful rearing of the young would have required female nurturing and male provisioning/protecting, both of which would have been served by bonding of breeding pairs—a pair bonding that might well be a precursor of what we call love (for related material, see Buck, 1989).

Although the "purpose" of love would thus be the strengthening of pair bonds and ensuing increases in sexual fidelity (and thus assurance of paternity for men) and consistent provisioning of the young for women (Buss, 1995), love becomes rewarding in and of itself to the extent that love is associated with strong emotions (Buck, 1989) and powerful sexual feelings (S. S. Hendrick & Hendrick, 1995).

The evolutionary perspective not only provides a niche for love, but offers explanations for sexual jealousy, gender differences in love and sexual strategies, and so on. Taking this perspective, we might expect certain aspects of love to be more nearly universal, and thus potentially more strongly related to relationship satisfaction, which can be reasoned to be central to the pair bonding discussed earlier. And by the same token, other, more culturally bound or constructed aspects of love might be less relevant for relationship satisfaction, as we discuss more fully later in this chapter.

Of course the evolutionary perspective is not the only viable one, and indeed the social-constructivist approach to love makes a strong case for the particularity rather than the universality of love (see Beall & Sternberg, 1995, for a detailed presentation). Although metatheoretical approaches such as evolutionary psychology or social constructionism are both useful and compelling, there are a number of approaches to love that function at more specific theoretical and empirical levels.

Theories of Love

Early social-scientific research on love categorized it into two major types: passionate and companionate (Berscheid & Hatfield, 1978; Hatfield & Walster, 1978). Whereas we might expect the roaring fires of passionate love to be related to satisfaction at the beginning of a romantic relationship, the steadily glowing embers of companionate love might be expected to relate to satisfaction in a long-term, committed relationship. Although the dual concepts of passionate and companionate love appear somewhat limiting, they are very resilient and have re-emerged in a new guise, as we show later in this chapter. Sternberg (1986, 1987) broadened conceptions of love to include three central components of intimacy, passion, and commitment, out of which eight types of love may be composed (see Barnes & Sternberg, Chapter 4, this volume). Hazan and Shaver (1987) explored love in the context of basic attachment styles (see Koski & Shaver, Chapter 2, this volume), and more recently Fehr (1988, 1993) sought people's central prototypes about love. For example, what types of love are people able to think of, and of these types, which do people view as most centrally representative of love? Also, what characteristics or qualities do people view as most representative of love? Fehr's painstaking work has added much richness to our understanding of love.

Because notions of love as two-dimensional seemed too limiting, at an early stage we embraced the work of Lee (1973), a sociologist whose multidimensional approach to love was more inclusive of human differences in loving. Lee articulated six major ways or styles of loving; he viewed them as equally viable. These six love styles include Eros (passionate love characterized by intensity and commitment), Storge (friendship love characterized by companionability), Ludus (game-playing love characterized by playfulness but insularity), Pragma (practical love characterized by rational choice making), Mania (possessive, dependent love characterized by emotional lability), and Agape (altruistic love characterized by giving more than receiving). Items representative of these orientations to love were developed and refined, and currently constitute the Love Attitudes Scale (C. Hendrick & Hendrick, 1986, 1990).

These six love styles (as measured by the Love Attitudes Scale) have been explored from a number of different directions over the past decade. For example, gender differences in love styles have appeared rather consistently, with men more ludic (game-playing) and women more storgic (friendship-oriented), pragmatic, and manic (C. Hendrick & Hendrick, 1986; S. S. Hendrick & Hendrick, 1995). Yet women and men produce relatively similar patterns of correlations between love and other relationship variables such as self-disclosure (S. S. Hendrick & Hendrick, 1987) and sexual attitudes (S. S. Hendrick & Hendrick, 1995). The love styles have also been related to various dimensions of personality (Richardson, Medvin, & Hammock, 1988; Woll, 1989), though it is arguable whether love styles are more nearly manifestations of personality, and therefore relatively enduring, or expressions of attitudes, and therefore more transient and influenced by life events. Are they to be found in people, in a relationship, or in both? Our approach has been to consider the styles as attitudinal, not trait-like, and thus as changeable both within and across relationships. However, people may have relatively consistent love styles throughout their lives, expressing their own individual relationship "theme." Only extensive longitudinal research will answer these questions. Meanwhile, a basic premise of the whole love style approach is that different styles "fit" different people, and that these differences should be accepted.

A related issue involves the relative dependence–independence of the love styles. Although it is convenient to describe the love styles as six different approaches to love, and they are statistically independent, they are in fact not mutually exclusive within an individual. Several of the love styles can be expressed to a greater or lesser degree with one relationship partner; different love styles may predominate at different points in time with the same partner; and different styles are potentially important with different partners (as noted above). A person is seldom if ever just one type of lover.

An important component of our own research program on love attitudes has involved the linkages between love styles and relationship satisfaction. Beginning with some of our earliest work on relationships (S. S. Hendrick, 1981), a central concern has been the prediction of relationship satisfaction.

THE LINKS BETWEEN SATISFACTION AND LOVE

Although we have described satisfaction as an important indicator for relationship continuance, and have introduced love as a significant construct in the general gestalt of a relationship, it still remains for us to link the two areas. Of course we realize that love is far from being the only predictor of relationship satisfaction. In fact, in a recent discussion of partners' unrealistic beliefs about selecting a mate, Larson (1992) noted that love was only one of over two dozen factors proposed as correlates of marital satisfaction by Lewis and Spanier (1979). Nevertheless, we propose that love, construed more broadly than romantic love, is one of the most important predictors of relationship satisfaction. However, before examining how love (in this chapter, represented typically by the six love styles) might predict satisfaction, it will be useful to understand more about the love styles themselves.

Approaches to Love

Eros, described earlier as passionate love characterized by intensity and commitment, is related to idealism in sexuality, to self-disclosure to a partner, and to the ability to elicit disclosure from a partner, and is generally unrelated to sensation seeking (S. S. Hendrick & Hendrick, 1987). Eros is also linked to solid self-esteem (C. Hendrick & Hendrick, 1986). Ludus (or game-playing love), is generally related to nondisclosure to a partner, to sensation seeking, and to casual and sometimes manipulative sexuality (S. S. Hendrick & Hendrick, 1987). In research by Woll (1989), Ludus was also related to greater extraversion, aggressiveness, dating variety, and playfulness. Storge (friendship-oriented love) is stable and steady; it is somewhat related to idealism about sexuality, and is also linked to eliciting disclosure from a partner and to not easily becoming bored or restless (S. S. Hendrick & Hendrick, 1987; Richardson et al., 1988). Pragma, the practical love style characterized by rational choice, is also related to practicality in sexual attitudes (S. S. Hendrick & Hendrick, 1987) and is not oriented to sensation seeking (Richardson et al., 1988). Mania, possessive, dependent love characterized by mood swings, also manifests some sexual idealism, inclinations both to give and to receive disclosure, and lower self-esteem (S. S. Hendrick & Hendrick, 1987). Mania is not oriented to sensation seeking, but needs social recognition (Woll, 1989). Finally, Agape is linked to altruism, to idealism about love, to disclosure to a partner, and to good listening; it is not oriented to casual sexuality or sensation seeking (S. S. Hendrick & Hendrick, 1987). If we subscribe to Lee's theory that the six love styles are valid but very different representations of how people love each other, then we might expect them all to be somewhat similar predictors of relationship satisfaction. However, they are not.

Predicting Relationship Satisfaction

Our research has often focused on how love and other relationship variables predict couples' relationship satisfaction, typically as measured by the Relationship Assessment Scale. In the first study in this genre (S. S. Hendrick et al., 1988), a sample of 57 heterosexual college couples completed measures of several constructs, including love attitudes, sexual attitudes, self-disclosure, commitment, investment, and relationship adjustment/satisfaction (two measures). First, partners were highly correlated on numerous variables, including the love attitudes of Eros, Storge, and Mania; commitment to and investment in the relationship; and adjustment/satisfaction (both measures). Regression analyses (separate for women and men) focusing on satisfaction showed that Eros was a positive predictor and Ludus a negative predictor of satisfaction for both men and women. In addition, Mania was a modest negative predictor for women and Storge a positive predictor. Discriminant analyses enabled comparisons between a subset of couples that had terminated their relationships over approximately a 2-month period from the initial assessment, and the remaining couples that were still together (30 couples total). The results of this comparison showed significantly more self-disclosure, higher self-esteem, greater commitment and investment, and higher relationship adjustment for the couples that had remained intact than for the couples that had terminated their relationships. More germane to our purposes, the intact couples were also higher on Eros and lower on Ludus. Thus our initial exploration of satisfaction indicated that love—although not the only important aspect of relationship satisfaction—was nevertheless well worth studying.

In another study, Davis and Latty-Mann (1987) assessed 70 couples on love attitudes and relationship characteristics (as measured by the Relationship Rating Form [Davis & Todd, 1982, 1985]); they found partner similarity on several love styles, and numerous correlations between love and subscales of their rating form. Although Middleton (1993) sought to explore dating partners' personality similarities and their associations with relationship satisfaction, he found the love styles to be more highly correlated with satisfaction than were personality characteristics. Eros, Storge, and Agape were strongly and positively correlated with satisfaction for both partners, and Ludus was negatively correlated with satisfaction for both. (Although partner similarity as a contributor to relationship satisfaction is not a focus of this chapter, we note similarity findings in passing and refer readers to recent studies addressing issues of similarity and satisfaction [e.g., Burleson & Denton, 1992; Deal, Wampler, & Halverson, 1992].)

Predicting satisfaction for dating couples is certainly important, but we have also sought to explore satisfaction in marital relationships. Another study (Contreras, Hendrick, & Hendrick, 1996) examined cultural and gender differences in predictors of relationship satisfaction among Mexican American and Anglo couples (n's = 54 and 30 couples, respectively). There were few ethnic differences, and the gender differences were consistent with previous research. However, a particularly interesting finding was that although one or another of the love styles predicted satisfaction for men or women, or for one or another of the ethnic groups, Eros (passionate love) was the strongest consistent predictor of relationship satisfaction for both women and men and for all ethnic groups (Anglos, and more and less acculturated Mexican Americans).

In yet another study (Inman-Amos, Hendrick, & Hendrick, 1994), we examined correlations among the love styles and other measures for mothers and fathers of college students, using a sample of 84 couples. We found a high match between partners, with correlations significant for relationship satisfaction and for all six love styles. Finally, several love styles were highly and positively correlated with relationship satisfaction, including Eros (.64 for mothers and .74 for fathers), Agape and Mania (modestly for women only), and Storge (modestly for men only). In addition, Ludus was strongly but negatively correlated with satisfaction for both partners (Inman-Amos, Hendrick, & Hendrick, 1995).

Most recently, Sokolski (1995) explored how a variety of variables (e.g., communication, physical intimacy, expectations of partner, social support, financial and general stress, presence of children, and love styles) might predict relationship satisfaction for 161 married couples in which at least one partner was a student in medical school, law school, or another graduate program. Not unexpectedly, several of the love styles were related to satisfaction, including Eros (highly and positively for both spouses), Ludus (highly and negatively for both spouses), Storge (modestly positively for men only), and Agape (modestly positively for both). Finally, regression analyses using the total sample and employing a number of demographic and relationship variables indicated that Eros was the strongest predictor of satisfaction.

To understand why Eros would be such a strong positive predictor of relationship satisfaction and Ludus such a strong negative predictor, one need only reexamine the basic orientation of each of these love styles (and the Love Attitudes Scale items composing them). Eros is a passionate, intense, communicative style, consistent with prevailing Western notions of love. Ludus is exemplified by game playing, distance, and reluctance to commit oneself to another—qualities not calculated to improve an intimate relationship. Ludus's potential for positive relating is probably greatest when both partners are ludic. It is possible that playfulness and excitement will characterize such a relationship.

After we and our students conducted a series of studies, we began to realize that although the love styles were indeed related to satisfaction, they were related differently. Without exception, we found Eros to be the strongest of all the love styles as a positive predictor of satisfaction, though Ludus also proved to be a consistent negative predictor. Less consistent were positive relations between Storge and satisfaction and between Agape and satisfaction, and some mixed findings for Mania. Although we espouse a multidimensional approach to love, Eros certainly seemed to be the "first among equals" when it came to predicting relationship satisfaction. Thus we felt compelled to reexamine the concept of passionate love.

PASSIONATE AND COMPANIONATE LOVE REVISITED

Although much of our early love research focused on an attempt to broaden concepts of love beyond passionate and companionate, our own findings began to convince us that the passionate–companionate distinction deserved more attention. In an attempt to compare several theoretical and empirical approaches (C. Hendrick & Hendrick, 1989), an extensive questionnaire was developed that included the three attachment measures developed by Hazan and Shaver (1987), the Passionate Love Scale (Hatfield & Sprecher, 1986), the Sternberg Triangular Theory of Love Scale (measuring intimacy, passion, and commitment; Sternberg, 1986, 1987), the Relationship Rating Form (measuring viability, intimacy, passion, care, satisfaction, and conflict; Davis & Todd, 1982, 1985), and the Love Attitudes Scale (C. Hendrick & Hendrick, 1986).

A factor analysis resulted in five factors, with two that seemed most compelling. The first and largest factor included 12 of the various scales and subscales and was described as Passionate Love. The second factor included five measures (and negative loadings by three other measures) and seemed to typify Caring Love without conflict. In our conclusion to that paper (C. Hendrick & Hendrick, 1989), we acknowledged the similarity of our two primary factors to Hatfield and Walster's (1978) description of passionate and companionate love.

In related research, we used the five factors from our measurement study as five "superscales" measuring love, grounded our theoretical predictions in an evolutionary perspective, and explored a number of findings, including the prediction of relationship satisfaction (C. Hendrick & Hendrick, 1991). Two of the love superscales, Passion and Closeness (along with Manic Love, a very modest predictor) were potent predictors of satisfaction, accounting for 65% of the variance. These findings were consistent with evolutionary explanations:

> Passion and closeness (or intimacy) are easily seen as pair-bonding attitudes. For the formation of sexual relationships, they guide the underlying needs that propel a pair into a relationship. Further, satisfaction of the needs represented by these attitudes should promote relationship satisfaction, a result demonstrated by the regression analyses. Consummation of passion requires physical proximity, and the existence of physical proximity implies the possibility of consummation of passion. Thus, the two attitudes of passion and closeness should covary. They are separate constructs (as the factor analysis demonstrated), but empirically the two should be substantially correlated, as indeed they were in this data set. (C. Hendrick & Hendrick, 1991, p. 225)

And passion and closeness are both potentially very important to reproduction, as we have noted. The passion fuels and is fueled by sexual union, and may serve both a short-term courtship function and a longer-term bonding one. Closeness and companionability are more likely to serve the long-term bonding, but also contribute to the development of intimacy, which is part of the initial courtship process. If passionate and companionate love are really as important as we have portrayed them, then there should be intercultural and intergenerational manifestations of these love orientations that supersede those of other love styles and that go well beyond our own work.

Love across Cultures

Hatfield (e.g., Hatfield & Rapson, 1987) has maintained for some time that passionate love is universal, found across cultures and across age groups. In recent research comparing Hawaiian residents representing European American, Japanese American, Pacific islander, and Chinese American ethnic backgrounds, Hatfield and her colleagues (Doherty, Hatfield, Thompson, & Choo, 1994) produced a number of interesting findings. As expected, the groups differed in individualism–collectivism, with the European Americans the most individualistic, Japanese Americans and Pacific islanders intermediate, and Chinese Americans the most collectivistic. What the authors did not find, however, was an impact of individualism–collectivism either on passionate and companionate love or on attachment styles. This led the authors to state that "we have been forced by this and other research to the conclusion that, when it comes to love, men and women from the various cultural and ethnic groups seem to possess very similar attitudes and behaviors" (Doherty et al., 1994, p. 396).

In another recent cross-cultural comparison, Sprecher et al. (1994) examined young people's orientations to love in Japan, Russia, and the United States. The authors found some significant cross-cultural differences (e.g., a greater proportion of U.S. respondents reported a secure attachment style; Japanese respondents were less romantic overall). However, the respondents from the different cultures were similar in several ways: Most had been in love at least once, most were somewhat romantic, and a majority believed that love should be the basis for marriage. Central to our concern here is that across cultures, the Eros love style "was the most common love style endorsed" (p. 363). As for the second most preferred love style, Storge was highest for the U.S. respondents, Agape for the Russians, and Mania for the Japanese. The authors noted that the cultural differences were less obvious than might have been expected from the political, economic, social, and psychological (e.g., individualistic vs. collectivistic) differences among the three countries. Again we see the seeming universality of love, particularly passionate love. In addition to certain intercultural similarities in love, there are also intergenerational similarities.

Love across Ages

Tucker and Aron (1993) assessed passionate love and marital satisfaction in 59 couples who were experiencing one of three major life transitions: (1) from engagement to marriage, (2) from childlessness to parenthood, and (3) from children at home to the empty nest. Though passionate love declined somewhat across the three transitions (i.e., as age and length of marriage ostensibly increased), and from pre- to post-transition at each stage, the decreases were slight. And the authors noted that the overall level of reported passionate love was high for all groups, both before and after the transitions. The authors were quick to note that "passionate love appears to remain fairly high over much of the course of marriage" (p. 144). Consistent with Tucker and Aron's results was the finding in the study of Mexican American and Anglo couples discussed earlier (Contreras et al., 1996) that Eros was the strongest consistent predictor of relationship satisfaction for both husbands and wives across the ethnic groups (thus highlighting passionate love's importance both intergenerationally and cross-culturally).

Companionate love is of course also important. As noted earlier, Storge was the second most frequently endorsed love style for the U.S. sample in Sprecher et al.'s (1994) cross-cultural study, and Hecht, Marston, and Larkey (1994) found that partners jointly experiencing higher levels of companionate love reported higher relationship quality, as did partners who were similar in companionate and/or secure love. In addition, Kamo (1993) found that for both Japanese and U.S. wives and husbands, such things as sharing friends and sharing time with friends were related to marital satisfaction.

Another study documenting the importance of companionate/friendship love (S. S. Hendrick & Hendrick, 1993) focused on college-age participants. In this research, some 84 participants (across three different studies) provided information through written accounts as well as rating scale responses in a study of love. In the written accounts, Storge was the most frequently noted theme. Furthermore, there was good correspondence between love themes in the free-form accounts and the love styles as measured by the Love Attitudes Scale. In one of the studies, participants generated free-form accounts of their closest friendship; almost half the respondents named their romantic partner as their closest friend. The results of this study suggested the substantial importance of friendship (as measured by Storge and linked closely to companionate love) in young adults' ongoing romantic relationships. Given passion's importance for mature couples (e.g., Contreras et al., 1996; Sokolski, 1995), and companionship's importance for younger couples, both types of love appear to be *concurrently* important in close relationships and in relationship satisfaction; this idea is contrary to previous notions that passionate love is gradually transformed into companionate love.

If, as has been proposed in this chapter, love has a central place in relationship satisfaction, then how can people increase their likelihood of finding partners with whom they can have the kind of love most likely to lead to relationship success? And once they have found such partners, how can love (and by implication, satisfaction) be maintained and increased?

STAYING SATISFIED

Looking for Love in the Right Places

A once-popular country and Western song talked about "looking for love in all the wrong places," and indeed there are some wrong places and right places in which to look for the love that leads to satisfying relationships.

If we go back to our theoretical basics (Lee, 1973), then we must maintain that there are at least six options for love: passionate love, game-playing love, friendship-based love, practical love, possessive love, and altruistic or giving love. Yet considerable research across cultures and age groups indicates that some love types are more preferred than others, particularly passionate love (as measured by us with the Eros subscale of the Love Attitudes Scale). If we examine the individual items that measure Eros, we find that they refer to more than passion; they also capture emotional involvement, a feeling of understanding, and a sense of "being meant for each other." So someone seeking this kind of love would do well to look for physical attraction and "chemistry" in a relationship, but then to look beyond—to a depth of understanding and sense of "at homeness" with the partner.

Of course passionate love is not the only type of love, and perhaps recognizing this fact early on is as important to relational well-being as is anything else. Lee (1973) found several other viable love approaches as he assessed and interviewed people, so if someone is more interested in friendship and shared interests or wants a sensible partner who will share in constructing a satisfying lifestyle, it is important not to discount those thoughts and feelings because they may not be laced with passion. Eros is the most frequently endorsed of the love styles, but all the other styles (except Ludus) are identified to some extent as representative of some people's approach to love.

Ludus, on the other hand, at least as it is measured by the Love Attitudes Scale, is a good love style to avoid, since it is negatively implicated in relationship satisfaction and was found in one study to be higher in couples that broke up than in couples that stayed together (S. S. Hendrick et al., 1988). It is certainly possible that there are playful and positive elements to a ludic love style that are not captured by our measure; given that caveat, if relationship partners engage in game playing, deception, or efforts to avoid disclosure to or intimacy with each other, then this love is not likely to be an enduring one. Contrary to another once-popular country and Western ballad, a bad love is *not* better than no love at all.

One last hint in looking for love is that similarity has long been recognized as a plus for relationships (Hecht et al., 1994; S. S. Hendrick & Hendrick, 1992a). So to the extent that an individual recognizes himself or herself as resonating to one or more love styles (e.g., an Eros–Storge combination), it would probably be wise to seek a partner with a similar style. Most matches could undoubtedly work to an extent, but some element of passion, excitement, or intensity is probably optimal for a lasting love.

Keeping Love

One way to stay satisfied is to keep love alive, though trying to figure out how exactly to do that is a challenge for many couple therapists and a topic for countless daytime talk shows. But it may be less of a priority for partners in ongoing relationships, at least until something goes amiss. Perhaps the first strategy for people who want to keep love alive is to remember that a relationship is not a static entity. It is not like a piece of artwork that, once acquired, is hung in a quiet corner of the living room and both admired and dusted periodically. Rather, it is like a garden that, if left untended, will at best be a riotous overgrowth of flowers and weeds, and at worst a barren patch of lifeless earth. Gardens of course differ in the amount of tending they require—some are clearly higher-maintenance than others—but all require at least some of the gardeners' attention. Love is a particularly beautiful part of the garden, with flowers that may be brilliantly colored and showy, or blooms that may be less dramatic but no less pleasing in quality.

Passion Strategies

Passionate love (or what we call Eros) has evolutionary utility, as we have discussed, and it is valued by people across cultures and age groups. But it can be difficult to maintain. Fortunate are the partners who remain attractive and interesting to each other after years of familiarity and adaptation. Of course many aspects of modern life, such as work pressures, family responsibilities, or just the sheer volume of today's sensory bombardments, seem to act continually to erode or wear down love. So it is necessary to make concerted efforts to protect passion, whether through weekly dinner "dates," periodic "adults-only" vacations, or some quiet time every evening during which partners talk about whatever is important to them at that moment.

Passion is much more than sexuality, but sexuality is important in most passionate relationships. It is essential to create a positive context for sexuality. Communicating in general and about sexuality in particular, expressing affection in physical and nonphysical ways, touching in sexual and nonsexual ways, and being aware of each other's presence—these are all conducive to sexual warmth in a relationship, as demonstrated by Maria's grandparents and their physical affection with each other throughout their 50-year marriage.

There is still more to passionate love than taking time for each other and being physically affectionate and expressive with each other. We have referred just above to fortunate partners who remain "attractive and interesting" to each other. Although everyone may want to be seen by his or her partner through the eyes of love, those eyes should not be expected to have X-ray vision. To put this another way, part of tending the garden of a relationship is for the partners to tend to themselves—their appearance, health, mental alertness, emotional responsiveness, altruism, humor, and on and on. Fit or fat, sober or drunk, supportive or snarly—every day people make choices about nurturing passionate love in their relationships or neglecting it until it withers and perhaps dies.

When many people ask the question "How do I keep passionate love alive?", what they really desire is an easy answer—for example, "Turn around three times, click your heels together, and you will live happily ever after." But if nature hard-wired humans to some extent for passionate love, the purpose of that hard-wiring was for dating and mating, and was thus tied to youth and reproduction. If passionate love is to last well beyond youth and the reproductive years, then people have to take some responsibility for it themselves. Everyone knows a few individuals who are almost middle-aged parodies of youth—who experience a midlife crisis and believe that its resolution lies in a facelift, a tan, and a new wardrobe. That is not what we are talking about in this chapter. We are talking not about people's trying to be something that they are not, but trying to be the very best that they are. Trite though it may sound, partners' taking good care of themselves physically, mentally, and emotionally may be one step toward taking care of the passionate love in their relationship. Keeping companionate love alive, while no less important, requires somewhat different strategies.

Friendship Strategies

In one study, as noted earlier, nearly half the respondents named their romantic partner as their "best friend" (S. S. Hendrick & Hendrick, 1993); moreover, the characteristics they ascribed to their relationships with both romantic *and* nonromantic partners included communication, support, and similarity. Although some people are proud of treating their friends "just like family," we are not aware of many people who boast about treating their family members "just like friends." Yet treating romantic partners as people do their friends might not be a bad idea. People are likely to extend certain courtesies to friends that they might not think of extending to relationship partners, yet these courtesies are part of what keeps friendships positive. Because friendships are voluntary (Fehr, 1993), and people are not bound to their friends by legal commitments (such as those that occur in marriage), they may indeed sometimes work harder at their friendships.

For example, it may be that a person is never too busy to listen to a friend's problems, but is sometimes unavailable to his or her partner. What if this person were as responsive to the partner as to the best friend, dropping everything when the partner was in need? And it is not just availability to the partner that is important, but also the quality of the communication and support that are part of that availability. When a friend has a problem with a coworker, for instance, a person may be inclined to take the friend's point of view and support his or her position. However, when the person's partner has difficulty with a coworker, the person may be more like an acquaintance of ours who never misses the opportunity to lecture his wife on how she could improve her relations at work by being a better manager. It is not hard to imagine how she responds to her husband's "helpful" suggestions. Had he maintained the modicum of tact and courtesy that he reserves for his friends, his marriage might have prospered instead of deteriorated.

Also, what about "similarity," mentioned by our research participants as a significant characteristic in their close friendships? People often value their similarities with friends, whether they are similarities in food preferences, movie preferences, or political views. But they are also typically tolerant of differences, tucking them off to one side, while they keep the similarities front and center. With relationship partners, however, people sometimes take similarities for granted—the result of some courtship filtering process (e.g., Murstein, 1976)—while they exaggerate differences (see Felmlee, 1995, for a relevant discussion). Perhaps if people were to honor, or at least accept, the differences between themselves and their relationship partners as gracefully as they accept those between themselves and close friends, they might move in the direction of better companionate love.

This small sampling of strategies for maintaining passionate and companionate love—and, by implication, relationship satisfaction—is only representative of the strategies offered throughout this volume and in dozens of useful books and articles geared toward improving people's love relationships. Although people often take their love relationships for granted, these relationships are so central to human existence that they are never far from consciousness. Love brings human beings their greatest joys and deepest sorrows, and it motivates much of how they live their lives.

CONCLUSIONS

There is an old song that affirms, "If we are lovers, we can't be friends." In past generations, many people subscribed to this either–or philosophy: Friendship was friendship, passionate love was passionate love, and the two could not be mixed. Increasingly, however, they are being mixed. Our own research suggests that both friendship (via Storge) and passion (via Eros) are important considerations for today's adults. People want not only passion, but also friendship to accompany that passionate love.

When we look at the situation from the standpoint of relationship satisfaction, these conclusions are doubly affirmed. Considerable research, including our own, has shown that passionate love strongly predicts relationship satisfaction. These results hold true for middle-aged couples as well as for young courting couples, and they hold across different cultural groups. The data also suggest that friendship, or Storge, is an important predictor of relationship satisfaction, though perhaps not quite as important as passionate love. These findings, along with data gathered by Hatfield and Rapson (1987) suggesting the universality of passionate love, begin to cinch the case for both passion and friendship as the two major predictors for relationship satisfaction. The data are rapidly converging on such a conclusion. This is not to say that there are not other relevant predictors of relationship satisfaction, at least within specific groups of people; rather, passionate love and friendship love are the most important predictors.

We have argued in previous publications, following Lee (1973), that the six love styles are all equally valid ways of loving. It now appears that we need to qualify this assertion. Clearly, Ludus is a negative predictor of relationship satisfaction; it has been shown to be so in several studies. If anything, Ludus is the opposite of a satisfactory style of love. Whether this is attributable to problems in our particular scale or to a misapplication of the concept is not at present clear. However, we can safely conclude that Ludus, as we measure it, is not a precursor to a satisfying relationship.

It also appears that conceptions such as Agape may be integrated with the concepts of passionate love and friendship love. A touch of the all-giving unselfish love style that is Agape would seem to lend potency to both Storge and Eros. Thus, we suspect that Agape is a contributor to the strength of these two important predictors of satisfaction, and occasionally is even an independent predictor. Likewise, Pragma seems not to be a powerful predictor of satisfaction, but may work indirectly through the effect of two people's selecting each other for similarity on various attributes. Pragmatic concerns are clearly important in some contexts, but equally clearly, Pragma is not a powerful predictor of relationship satisfaction. It is mediate in ways yet to be determined, rather than immediate, in its predictive power. In one or two samples, Mania has had minor predictive success for relationship satisfaction. Because Mania contains both happiness and unhappiness, we would not expect it to be powerfully related to ongoing relationship satisfaction. It may also work in mediate ways, picking up a small bit of the power of Eros, and is perhaps thus linked to relationship satisfaction indirectly through Eros. However, one would expect a relationship between two partners high in Mania to be volatile and problematic at best.

We conclude, from our data as well as those of other researchers, that the predominant styles of love embodied in Eros and Storge (or passion and friendship) are the most important predictors of relationship satisfaction in heterosexual couples. It will be interesting to explore this conclusion in future research, as well as to determine what other variables might have predictive power approaching that of passion and friendship.

REFERENCES

Attridge, M., & Berscheid, E. (1994). Entitlement in romantic relationships in the United States: A social-exchange perspective. In M. J. Lerner & G. Mikula (Eds.), *Entitlement and the affectional bond: Justice in close relationships* (pp. 117–147). New York: Plenum Press.

Beall, A. E., & Sternberg, R. J. (1995). The social construction of love. *Journal of Social and Personal Relationships, 12,* 417–438.

Berscheid, E., & Walster, E. (1978). *Interpersonal attraction* (2nd ed.). Reading, MA: Addison-Wesley.

Buck, R. (1989). Emotional communication in personal relationships: A developmental–interactionist view. In C. Hendrick (Ed.), *Close relationships* (pp. 144–163). Newbury Park, CA: Sage.

Burleson, B. R., & Denton, W. H. (1992). A new look at similarity and attraction in marriage: Similarities in social-cognitive and communication skills as predictors of attraction and satisfaction. *Communication Monographs, 59*, 268–287.

Buss, D. M. (1995). Evolutionary psychology: A new paradigm for psychological science. *Psychological Inquiry, 6*, 1–30.

Contreras, R., Hendrick, S. S., & Hendrick, C. (1996). Perspectives on marital love and satisfaction in Mexican American and Anglo couples. *Journal of Counseling and Development, 74*, 408–415.

Davis, K. E., & Latty-Mann, H. (1987). Love styles and relationship quality: A contribution to validation. *Journal of Social and Personal Relationships, 4*, 409–428.

Davis, K. E., & Todd, M. J. (1982). Friendship and love relationships. In K. E. Davis (Ed.), *Advances in descriptive psychology* (Vol. 2, pp. 79–122). Greenwich, CT: JAI Press.

Davis, K. E., & Todd, M. J. (1985). Assessing friendship: Prototypes, paradigm cases and relationship description. In S. Duck & D. Perlman (Eds.), *Understanding personal relationships: An interdisciplinary approach* (pp. 17–38). London: Sage.

Deal, J. E., Wampler, K. S., & Halverson, C. F. (1992). The importance of similarity in the marital relationship. *Family Process, 31*, 369–382.

Doherty, R. W., Hatfield, E., Thompson, K., & Choo, P. (1994). Cultural and ethnic influences on love and attachment. *Personal Relationships, 1*, 391–398.

Fehr, B. (1988). Prototype analysis of the concepts of love and commitment. *Journal of Personality and Social Psychology, 55*, 557–579.

Fehr, B. (1993). How do I love thee? Let me consult my prototype. In S. Duck (Ed.), *Individuals in relationships* (pp. 87–120). Newbury Park, CA: Sage.

Felmlee, D. H. (1995). Fatal attractions: Affection and disaffection in intimate relationships. *Journal of Social and Personal Relationships, 12*, 295–311.

Fowers, B. J., Applegate, B., Olson, D. H., & Pomerantz, B. (1994). Marital conventionalization as a measure of marital satisfaction: A confirmatory factor analysis. *Journal of Family Psychology, 8*, 98–103.

Glenn, N. D. (1990). Quantitative research on marital quality in the 1980s: A critical review. *Journal of Marriage and the Family, 52*, 818–831.

Guldner, G. T., & Swensen, C. H. (1995). Time spent together and relationship quality: Long-distance relationships as a test case. *Journal of Social and Personal Relationships, 12*, 313–320.

Hatfield, E., & Sprecher, S. (1986). Measuring passionate love in intimate relations. *Journal of Adolescence, 9*, 383–410.

Hatfield, E., & Rapson, R. (1987). Passionate love: New directions in research. In W. H. Jones & D. Perlman (Eds.), *Advances in personal relationships* (Vol. 1, pp. 109–139). Greenwich, CT: JAI Press.

Hazan, C., & Shaver, P. (1987). Romantic love conceptualized as an attachment process. *Journal of Personality and Social Psychology, 52*, 511–524.

Hecht, M. L., Marston, P. J., & Larkey, L. K. (1994). Love ways and relationship quality in heterosexual relationships. *Journal of Social and Personal Relationships, 11*, 25–43.

Hendrick, C., & Hendrick, S. S. (1986). A theory and method of love. *Journal of Personality and Social Psychology, 50*, 392–402.

Hendrick, C., & Hendrick, S. S. (1989). Research on love: Does it measure up? *Journal of Personality and Social Psychology, 56*, 784–794.

Hendrick, C., & Hendrick, S. S. (1990). A relationship-specific version of the Love Attitudes Scale. *Journal of Social Behavior and Personality, 5*, 239–254.

Hendrick, C., & Hendrick, S. S. (1991). Dimensions of love: A sociobiological interpretation. *Journal of Social and Clinical Psychology, 10*, 206–230.

Hendrick, S. S. (1981). Self-disclosure and marital satisfaction. *Journal of Personality and Social Psychology, 40*, 1150–1159.

Hendrick, S. S. (1988). A generic measure of relationship satisfaction. *Journal of Marriage and the Family, 50*, 93–98.

Hendrick, S. S. (1995). *Close relationships: What couple therapists can learn.* Pacific Grove, CA: Brooks/Cole.

Hendrick, S. S., & Hendrick, C. (1987). Love and sexual attitudes, self-disclosure, and sensation seeking. *Journal of Social and Personal Relationships, 4*, 281–297.

Hendrick, S. S., & Hendrick, C. (1992a). *Liking, loving, and relating* (2nd ed.). Pacific Grove, CA: Brooks/Cole.

Hendrick, S. S., & Hendrick, C. (1992b). *Romantic love.* Newbury Park, CA: Sage.

Hendrick, S. S., & Hendrick, C. (1993). Lovers as friends. *Journal of Social and Personal Relationships, 10*, 459–466.

Hendrick, S. S., & Hendrick, C. (1995). Gender differences and similarities in sex and love. *Personal Relationships, 2*, 55–65.

Hendrick, S. S., Hendrick, C., & Adler, N. L. (1988). Romantic relationships: Love, satisfaction, and staying together. *Journal of Personality and Social Psychology, 54*, 980–988.

Inman-Amos, J., Hendrick, S. S., & Hendrick, C. (1994). Love attitudes: Similarities between parents and between parents and children. *Family Relations, 43*, 456–461.

Inman-Amos, J., Hendrick, S. S., & Hendrick, C. (1995). *Love attitude correlations between college students' parents.* Unpublished raw data.

Kamo, Y. (1993). Determinants of marital satisfaction: A comparison of the United States and Japan. *Journal of Social and Personal Relationships, 10*, 551–568.

Larson, J. H. (1992). "You're my one and only": Premarital counseling for unrealistic beliefs about mate selection. *American Journal of Family Therapy, 20*, 242–253.

Lee, J. A. (1973). *The colors of love: An exploration of the ways of loving.* Don Mills, Ontario: New Press.

Lewis, R. A., & Spanier, G. B. (1979). Theorizing about the quality and stability of marriage. In W. Burr, F. I. Nye, & I. R. Reiss (Eds.), *Contemporary theories about the family* (Vol. 1, pp. 268–294). New York: Free Press.

Mellen, S. L. (1981). *The evolution of love*. San Francisco: Freeman.

Middleton, C. F. (1993). *The self and perceived-partner: Similarity as a predictor of relationship satisfaction*. Unpublished doctoral dissertation, Texas Tech University.

Morris, C. (1972). *The discovery of the individual: 1050–1200*. New York: Harper & Row.

Murstein, B. I. (1976). *Who will marry whom?* New York: Springer.

Richardson, D. R., Medvin, N., & Hammock, G. (1988). Love styles, relationship experience, and sensation seeking: A test of validity. *Personality and Individual Differences, 9,* 645–651.

Russell, R. J. H., & Wells, P. A. (1992). Social desirability and the quality of marriage. *Personality and Individual Differences, 13,* 787–791.

Sabatelli, R. M. (1988). Measurement issues in marital research: A review and critique of contemporary survey instruments. *Journal of Marriage and the Family, 50,* 891–915.

Sacher, J. A., & Fine, M. A. (1996). Predicting relationship status and satisfaction after six months among dating couples. *Journal of Marriage and the Family, 58,* 21–32.

Schumm, W. R., Paff-Bergen, L. A., Hatch, R. C., Obiorah, F. C., Copeland, J. M., Meens, L. D., & Bugaighis, M. A. (1986). Concurrent and discriminant validity of the Kansas Marital Satisfaction Scale. *Journal of Marriage and the Family, 48,* 381–387.

Simpson, J. A., Campbell, B., & Berscheid, E. (1986). The association between romantic love and marriage: Kephart (1967) twice revisited. *Personality and Social Psychology Bulletin, 12,* 363–372.

Singer, I. (1984). *The nature of love: Vol. 2. Courtly and romantic.* Chicago: University of Chicago Press.

Snyder, D. K. (1979). *Marital Satisfaction Inventory*. Los Angeles: Western Psychological Services.

Sokolski, D. M. (1995). *A study of marital satisfaction in graduate student marriages*. Unpublished doctoral dissertation, Texas Tech University.

Spanier, G. B. (1976). Measuring dyadic adjustment: New scales for assessing the quality of marriage and similar dyads. *Journal of Marriage and the Family, 38,* 15–25.

Sprecher, S., Aron, A., Hatfield, E., Cortese, A., Potapova, E., & Levitskaya, A. (1994). Love: American style, Russian style, and Japanese style. *Personal Relationships, 1,* 349–369.

Sternberg, R. J. (1986). A triangular theory of love. *Psychological Review, 93,* 119–135.

Sternberg, R. J. (1987). Liking versus loving: A comparative evaluation of theories. *Psychological Bulletin, 102,* 331–345.

Tucker, P., & Aron, A. (1993). Passionate love and marital satisfaction at key transition points in the family life cycle. *Journal of Social and Clinical Psychology, 12,* 135–147.

Walster, E., & Walster, G. W. (1978). *A new look at love*. Reading, MA: Addison-Wesley.

Woll, S. B. (1989). Personality and relationship correlates of loving styles. *Journal of Research in Personality, 23,* 480–505.

CHAPTER 4

————•◆•————

A Hierarchical Model of Love and Its Prediction of Satisfaction in Close Relationships

MICHAEL L. BARNES
ROBERT J. STERNBERG

Forty years ago, psychological theories of love were few and far between. In his presidential address to the American Psychological Association in 1958, Harry Harlow declared: "So far as love or affection is concerned, psychologists have failed in their mission. The little we know about love does not transcend simple observation, and the little we write about it has been written better by poets and novelists" (quoted in Rubin, 1988). Today, however, the situation has changed dramatically. Psychologists have studied the differences between loving and liking (Davis & Todd, 1982; Duck, 1983; Rubin, 1970, 1973; Sternberg, 1987), have applied theories of emotion toward the understanding of passionate love (Berscheid, 1983; Berscheid & Walster, 1978; Dutton & Aron, 1974), and have derived several unidimensional formulations of specific aspects of love (Hatfield & Sprecher, 1985; Sperling, 1986; Sternberg & Barnes, 1985; Tennov, 1979). Theoretical conceptions of love have included the following: love as self-expansion (Aron & Aron, 1986); love as emotion and attachment (Hazan & Shaver, 1987; Shaver, Hazan, & Brad-

79

shaw, 1988); love as reinforcement (Clore & Byrne, 1974); analogies to a color wheel (Lee, 1973, 1988); love as addiction (Peele & Brodsky, 1976); a three-component model of intimacy, passion, and commitment (Sternberg, 1986, 1988); love as a story (Sternberg, 1994, 1995); and even a model based on evolutionary biology (Buss, 1988, 1989).

Theorizing about love has reached a "critical mass." More theories and more empirical studies are being produced than ever before. How might these theories and the empirical results they have generated be unified in a larger framework? One such larger theoretical framework might be a hierarchy. In this hypothetical hierarchy, some of the differences among theories could be explained in terms of differences in the levels of the hierarchy to which they apply. For example, there are theories that describe love in terms of a single dimension. However, other theories of love attempt to carve the overall emotion into smaller, though related, components. Finally, there are theorists who believe that love is an assortment of smaller affects, cognitions, motivations, and behaviors that sum together to produce the overall feeling. One way to account for these differences is to posit that each type of theory is merely speaking to the phenomenon at a different level in the hierarchy.

A similar evolution has occurred in theories of intelligence. To account for the differences between Spearman's (1927) general ability (g), Thomson's (1939) theory of "bonds," and Thurstone's (1938) theory of primary mental abilities, some theorists began to conceptualize intelligence in terms of a hierarchy (Carroll, 1993; Cattell, 1971; Holzinger, 1938; Horn, 1968; Vernon, 1971). For example, the Cattell–Horn theory divided Spearman's g into fluid intelligence and crystallized intelligence. Vernon broke the general factor down into verbal/educational ability and practical/mechanical ability. Furthermore, each of these subfactors of g was itself theoretically decomposable into still smaller components of intelligence. Thus, advances in theories of intelligence utilized a hierarchical arrangement of the phenomenon to resolve some of the theoretical and empirical conflicts (Sternberg & Powell, 1982).

Sternberg and Grajek (1984) sought to distinguish among these alternative structural models as applied to the domain of love. Our collaborative research, in contrast, has sought to integrate these models. It has addressed, in part, the utility of a hierarchical structural account of love in order to resolve the numerous conflicts in theory and research on love, and also to understand the relation of love to satisfaction in close relationships.

There are two main classes of theories of love: "explicit" and "implicit." We now consider each of these.

EXPLICIT THEORIES OF LOVE

Explicit theories of love are those of psychological researchers. They may be classified into "structural" and "process" theories. Of course, the assignment of any one theory to a category can always be debated, but we believe that our assignments capture some of the major concepts underlying the various theories.

Structural Theories

Structural theories attempt to capture the main elements of love. Such theories have a certain static quality, their goal is to analyze the dimensions or other elements that jointly constitute love. There are three main kinds of structural theories: "unifactorial," "multifactorial," and "multiple-cluster."

Love as a Unifactorial (Spearmanian) Entity

The first type of theory proposes that love is best characterized as a single dimension—an undifferentiated whole (as in Spearman's [1927] theory of general intelligence). In this category we find theorists such as Rubin (1970), who believes that love is largely a unidimensional entity, with the possibility that subfactors might exist underneath the general factor. Although this theory could be conceived of as hierarchical in nature, the emphasis in Rubin's writing is on the notion that love is a unifactorial phenomenon. Rubin's factor analysis of his liking and loving scales demonstrated support for this conceptualization of love.

Many other psychometric approaches to the discovery of love's internal structure have also revealed support for a single underlying dimension of love (Dion & Dion, 1973; Mathes, 1980; Sternberg & Grajek, 1984; Swensen, 1961, 1972; Swensen & Gilner, 1964). All of these studies have concluded that love consists of a single factor comprising many different but highly correlated feelings, behaviors, attitudes, and motivations. This view—that love consists of a single factor dwarfing all subsequent factors—is nearly ubiquitous throughout psychometric studies of love (Murstein, 1988).

Freud also conceived of love in a unidimensional framework. He defined love as aim-inhibited sexual desire (Freud, 1921/1952); thus, the core of love is the sexual urge, or the desire for sexual union with another person. In order to compensate for the fact that such sexual desire usually cannot be expressed, one idealizes the love object and falls in love. This definition of love may be captured in a single dimension—that of sexual desire—and therefore represents the structural na-ture of love as a unitary concept.

Reik (1944, 1949) defined love as a substitute for another desire in the unsuccessful struggle toward self-fulfillment and the reaching of one's ego-ideal. For Reik, love is born from deficiency, and one is almost compelled to love another person in order to obtain from the relation-ship with that person the very qualities one lacks. The structural repre-sentation of Reik's view of love, therefore, may also be that of a single dimension: deficiency. Love, then, for Reik, is a singular phenomenon deriving from a person's shortcomings.

Another one-dimensional conceptualization of love may be found in the theoretical work of Tennov (1979). Tennov has defined love in terms of "limerance," a concept that involves acute longing for and dependency on the loved one (referred to as the "limerant object"). This form of love involves a high degree of intrusive cognitive activ-ity, preoccupation with the loved one, and extreme emotional attach-ment to another individual. Although this definition of love may seem to stress the negative aspects of a love relationship, there is also an emphasis on the exquisite feelings one can experience when the limerant object fulfills the needs and expectations of the person in love.

Support for a unidimensional formulation of love was also obtained by Bentler and Huba (1979), who proposed two alternative causal models to a model proposed by Tesser and Paulhus (1976). The causal model proposed by Tesser and Paulhus was based on a path analysis of the internal relationships between behaviors characterizing love. Tesser and Paulhus found that thinking about the other person and frequently dating him or her had a positive impact on love. In contrast, "reality con-straints," defined as "knowledge that is inconsistent with one's own thought-produced expectations" (Tesser & Paulhus, 1976, p. 1095), were found to have a negative impact on love. Bentler and Huba, however, found that a unitary view of love provided a better account of their data than did more complicated models based (in part) on the Tesser and Paulhus model.

These unidimensional approaches of love posit that love should be conceptualized in terms of a single entity, comprised of an undif-ferentiated mass of both positive and negative feelings that are not readily decomposed. According to these theories, an individual should label an experience as "love" when the experience consists of this huge mass of undifferentiated positive or negative feelings. Perhaps this structure of love has created the popular notion that "love is blind."

Love as a Multifactorial (Thurstonian) Entity

A second category of theories of love proposes that love consists of a few primary, and equally important, factors of love. These "primary-factors" theorists include Hatfield (1988) and Walster and Walster (1978), who have proposed that love consists of two factors, passionate and companionate love. Passionate love has been defined as follows: "A state of intense longing for union with another. Reciprocated love (union with the other) is associated with fulfillment and ecstasy. Unrequited love (separation) [is linked] with emptiness, anxiety, or despair. A state of profound physiological arousal" (Hatfield, 1988, p. 193). Companionate love, on the other hand, has been defined as "the affection we feel for those with whom our lives are deeply entwined" (Hatfield, 1988, p. 205). Although both passionate and companionate love are described as having cognitive, emotional, and behavioral components, those components are viewed as important, primary factors of love (Sullivan, 1985). Perhaps the most distinguishing characteristic of these two primary factors of love is that both ecstasy and misery intensify passionate love, whereas only pleasure increases companionate love (Hatfield, 1988).

Sternberg (1986) has also proposed a primary-factors theory of love. The triangular theory of love defines love in terms of three components: intimacy, passion, and commitment. The intimacy component comprises the bonded, connected, and close feelings people have toward each other in loving relationships. Intimacy is responsible for the warmth people feel toward the ones they love. The passion component refers to drives and motivations; this component is responsible for the romantic, physical attraction, and sexual aspects of loving relationships. Finally, the commitment component consists of the decisions one makes about being in love and staying in love. These three components, both individually and in combination, are assumed to cover the entire phenomenon of love. For example, because there are three components, each of which is either present in some degree or absent, there are eight (i.e., $2 \times 2 \times 2$) limiting possibilities: nonlove (all three components absent), liking (intimacy only), infatuated love (passion only), empty love (commitment only), romantic love (intimacy and passion), companionate love (intimacy and commitment), fatuous love (passion and commitment), and finally, consummate love (intimacy, passion, and commitment).

Maslow (1970) described two types of love, both of which are conceptualized as being of nearly equal importance in terms of accounting for the phenomenon. A person who falls in love because of deficiency (D-love) "falls in love because he needs and craves love, because he lacks it, and is impelled to make up this pathogenic deficiency" (p. 198). Being love (B-love), on the other hand, "tends to be a free giving of oneself, wholly and with abandon, without reserve, withholding or calculation" (p. 183). Maslow's D-love relates strongly to Reik's account of love as relating to deficiency; however, Maslow then moves on to describe a wholly separate love experience—one of freedom from demand and dependent need of the other person. This two-factor theory of love fits into the primary-factors category of theories of love. Primary-factors accounts of love also have a long history. St. Augustine (1961), writing about 400 A.D., drew a distinction between two forms of love: *Cupiditas*, the ill-fated love one person has for another, and *Caritas*, the universal, ultimate, pure love for God. For St. Augustine, as well as for the thousands of Christians to follow, love was conceptualized as being of either one or the other of these forms, although only the latter (*Caritas*) form was considered "true" love.

These primary-factor theories of love suggest that the structure of love consists of a small set of emotions, cognitions, motivations, and behaviors that are all of nearly equal importance. Love must be viewed as a set of primary structures, regardless of the possibility that a higher-order factor unifying these structures may or may not exist. The structure of love is best viewed as a small set of separate components rather than as a single entity.

Love as a Multiple-Cluster (Thomsonian) Entity

The third category of theories of love includes those that describe love as involving a set of characteristic features—that is, a set of affects, cognitions, motivations, and even behaviors that, when sampled in sufficient quantity, produce the overall feeling referred to as "love." One such theory is that of Murstein (1988). Murstein has explicitly described the structure of love as a highly complex phenomenon. Murstein defines love as "an Austro-Hungarian Empire uniting all sorts of feelings, behaviors, and attitudes, sometimes sharing little in common, under the rubric of *love*" (Murstein, 1988, p. 33). For Murstein, the structure of love consists of a nearly limitless number of aspects.

In her theory of emotion, Berscheid (1983) has described the structure of love in terms of the interconnectedness of numerous clusters or "bonds." The number and intensity of these bonds are what characterize an emotional relationship. In this theory, "the affective phenomena that occur in a relationship are a direct function of, and therefore predictable from the various properties of interdependence that characterize the relationship" (Berscheid, 1983, p. 118). Each person in the relationship is assumed to be participating in a chain of events (behaviors, expectations, attitudes, etc.) to which the other person in the relation-ship is subjected. The degree to which each of the two individuals par-ticipates, causes, or reacts to the other's chain of events is the defining feature of an emotional relationship. Thus, Berscheid believes that the structure of love consists of a large number of entities or aspects (clusters or "bonds"). Empirical support for this theoretical treatment of love has also been obtained by Sternberg and Grajek (1984).

These cluster-based theories of love propose that love is best described in terms of a large number of characteristic features, includ-ing feelings, cognitions, attitudes, and behaviors. The various features must be sampled together to yield love. Although the experience of love may feel unitary in nature, the underlying structure of love is the sampling of a sufficient number of elements to yield, jointly, the ex-perience. The combination of elements is not, then, viewed as an un-differentiated mass. Rather, love is viewed as a combination of a large number of underlying and interrelated elements that tend to covary in close relationships.

Process Theories

The theories described above all emphasize the structure of love. Although the emphasis in our chapter is on structural theories, it is important to note that other theories emphasize the processes of love.

One process theory is that of Lee (1977), who proposes six love styles that together provide an account of most of the ways people interact with each other within the context of loving relationships. The six love styles are (1) Eros—erotic/passionate love; (2) Ludus—game-like, playing-the-field love; (3) Storge—companionate, friendship-based love; (4) Mania—obsessive/jealous love; (5) Agape—selfless love; and (6) Pragma—practical love.

Hazan and Shaver (1987; Shaver & Hazan, 1993) proposed three attachment styles that purportedly account for the different behavior patterns people display in love relationships. The three attachment styles derive from the attachment styles people develop as infants toward their mothers. The attachment styles derive from an extension of work on infant attachment. The three attachment styles are avoidant, ambiva-lent, and secure. These styles have proven to be useful conceptions of the ways in which people relate to each other (Davis & Latty-Mann, 1987; Hazan & Shaver, 1987; Hendrick & Hendrick, 1986; Shaver et al., 1988).

Finally, Sternberg (1994, 1995, 1996) has proposed a process ac-count of love as a story. The basic idea is that everyone, from the time of birth, begins to form a story of what love should be. These stories result from the interaction of personality attributes with experience. Each story involves two complementary slots or roles. For example, in a fantasy story, the complementary roles are of prince and princess; in a business story, of business partners; in a horror story, of the individual who inflicts and of the one who receives pain. According to this view, people construct their own notions of love (see also Beall & Sternberg, 1995). Moreover, everyone has a hierarchy of stories, ranging from most to least preferred.

IMPLICIT THEORIES OF LOVE

An investigation into the structure of love need not be limited to explicit theories. It is quite possible (and indeed likely) that people maintain conceptions of love, or implicit theories, that define their own notions of what love is. As defined by Sternberg (1985), implicit theories are "constructions by people . . . that reside in the minds of these individuals. Such theories need to be discovered rather than invented because they already exist, in some form, in people's heads" (p. 608).

Fehr (1988) took a social-cognitive prototype-based approach to the study of love to ascertain whether the concepts of love and commitment could be viewed as containing a set of features that are typical but not defining. Drawing on the work of Rosch (1975), Fehr demonstrated that the concepts of love and commitment are in fact organized around a prototype; that some aspects of love and commitment are more central than are others (see also Kelley, 1983); and, finally, that people's conceptions of love and commitment are partially though not completely overlapping. This research by Fehr suggests that even though people's conceptions of love are organized around a prototype, its features are easily decomposed into a collection of smaller aspects, some of which are better indicators of love than are other aspects (see also Aron & Westbay, 1996; Fehr, 1993).

In similar work, Fehr and Russell (1991) undertook six studies to provide further evidence that the basic-level concept of love can be better understood from a prototype perspective than from a classical perspective. The series of experiments indicated that love has an internal structure such that types of love (e.g., maternal, friendship, affection, infatuation, etc.) can be reliably ordered from better to worse instances of love.

Across six experiments, eight separate methods for measuring the internal structure of the concept of love were generated. The internal structure of love was demonstrated via converging operations among these eight measures. The median correlation for the 28 correlations obtained was .53, indicating high agreement among the eight measures. Thus, love fits a prototype-based approach to definition rather than a classical approach, indicating support for the notion that the structure of love is consistent with numerous co-occurring aspects. Especially strong elements of it appear to be intimacy, passion, and commitment (Aron & Westbay, 1996)—the same elements that form the core of the triangular theory of love (Sternberg, 1986). The prototype may differ somewhat, however, from one culture to another (Sprecher et al., 1994) and from one time to another (Beall & Sternberg, 1995).

AN INTEGRATIVE HIERARCHICAL MODEL

Our own model suggests that the various kinds of structural theories described above—explicit and implicit—may be, in some respects, compatible with each other. In particular, unifactorial, multifactorial, and multiple-cluster theories may represent three successive and more specific levels of a hierarchy. On this view, the question would not be, as in the Sternberg and Grajek (1984) study, "Which structure is correct?" Rather, it would be "How do these various structures relate to each other?"

Methodological Overview

We conducted three studies in order to explore various aspects of the hierarchical model. We combined factor analysis and hierarchical cluster analysis, because each method elucidates different aspects of structure. Our approach was primarily implicit-theoretical.

In a prestudy, we asked 40 laypersons to write down, in any form they chose, what was important to them in their romantic relationships (both good and bad). The resulting list was then content-analyzed and reduced to 80 statements of behavior or attitude. In Study 1, we investigated the extent to which the statements obtained in the prestudy could be understood in terms of a hierarchical model. Subjects provided ratings on a 1–9 scale of the various statements. We also examined the relation of the hierarchical attributes of love to various aspects of satisfaction. In Study 2, we used a sorting procedure to examine aspects of love. Subjects sorted statements into piles. In Study 3, we were concerned primarily with whether and how people would actually use their implicit theories of love in evaluating hypothetical scenarios describing close relationships (see Sternberg, Conway, Ketron, & Bernstein, 1981). We report in detail on Study 1, and in less detail on the Prestudy as well as Studies 2 and 3.

Prestudy

A brief questionnaire was distributed to 40 individuals, 20 men and 20 women. Participants were residents of the New Haven, Connecticut, area, and were recruited through newspaper advertisements. Their ages ranged from 18 to 66 years, with a mean of 31 years. Participants were asked to list "the thoughts and feelings (both positive and negative) [they] have toward [their] partner which [they] feel are distinctive of [their] romantic involvement." Participants were encouraged to list as many thoughts and feelings as they wished.

Responses to the survey ranged from barely one sentence to a few pages. We reduced the statements by combining any statements across participants that we viewed as essentially synonymous, and by wording the statements as clearly and concisely as possible, with the constraint that edited statements retained their original meaning. Obviously, there was some subjectivity in the reduction process. Reduction of the responses produced 80 statements.

Study 1

Methodology

In our first study, 172 adults were recruited via advertisements in two local newspapers and via flyers and posters. In order to participate, individuals had (1) to be at least 18 years of age, (2) to be currently involved in a heterosexual close relationship, and (3) to have graduated from high school. Thus, this and subsequent studies pertain only to adult heterosexual love. The participants ranged in age from 18 to 73 years, with a mean of 31 years. There were 79 males and 93 females, whose average age did not differ significantly. There were 105 never-married people, 47 married people, and 20 people who were either divorced or separated. The sample was primarily Caucasian (85%).

Participants received a number of measures (see Barnes, 1990, for a description of the full set). The measures of primary interest here were the implicit-theoretical questionnaire from the Prestudy, and a relationship satisfaction questionnaire. All questions were answered on a 9-point rating scale with anchors on odd-numbered points (1 = "not at all," 3 = "somewhat," 5 = "moderately," 7 = "quite," 9 = "extremely").

Factor Analysis

In order to ascertain the structure of love emanating from these data, the 80 implicit-theoretical items were subjected to both principal-component and principal-factor analysis. Both of these methods look at the structure underlying a set of correlational data. The idea is to chart a "map of the mind." The first method has no provision for separating the unique (unshared) variance in individual statements from the common (shared) variance across statements, whereas the second method attempts to separate out unique variance. Because the two types of factor analyses produced highly similar results, only the results from the principal-component analysis are reported here. However, the relatively low participant–item ratio in this study (2.2:1) requires that the conclusions drawn from these analyses remain tentative.

Our hierarchical conception of love suggested the appropriateness of an oblique rotation of the principal components initially obtained. Rotation essentially takes an initial factor solution, and assigns the position of axes in the geometric space. An oblique rotation allows correlations among the axes. In other words, the axes are not orthogonal (at right angles) to each other.

Thus, we followed the principal-component analysis with an oblique rotation, which could yield a set of correlated factors. These in turn could, in principle, be factored to yield a higher-order general factor (the apex of the hierarchy), if one existed. Promax rotation was chosen because of its relative conceptual simplicity and applicability, given our theoretical framework. In promax rotation, exponentiation is used to create dependence among initially orthogonal axes.

The oblique rotation produced a five-factor solution that accounted for 71% of the variance in the data. Correlations among the five factors ranged from .35 to .65, with a median of .55. The five factors, respectively, could be interpreted as Intimacy, Sexuality, Mutual Need, Congeniality, and Sincerity.

In factor analysis, each item is assigned a correlation with, or loading on, a factor. The loading refers to the strength of relation between the item and the factor. Loadings of over .40 (or sometimes .30) are viewed as sufficiently high to be worthy of note. The loadings do not, however, lend themselves to formal tests of statistical significance.

Items showing a loading of .40 or greater on Factor I, Intimacy, were as follows (in descending order): (1) have a partner who makes you feel wanted, (2) have a partner who encourages and praises you, (3) have a partner who is willing to put his or her problems on hold and listen to yours, (4) feel equally important to your partner, (5) have a partner who is considerate of and sensitive to your needs, (6) have a partner who makes you feel special, (7) have a partner who is observant of your needs, (8) have a partner who has compassion, (9) feel loved by your partner, (10) have a partner who tries to make you happy, (11) have a partner who supports you more than anyone else, (12) have a partner who understands your hopes and dreams, (13) have a partner who accepts you, (14) have a partner who stimulates you intellectually, (15) cheer each other up when one or both of you feel down, (16) respect each other's differences, (17) treat each other as special, (18) have a partner who is not afraid to share his or her innermost feelings with you, (19) have a partner who brings out the best of what you're capable of being.

Items loading at .40 or greater on Factor II, Sexuality, were as follows (in descending order): (1) be sexually attracted to your partner, (2) have a partner who stimulates you sexually, (3) be very physically attracted to your partner, (4) have a partner who is good sexually, (5) be close to your partner sexually, (6) experience love making that is very emotional, (7) have a partner who is easily aroused sexually, (8) feel very happy and warm through touching each other, (9) have a partner who lets you have your own time.

Items loading at .40 or greater on Factor III, Mutual Need, were the following (in descending order): (1) feel unhappy when you and your partner are apart for long, (2) have similar attitudes about marriage and money and children, (3) want to be with your partner more than anyone else, (4) feel that the love you have for your partner outweighs any faults he or she may have, (5) receive feelings of security through your partner's care.

Items loading at .40 or greater on Factor IV, Congeniality, were as follows (in descending order): (1) have a partner who is good with children, (2) have a partner who gets along well with people, (3) have a partner who is strong morally.

Finally, items loading at .40 or greater on Factor V, Sincerity, were the following (in descending order): (1) never lie to your partner, (2) be honest with your partner, (3) be faithful to your partner.

Given the moderate correlations among the five factors, and consistent with our search for a hierarchical structure, we submitted the five factors to a second-order factor analysis, which would reveal a general factor if one existed. Second-order factor analysis basically involves factoring the (first-order) factors; it is thus a factor analysis of a factor analysis. The principal-components analysis of the five factors produced a single factor. This factor accounted for 63% of the total variance among the factors, and was interpreted as an overall general factor of Love.

Thus, the principal-components analysis of the 80 implicit-theoretical items indicated some support for the proposed overall hierarchical structure of love. We conducted a further analysis in order to confirm our interpretation.

Hierarchical Cluster Analysis

The correlation matrix of the 80 implicit-theoretical items was submitted to a hierarchical cluster analysis to determine whether the items formed an interpretable hierarchical structure. The method we used is called the "complete-linkage method" (Hartigan, 1975). This method tends to produce relatively compact and internally coherent clusters.

At a low level in the hierarchy, eight interpretable clusters were found: (1) Fulfillment, (2) Compatibility, (3) Mutual Understanding, (4) Sincerity with Your Partner, (5) Trusting Your Partner, (6) Sexuality, (7) Intimacy, and (8) Mutual Need. (Each of these clusters could be decomposed into even smaller clusters. For example, the Fulfillment cluster contained subclusters of Need Fulfillment and Reciprocity. But such very fine clusters were not of particular interest to us in this analysis.)

At a higher level in the hierarchy, two clusters could be identified. The clusters were formed by the combination of the Trust, Sincerity, Mutual Understanding, Fulfillment, and Compatibility clusters on the one hand, and the Sexuality, Intimacy, and Mutual Need clusters on the other. These two superordinate clusters can be described as Companionate Love and Passionate Love, as proposed by the theory of Hatfield (1988).

In a hierarchical cluster analysis, it is always possible to view all lower-level clusters as merging at a unitary, highest level. The question is whether there are any interpretable lower-level clusters. We obtained such clusters.

These results suggest that there are interpretable clusters at various hierarchical levels in people's conceptions of love. Moreover, the clusters we obtained are similar and even nearly identical, in several cases, to clusters obtained in a similar analysis by Sternberg and Grajek (1984). Thus, there is reasonable evidence from the current and past work to suggest that although people may experience love as an overall, general factor, love can be further decomposed structurally. Our results suggest that various theories of love may be integrated through a hierarchical model.

Relationship Satisfaction

All participants also received a two-part questionnaire querying them about their satisfaction with their intimate relationship. The first part pertained to emotional satisfaction; the second part covered behavioral satisfaction. The emotional questionnaire asked participants such things as "How satisfied are you in the relationship?", "Do you feel fulfilled by the relationship?", "To what extent are your needs met by the relationship?", and "How happy do you feel in the relationship?" A principal-component analysis of the emotional questionnaire revealed a single Emotional Satisfaction factor, with 19 of 20 items loading over .40 on this single factor.

The behavioral questionnaire asked participants such things as whether they had "considered ending [their] relationship," "told [their] partner, 'I love you,'" and "worked together to try to solve a problem in [their] relationship." A principal-component analysis of the behavioral questionnaire revealed three factors, which were labeled (1) Togetherness, (2) Absence of Tension and Fighting, and (3) Shared Intimacy. All items except one loaded at least .40 on (at least) one of these three components.

Relationship of Love Clusters to Relationship Satisfaction

Finally, we computed scores for each of the love clusters (Fulfillment, Compatibility, Mutual Understanding, Sincerity with Your Partner, Trusting Your Partner, Sexuality, Intimacy, and Mutual Need) and each of the satisfaction indices (Emotional Satisfaction, Togetherness, Absence of Tension and Fighting, and Shared Intimacy). All of these computed scores were found to be statistically reliable: Reliability indices ranged from .75 to .97, with a median of .89.

The question of interest was the extent to which each of the love clusters related to each of the aspects of satisfaction. These data are shown in Table 4.1. Three main patterns in the results are worth noting. First, the correlations were all highly statistically significant in the expected direction, both for the Emotional Satisfaction factor and for the three behavioral satisfaction factors. Second, the correlations with the Emotional Satisfaction factor were noticeably higher than the correlations with the three behavioral indices. Third, the eight clusters did not vary considerably in their overall level of correlation with the satisfaction composites. Sincerity with Your Partner showed the lowest correlation overall, and Fulfillment the highest, but the differences were not large. Thus, the clusters "passed" the validation test: All 32 correlations were significant, suggesting that all of the clusters of love are related to satisfaction at some nontrivial level.

Study 2

Methodology

Our second study had a similar goal to the first, but employed a different methodology. In this study, 50 adults from the New Haven area

TABLE 4.1. Correlations between Clusters and Satisfaction Indices

	Emotional Satisfaction	Togetherness	Absence of Tension and Fighting	Shared Intimacy
Trusting your Partner	.70	.37	.55	.34
Sincerity with Your Partner	.59	.44	.34	.42
Mutual Understanding	.82	.48	.55	.51
Compatibility	.76	.42	.56	.49
Fulfillment	.91	.56	.51	.60
Sexuality	.65	.43	.23	.60
Intimacy	.88	.59	.44	.63
Mutual Need	.84	.68	.29	.56

Note. All correlations are significant beyond the .002 level.

were recruited through flyers. There were 23 males and 27 females in the sample, ranging in ages from 18 to 56 years with an average of 29 years. The majority of participants were Caucasian (90%).

Participants were given the items in the implicit-theoretical inventory, but this time the items were each printed on a 3″ × 5″ index card. The participants were asked to sort the cards so that each pile of cards they created would represent statements that somehow "go together." It was emphasized that there was no one correct way to sort the cards, and that participants could create as many or as few piles as they wished.

Hierarchical Cluster Analysis

An overall similarity matrix linking the 80 statements was created by counting the number of times each statement was sorted with every other statement. We then used the complete-linkage method (the same method used in Study 1) to subject this matrix to hierarchical cluster analysis.

The data seemed to fit the hierarchical model well. At a relatively lower level of the hierarchy, we identified eight clusters: Sexuality, Compatibility, Happiness, Companionate Love, Valuing of Partner, Mutual Need, Trust/Sincerity, and Mutual Respect. A comparison of these eight clusters with those obtained from the first study indicated notable similarities. Four clusters from Study 1 were readily identifiable in Study 2. Both solutions revealed a Sexuality cluster consisting of exactly the same items, with one exception. Both solutions also revealed the importance of trust and sincerity. However, in Study 2 these two clusters were combined, whereas in Study 1 they were separate. The Compatibility cluster from Study 1 was also evident in Study 2. One cluster from Study 1, Fulfillment, was widely scattered throughout the clusters in Study 2.

Two additional clusters in Study 2 bore some resemblance to the clusters from Study 1. The Mutual Need cluster from Study 2 resembled the comparable cluster from Study 1. Both clusters comprised a sense of needing and of being needed by the other member of the couple. Whereas the Intimacy cluster from Study 2 bore the same name as a cluster from Study 1, there was incomplete overlap in underlying items. In Study 2, the intimacy cluster also contained some items pertaining to feeling happy in the relationship and needing the other. Finally, there was a cluster in Study 2 that occurred in Study 1, but at a higher level in the hierarchy than in Study 2: Companionate Love.

In sum, the second study, like the first, revealed a sensible and interpretable hierarchical structure underlying the data, except that in this study we used sorting rather than rating data. The clusters were quite similar, although not identical, to those that emerged in Study 1. Given the relatively small numbers of cases and the difference in methodologies, the results of the two studies seem to us to be largely, although not totally, mutually supportive.

Study 3

Our goal in the third study was to see whether the relation between the aspects of love revealed in cluster analysis and the measures of satisfaction would show up when participants were asked to rate various aspects of hypothetical relationships. Participants were presented with scenarios about 48 fictitious relationships, constructed on the basis of the results of the hierarchical cluster analysis conducted in Study 1 (see Barnes, 1990; see also Sternberg et al., 1981, for details on the method). We used a three-step process to construct each scenario. First, we selected between five and seven items according to a rather elaborate set of rules for combining these items, which ensured that each scenario would include a balanced set of items across the eight clusters and would potentially reflect both positive and negative aspects of each item. Second, we randomly selected a male first name and a female first name, and then used the selected items to describe a fictitious close relationship. Third, we wrote descriptions from both the male and the female points of view. This procedure created 96 descriptions of fictitious relationships, 48 from the male point of view and 48 from the female point of view. Here is the male version of one such scenario:

Rick is sexually attracted to Rita. Knowing that Rita loves and cares for him does not really affect Rick's self-image in any way. Rick does not feel more secure just because Rita takes care of him, and she does not really need him either. He feels content just being with her, and they often make time to spend alone together. Rita is good with children.

Now here is the female version of the same scenario:

Rita is sexually attracted to Rick. Knowing that Rick loves and cares for her does not really affect Rita's self-image in any way. Rita does not feel more secure just because Rick takes care of her, and he does not really need her either. She feels content just being with him, and they often make time to spend alone together. Rick is good with children.

Each participant received 48 different descriptions, 24 from the male point of view and 24 from the female point of view. Thus, participants would read one, but not both, versions of the same scenario. Following each description of a relationship, participants were asked to rate the following on a scale of 1 (low) to 9 (high): (1) how good the relationship is, (2) how long the relationship will last, (3) how satisfied the male partner is, and (4) how satisfied the female partner is.

We found very high levels of internal-consistency reliability across scenarios (generally in the .80s) and across participants (generally in the .90s). In other words, to the extent that there were individual differences in how people used the information, they were unlikely to have an effect on our results.

In this third study, 40 adults from the New Haven area, 22 women and 18 men, were recruited through flyers. Participants ranged in age from 19 to 50 years, with a mean of 32 years. Just over 90% of the participants were Caucasian.

The question we were now ready to address was whether the number of items from a given cluster would predict the ratings of the relationships. In theory, the more items from a given cluster of love, the higher the predicted level of satisfaction should be. In contrast, fewer items from a cluster should predict less satisfaction. Because the four ratings of the relationships were extremely highly correlated (.96, on average), they were combined into an overall measure of "satisfaction."

All of the correlations were in the predicted direction, and most were statistically significant. The correlations between predicted and observed values (predicted values were based on the cluster analysis, and observed values on the ratings of satisfaction) were .39 for Fulfillment ($p < .01$), .28 for Compatibility ($p < .05$), .06 for Mutual Understanding ($p > .05$), .21 for Sincerity with Your Partner ($p > .05$), .33 for Trusting Your Partner ($p < .05$), .33 for Sexuality ($p < .05$), .37 for Intimacy ($p < .01$), and .21 for Mutual Need ($p > .05$).

It is hard to know what to make of the differences in the correlations, given that they were all in the predicted direction. At a minimum, we can say that for the hypothetical scenarios, levels of Fulfillment, Compatibility, Trusting Your Partner, Sexuality, and Intimacy were predictive of participants' ratings of satisfaction in the described close relationships.

In sum, this study helped to validate the hierarchical cluster model derived from the earlier studies. It also showed not only that people have an implicit hierarchical model, but also that they use their model when evaluating satisfaction in close relationships.

CONCLUSIONS

Our research was aimed at finding a structure of love that could begin to account for the many alternative theoretical conceptualizations of love that currently exist in the psychological literature (see Sternberg, 1987, for a review). In particular, some theoretical notions emphasize love as a single entity or factor; other notions emphasize a small number of entities (multiple factors) that overlap to some degree but nevertheless represent relatively separate and important aspects of love. Finally, there are theories of love that describe love in terms of many small clusters or bonds, the sufficient sampling of which produces the overall feeling of love.

The results of the three studies suggest that these three conceptualizations of love are not necessarily mutually exclusive. First, there is support for a single overall entity of love at the top of a hierarchical model. Underlying the single factor are multiple correlated entities. Our analysis suggested a "hot" cluster of passionate love and a "warm" cluster of companionate love. These two clusters can in turn be decomposed into even smaller entities or clusters.

The decomposition of love into "hot" passionate love and "warm" companionate love has a long history. Perhaps one of the oldest traditions in the long history of writing about love is the distinction between Eros and Agape (Nygren, 1952; Singer, 1984–1987; Soble, 1990).

In the Eros tradition, love is considered acquisitive, erotic, and centered on a specific individual or object of love. The phenomenon of love is explained in terms of the qualities of the loved one; that is, love is thought to be caused by these qualities. A love based on Eros is sexual and passionate. The Eros tradition is usually associated with Plato's *Symposium* (1970), written over 300 years before the birth of Christ.

Agape is often associated with Aristotle's *Ethics* (1953), in which love is defined as wishing good things for someone for the good of that person. Definitions of love based on Agape largely reject the idea that attributes of the lover are the grounds for the love. In fact, the definitions in this tradition often reverse the causal direction of the arrow between the qualities of the loved one and the feeling of love (Nygren, 1952; Soble, 1990). Definitions of Agape claim that the feeling of love one has for the loved one is what makes his or her qualities attractive to the lover. Where does love come from, then? These definitions retain the mystery of love, and generally claim that "love is its own reward." In the tradition of Agape, any attempt to explain love must look to the lover, not the loved one, for the reasons.

Of course, a more recent theory emphasizing this distinction is that of Hatfield (1988), who posits passionate and companionate forms of love. Our results seem to fit directly with her theory, as well as with the intimacy and passion components of Sternberg's (1986) triangular theory.

The hierarchical view proposed here provides a parsimonious summary of many of the existing formulations about the nature of love. Theories of love do not differ so much in their validity as they do in their respective emphases on different levels of the overall phenomenon of love. Some theories specify that the overall, global experience of love requires the most theoretical attention, whereas other theories specify the more particulate components.

Of course, our research has limitations. The numbers of participants were small; the research examined primarily Caucasian adults in a given place at a given time; our questionnaires were certainly not the most refined. Nonetheless, the results of our research demonstrate at least partial support for a hierarchical model of love. It provides at least a first approximation of a way in which love may be understood. Looking at love from a broad, intermediate level, we need at the very least to identify passion (Berscheid & Walster, 1978; Hatfield, 1988; Lee, 1988; Sternberg, 1986) and companionate love or intimacy (Berscheid, Snyder, & Omoto, 1989; Hatfield, 1988; McAdams, 1989; Rubin, 1970; Sternberg, 1986) as important parts of love.

ACKNOWLEDGMENTS

We wish to thank Robert Abelson, Elizabeth Barnes, Kelly Brownell, and Peter Salovey for their helpful feedback on our research. This research was supported in part by funds from the Department of Psychology, Yale University.

REFERENCES

Aristotle. (1953). *Ethics* (J. A. K. Thomson, Trans.). Harmondsworth, England: Penguin.

Aron, A., & Aron, E. N. (1986). *Love and the expansion of the self: Understanding attraction and satisfaction.* Washington, DC: Hemisphere.

Aron, A., & Westbay, L. (1996). Dimensions of the prototype of love. *Journal of Personality and Social Psychology, 70,* 535–551.

Augustine. (1961). *Confessions.* Harmondsworth, England: Penguin.

Barnes, M. L. (1990). *Love and common sense.* Unpublished manuscript, Yale University.

Beall, A., & Sternberg, R. J. (1995). The social construction of love. *Journal of Personal and Social Relationships, 2*(3), 417–438.

Bentler, P. M., & Huba, G. J. (1979). Simple minitheories of love. *Journal of Personality and Social Psychology, 37,* 124–130.

Berscheid, E. (1983). Emotion. In H. H. Kelley, E. Berscheid, A. Christensen, J. H. Harvey, T. L. Huston, G. Levinger, E. McClintock, L. A. Peplau, & D. R. Peterson, *Close relationships* (pp. 110–168). New York: Freeman.

Berscheid, E., Snyder, M., & Omoto, A. M. (1989). Issues in studying close relationships: Conceptualizing and measuring closeness. In C. Hendrick (Ed.), *Close relationships* (pp. 63–91). Newbury Park, CA: Sage.

Berscheid, E., & Walster, E. H. (1978). *Interpersonal attraction* (2nd ed.). Reading, MA: Addison-Wesley.

Buss, D. M. (1988). Love acts: The evolutionary biology of love. In R. J. Sternberg & M. L. Barnes (Eds.), *The psychology of love* (pp. 100–118). New Haven, CT: Yale University Press.

Buss, D. M. (1989). Sex differences in human mate preferences: Evolutionary hypotheses tested in 37 cultures. *Behavioral and Brain Sciences, 12,* 1–14, 39–49.

Carroll, J. B. (1993). *Human cognitive abilities: A survey of factor-analytic studies.* New York: Cambridge University Press.

Cattell, R. B. (1971). *Abilities: Their structure, growth, and action.* Boston: Houghton Mifflin.

Clore, G. L., & Byrne, D. (1974). A reinforcement–affect model of attraction. In T. L. Huston (Ed.), *Foundations of interpersonal attraction* (pp. 143–170). New York: Academic Press.

Davis, K. E., & Latty-Mann, H. (1987). Love styles and relationship quality: A contribution to validation. *Journal of Personal and Social Relationships, 4,* 409–428.

Davis, K. E., & Todd, M. J. (1982). Friendship and love relationships. In K. E. Davis & T. D. Mitchell (Eds.), *Advances in descriptive psychology* (Vol. 2, pp. 79–122). Greenwich, CT: JAI Press.

Dion, K. L., & Dion, K. K. (1973). Correlates of romantic love. *Journal of Consulting and Clinical Psychology, 4,* 51–56.

Duck, S. (1983). *Friends for life.* New York: St. Martin's Press.

Dutton, D. G., & Aron, A. P. (1974). Some evidence for heightened sexual attraction under conditions of high anxiety. *Journal of Personality and Social Psychology, 30,* 510–517.

Fehr, B. (1988). Prototype analysis of the concepts of love and commitment. *Journal of Personality and Social Psychology, 55,* 557–579.

Fehr, B. (1993). How do I love thee? Let me consult my prototype. In S. Duck (Ed.), *Individuals in relationships* (Vol. 1, pp. 87–120). Newbury Park, CA: Sage.

Fehr, B., & Russell, J. A. (1991). Concept of love viewed from a prototype perspective. *Journal of Personality and Social Psychology, 60,* 425–438.

Freud, S. (1952). Group psychology and the analysis of the ego. In *The major works of Sigmund Freud* (pp. 664–696). Chicago: Encyclopedia Britannica. (Original work published 1921)

Hartigan, J. (1975). *Clustering algorithms.* New York: Wiley.

Hatfield, E. (1988). Passionate and companionate love. In R. J. Sternberg & M. L. Barnes (Eds.), *The psychology of love* (pp. 191–217). New Haven, CT: Yale University Press.

Hatfield, E., & Sprecher, S. (1986). Measuring passionate love in intimate relations. *Journal of Adolescence, 9,* 383–410.

Hazan, C., & Shaver, P. (1987). Romantic love conceptualized as an attachment process. *Journal of Personality and Social Psychology, 52,* 511–524.

Hendrick, C., & Hendrick, S. (1986). A theory and method of love. *Journal of Personality and Social Psychology, 50,* 392–402.

Holzinger, K. J. (1938). Relationships between three multiple orthogonal factors and four bifactors. *Journal of Educational Psychology, 29,* 513–519.

Horn, J. L. (1968). Organization of abilities and the development of intelligence. *Psychological Review, 75,* 242–259.

Kelley, H. H. (1983). Love and commitment. In H. H. Kelley, E. Berscheid, A. Christensen, J. H. Harvey, T. L. Huston, G. Levinger, E. McClintock, L. A. Peplau, & D. R. Peterson, *Close relationships* (pp. 265–314). New York: Freeman.

Lee, J. A. (1973). *Colours of love.* Toronto: New Press.

Lee, J. A. (1977). A typology of styles of loving. *Personality and Social Psychology Bulletin, 3,* 173–182.

Lee, J. A. (1988). Love-styles. In R. J. Sternberg & M. L. Barnes (Eds.), *The psychology of love* (pp. 38–67). New Haven, CT: Yale University Press.

Maslow, A. H. (1970). *Motivation and personality.* Princeton, NJ: Van Nostrand.

Mathes, E. W. (1980). Nine colours or types of romantic love. *Psychological Reports, 47,* 371–376.

McAdams, D. P. (1989). *Intimacy: The need to be close.* New York: Doubleday.

Murstein, B. I. (1988). A taxonomy of love. In R. J. Sternberg & M. L. Barnes (Eds.), *The psychology of love* (pp. 13–37). New Haven, CT: Yale University Press.

Nygren, A. (1952). *Agape and Eros.* Chicago: University of Chicago Press.

Peele, S., & Brodsky, A. (1976). *Love and addiction.* New York: New American Library.

Plato. (1970). *The symposium* (S. Q. Groden, Trans.). Amherst: University of Massachusetts Press.

Reik, T. (1944). *A psychologist looks at love.* New York: Farrar & Rinehart.

Reik, T. (1949). *Of love and lust.* New York: Farrar, Straus.

Rosch, E. (1975). Cognitive representations of semantic categories. *Journal of Experimental Psychology: General, 104,* 192–233.

Rubin, Z. (1970). Measurement of romantic love. *Journal of Personality and Social Psychology, 16,* 265–273.

Rubin, Z. (1973). *Liking and loving: An invitation to social psychology.* New York: Holt, Rinehart & Winston.

Rubin, Z. (1988). Preface. In R. J. Sternberg & M. L. Barnes (Eds.), *The psychology of love* (pp. vii–xii). New Haven, CT: Yale University Press.

Shaver, P. R., & Hazan, C. (1993). Adult romantic attachment: Theory and evidence. In D. Perlman & W. H. Jones (Eds.), *Advances in personal relationships* (Vol. 4, pp. 29–70). London: Jessica Kingsley.

Shaver, P. R., Hazan, C., & Bradshaw, E. (1988). Love as an attachment process. In R. J. Sternberg & M. L. Barnes (Eds.), *The psychology of love* (pp. 68–99). New Haven, CT: Yale University Press.

Singer, I. (1984–1987). *The nature of love* (3 vols.). Chicago: University of Chicago Press.

Soble, A. (1990). *The structure of love.* New Haven, CT: Yale University Press.

Spearman, C. (1927). *The abilities of man.* New York: Macmillan.

Sperling, M. B. (1985). Discriminant measures for desperate love. *Journal of Personality Assessment, 49,* 324–328.

Sprecher, S., Aron, A., Hatfield, E., Cortese, A., Potapova, E., & Levitskaya, A. (1994). Love: American style, Russian style, and Japanese style. *Personal Relationships, 1,* 349–369.

Sternberg, R. J. (1985). Implicit theories of intelligence, creativity, and wisdom. *Journal of Personality and Social Psychology, 49,* 607–627.

Sternberg, R. J. (1986). A triangular theory of love. *Psychological Review, 93,* 119–135.

Sternberg, R. J. (1987). Liking versus loving: A comparative evaluation of theories. *Psychological Bulletin, 102,* 331–345.

Sternberg, R. J. (1988). *The triangle of love.* New York: Basic Books.

Sternberg, R. J. (1994). Love is a story. *The General Psychologist, 30*(1), 1–11.

Sternberg, R. J. (1995). Love as a story. *Journal of Social and Personal Relationships, 12*(4), 541–546.

Sternberg, R. J. (1996). Love stories. *Personal Relationships, 3,* 1359–1379.

Sternberg, R. J., & Barnes, M. L. (1985). Real and ideal others in romantic relationships: Is four a crowd? *Journal of Personality and Social Psychology, 49,* 1586–1608.

Sternberg, R. J., Conway, B. E., Ketron, J. L., & Bernstein, M. (1981). People's conceptions of intelligence. *Journal of Personality and Social Psychology, 41,* 37–55.

Sternberg, R. J., & Grajek, S. (1984). The nature of love. *Journal of Personality and Social Psychology, 55,* 345–356.

Sternberg, R. J., & Powell, J. S. (1982). Theories of intelligence. In R. J. Sternberg (Ed.), *Handbook of human intelligence* (pp. 975–1005). New York: Cambridge University Press.

Sullivan, B. O. (1985). *Passionate love: A factor analytic study.* Unpublished manuscript, University of Hawaii, Manoa.

Swensen, C. H. (1961). Love: A self-report with college students. *Journal of Individual Psychology, 17,* 167–171.

Swensen, C. H. (1972). The behavior of love. In H. Otto (Ed.), *Love today: A new exploration* (pp. 86–101). New York: Association Press.

Swensen, C. H., & Gilner, F. (1964). Factor analysis of self-report statements of love relationships. *Journal of Individual Psychology, 20,* 186–188.

Tennov, D. (1979). *Love and limerance.* New York: Stein & Day.

Tesser, A., & Paulhus, D. L. (1976). Toward a causal model of love. *Journal of Personality and Social Psychology, 34,* 1095–1105.

Thomson, G. (1939). *The factorial analysis of human ability.* London: University of London Press.

Thurstone, L. L. (1938). *Primary mental abilities.* Chicago: University of Chicago Press.

Vernon, P. E. (1971). *The structure of human abilities.* London: Methuen.

Walster, E., & Walster, G. W. (1978). *A new look at love.* Reading, MA: Addison-Wesley.

CHAPTER 5

Philosophy of Life as a Model of Relationship Satisfaction

MAHZAD HOJJAT

The question "What factors determine partners' satisfaction in their intimate relationship?" has challenged both past (Terman, Buttenweiser, Ferguson, Johnson, & Wilson, 1938) and present (Gottman, 1994; Gottman & Krokoff, 1989) generations of marital relationship researchers. The importance of this question is certainly reflected in the fact that approximately two-thirds of newlyweds in the United States are likely to get a divorce (Martin & Bumpass, 1989). Marital dissatisfaction is considered one of the main determinants of marital instability (Terman & Wallin, 1949), and as such is thought to be influential in the gradual dissolution of the relationship. Divorce has been shown to have adverse effects upon the psychological, physical, and emotional well-being of the spouses (Bloom, Asher, & White, 1978; McKay, Rogers, Blades, & Gosse, 1984) and their children (Amato & Keith, 1991; Dawson, 1991). Although all dissatisfied partners do not separate, those who do have certainly experienced dissatisfaction with their relationships. What factors promote satisfaction in relationships? Why do some people who once made a decision to stay together for life eventually separate? Why do other relationships last for decades?

The aim of this chapter is to put forth a model of satisfaction in intimate relationships whose basic premise is based upon the degree of similarity between partners' philosophies of life. It is postulated that the satisfaction of partners in an intimate relationship is primarily related to the similarity in their basic beliefs and assumptions about the world around them, and also to the similarity of their beliefs about themselves relative to the world. These beliefs constitute what is called one's "philosophy of life" (hereafter abbreviated as POL). Just as individuals may behave as naive scientists in their attempt to find causality for their own and other people's behavior, they also may think as naive philosophers and, overtime, create their own (POLs) based on personal, social, and cultural influences. Although a person's POL is constantly revised on the basis of everyday experiences, because it is shaped by early socialization throughout the years, some of its basic premises are resistant to change. Part of one's POL is the way one thinks about intimate relationships in general. Included in this philosophy are beliefs that the individual assumes to be true in regard to intimate relationships (e.g., "Men are more romantic"), qualities that the individual considers to be desirable or ideal in a relationship (e.g., "An ideal husband is someone who is caring"), and the individual's own behavioral preferences in regard to relationships (e.g., "It is better not to marry before the age of 25"). The perceptions of individuals concerning relationships, in turn, give rise to the way they view different aspects of their own relationships—in particular, their perceptions of the similarities and differences between themselves and their partners, and their attribution of these similarities and differences. It is proposed that the degree to which two partners are compatible in their POLs also shapes the degree to which they are likely to experience satisfaction in their relationship with each other (see Figure 5.1).

The chapter begins with an outline of the POL construct, in terms of both its theoretical background and its conceptualization in the present model. Next, POL is discussed as it relates to satisfaction in relationships and as a part of the proposed model. Different components of the model and their interrelations are then described and discussed in the context of the relevant research. The final section of the chapter considers the unique characteristics of the present model and its possible contributions to the present body of satisfaction literature.

WHAT IS A PHILOSOPHY OF LIFE?

Differing Constructs for Philosophy of Life

A person's value system or value orientation has been a "major focus of psychological research" as a construct (Zavalloni, 1980, p. 114), and

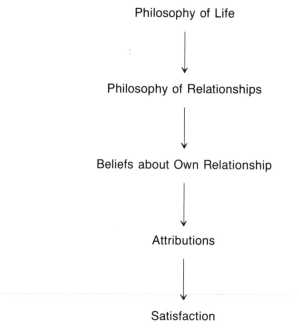

FIGURE 5.1. Model of the process by which philosophy of life (POL) shapes relationship satisfaction.

has been described as "occupying a position of central importance in social psychology" (Epstein, 1989, p. 3). Numerous theorists have identified and theorized about a system of beliefs or values that is essential to the interaction of individuals with their environment. Kelly (1955) referred to this system as "personal constructs," Kluckhohn and Strodtbeck (1961) as "value orientations," Rokeach (1973) as a "value system," Parkes (1975) as a "world model," Janoff-Bulman (1991) as "assumptive worlds," Ibrahim (1985) as a "philosophy of life," Sue (1978) and Ibrahim and Kahn (1987) as a "world view," and Epstein (1977, 1990) as "personal theories of reality" or "cognitive–experiential self-theory." As Janoff-Bulman (1991) points out:

> Whether termed "assumptive world," "world model," "structure of meaning," or "theory of reality," there is a congruence in the meaning of these phrases. In all cases the reference is to a basic conceptual system, developed over time, that provides us with expectations about ourselves and the world so that we might function effectively. This conceptual system is best represented by a set of assumptions, or theories, that generally prove viable in interactions with the world. (p. 101)

Anthropologists have long recognized the existence of a central core of meaning or a set of basic values that is common among individuals of all cultures, although cultures may vary among themselves in their patterns of response to each set. "There is a philosophy behind the way of life of each individual and of every relatively homogeneous group at any given point in their histories. Each personality gives to the philosophy an idiosyncratic coloring" (Kluckhohn, 1951, pp. 409–410). The construct presented in this chapter (POL) is influenced by Kluckhohn and Strodtbeck's (1961) conceptualization of a similar construct called "value orientations."

In an extensive review of the different world view models, Koltko-Rivera (1995) has described Florence Kluckhohn's approach as "the most articulated of any of the theories" (p. 39) and as one that "has had much influence on contemporary thought and research in this area" (p. 31). The framework offered by Kluckhohn and Strodtbeck (1961, 1973) considers "both philosophical and psychological dimensions" of individuals' basic beliefs (Ibrahim & Kahn, 1987, p. 164). It is assumed that individuals are endlessly seeking to unfold and evolve their views of the world around them. According to Kluckhohn and Strodtbeck (1961, 1973), the underlying principles of fundamental values "arise out of, or are limited by, the givens of biological human nature and the universalities of social interaction. The specific formulation is ordinarily a cultural product" (1961, p. 2).

The assumptions underlying this conceptualization are that there are circumscribed problems common to all humans for which people must find solutions. Although there is variability in the choice of problems and solutions, both are limited within a range. The key assumption is that all solutions are present in all individuals (or societies), but that they are preferred by people differentially.

Kluckhohn's Five Dimensions of Variation in Value Orientations

Kluckhohn and Strodtbeck (1961, 1973) have postulated five possible dimensions of variation in value orientations in response to common problems: human nature, the human–nature relationship, time, activity, and personal relationships. According to this classification, individuals may vary in their orientation toward human nature. Individuals may consider human nature either entirely evil, a combination of good and evil, or entirely good. In regard to their relationship to nature (and supernature), individuals may seek either to master it, to coexist with it in harmony, or to be in its control. The temporal focus of life for individuals may be in either the past, present, or future. Individuals may value an activity orientation that focuses either only on being (providing spontaneous self-expression), on being-in-becoming (developing an integrated inner self), or on doing (achieving external rewards). Finally, the relational orientation of individuals to other persons may be either lineal (hierarchical), collateral (collectivist), or individualistic.

Incorporated in the present model are Kluckhohn's basic assumptions about the impact of personal, social, and cultural factors on the formation of basic values, and about the universality of the dimensions across which values of individuals and societies may vary. Although the focus of Kluckhohn and Strodtbeck's model is very broad, I believe its underlying principles are quite useful for the construction of a specific model of satisfaction in close relationships. How individuals see the world and their place in it determines also how they see, think about, and respond to their intimate relationships. As Sue and Sue (1990) have pointed out, people's views of the world not only are reflected in their attitudes, values, and opinions, but also may influence how they define specific events in the context of their relationships, and thus how they behave in these situations.

I believe that the similarities and differences of individuals in their POLs may determine how they relate to each other. I would like to propose that the five dimensions offered by Kluckhohn and Strodtbeck (1961, 1973) as sources of variety in people's values across cultures may also be conceived, although on a smaller scale, as sources of variety among individuals and thus within couples. In the following sections, I first present a general outline and definition of the POL construct, and then discuss its usefulness for gaining a better understanding of the satisfaction process in close relationships.

PHILOSOPHY OF LIFE AS A CONSTRUCT IN THE PRESENT MODEL

The Construct and Three Fundamental Questions

POL may be defined as the collection of beliefs and assumptions that an individual holds about the world (i.e., nature, society, other people, etc.) and his or her place in it. Although the basic premises of POL are drawn from Kluckhohn's concept of value orientations, the construct is conceptualized somewhat differently in this chapter. The POL construct, as defined here, consists of three processes: "existential," "evaluative," and "directive." As such, individuals' views of any particular phenomenon are dependent on the ways they answer three fundamental questions: What is? What ought to be? And what must be done?

The first question pertains to the existential element of one's philosophy—that is, one's belief about the nature of the phenomenon, and essentially how one sees things as they stand. Statements such as "The world is not fair" or "Bad things always happen to good people" may be considered good examples of this category. The second question is related to the evaluative aspect of one's philosophy. It is concerned with moralistic issues, or how one believes things ought to be. Good examples are the statements "People should not be judged according to the color of their skin" or "The world should be fair." Finally, the third question is concerned with the directive aspect of the construct, which is the element that guides one's behavior. Statements such as "One must always help those who are less fortunate" or "It is foolish to try to make the world fair" reflect the directive element. For instance, some individuals' philosophy about justice in the world may be that past history has shown that justice is possible in the world (focus on past time). Individuals are by nature good (focus on human nature), and there should be justice for everyone, not just for a small group (collateral focus). It is important to work very hard to achieve justice (focus on doing), because only we determine our own destiny (focus on mastery over nature). Thus, one's philosophy in regard to any particular topic may be a function of the dimensions one selects to answer these three fundamental questions.

The Construct and Kluckhohn's Five Basic Dimensions

It is important to discuss in more detail the significance of the five basic dimensions that have been adopted from Kluckhohn's theory. As mentioned earlier, these dimensions arise out of the commonality of the problems humans face in their interaction with their environment and with each other. The conceptualization of humans as sharing a common set of problems and possible answers, and yet as different in their selection of responses, appears quite similar to the picture of humans drawn by psychologists. As McGuire (1980) points out, "the two great discoveries of psychology are: first, that basically everybody is the same; and second, that everybody is fundamentally different" (p. 180). Thus, the disciplines of philosophy and psychology concur in their portrayal of humans as essentially similar and as different. In the same vein, the five possible dimensions that are postulated as major sources of variation in one's POL reflect both philosophical and psychological elements of one's basic beliefs.

The question of whether human nature is good, evil, or a mixture of both is one that has preoccupied generation of philosophers. Although inquiry into this question has historically fallen into the philosophical domain, the implication associated with the choice of response is very much a psychological one. Sue and Sue (1990) discuss the differences in beliefs about human nature among diverse ethnic groups in the United States, and the implications of these differences for counseling. For instance, many minority groups, including Asian Americans, consider human nature as inherently good. The ancient philosophies of the East (Buddhism and Confucianism) emphasize "the original goodness of human nature" (Yum, 1988). Some European Americans, however, believe human nature to be neutral and basically a product of the environment, while others may believe in the genetic inferiority of some races or of particular individuals (Sue & Sue, 1990).

The question of the relationship between humans and nature or supernature is also an important one. Europeans and European Americans have historically sought mastery over nature, whereas members of many other cultures (e.g., Native Americans and Asians) believe it essential to live with nature in harmony (Benesch & Ponterotto, 1989; Kluckhohn & Strodtbeck, 1961). At an individual level, a belief in the supernatural (God, fate, etc.) has considerable implications for the way in which human beings view their world. A closely related concept is the "locus of control orientation" (Rotter, 1954), or the belief that the outcomes of one's behavior depend either on one's own behavior or on external factors that are beyond one's control. Those individuals with high internal locus of control may be more strongly motivated to achieve and earn external rewards, and may also possess superior coping strategies; they may therefore be less likely to become depressed (Rotter, 1975).

The concept of time in U.S. culture is hardly negligible. Differences in people's perception of its importance may not only be readily demonstrated across cultures and ethnicities, but also across urban versus rural settings. Sue and Sue (1990) compare the temporal focus of a future-oriented culture (dominant U.S. culture) with that of a past-oriented culture (Asian culture). U.S. culture is often characterized as preoccupied with the future, as reflected in the emphasis placed on the "American dream" and on achievement. Asian cultures, on the other hand, have a stronger belief in the traditions of the past (Marsella, 1993). "Historically, Asian societies have valued the past as reflected in ancestor worship and the equating of age with wisdom and respectability. Contrast this with U.S. culture in which youth is valued over the elderly, and the belief that once one hits the retirement years, one's usefulness in life is over" (Sue & Sue, 1990, p. 127). According to Zimbardo (1980), time perspective is "the single most important determinant of human behavior" (p. 204), and the one upon which all mechanisms of the social control of behavior rely.

The two dimensions of activity and personal relationships may be parallel to the concepts of "work and love" as conceptualized by Freud. A focus on "doing" emphasizes gaining external reward and achievement, which is valued highly by Western cultures (Benesch & Ponterotto, 1989; Yum, 1988). On the other hand, stress may be placed in Native American cultures on the spiritual state of "being," or, as Sue and Sue (1990) point out, on the concept of "noninterference" as manifested in the philosophy of living in harmony with nature. The "being-in-becoming" dimension may stress developing one's inner strength and a personal sense of achievement. In Asian cultures, although the focus on doing may be dominant, the sense of achievement becomes especially meaningful at the group or collective level (Marsella, 1993; Yum, 1988). Several studies have suggested that cultures may vary in their portrayal of the individual in relation to others (Markus & Kitayama, 1991).

Eastern cultures seem to view individuals as interconnected with their environment (collectivist), whereas Western cultures view individuals as more independent and separated from others (individualistic). On the other hand, societies such as Japan or England have been characterized as lineal systems in which hierarchies of power have traditionally belonged to certain classes or families (Marsella, 1993; Hong, 1989). At an interpersonal level, individuals with a lineal relation perspective may be those who are inclined to view others from a hierarchical perspective and thus to treat certain groups as inferior to themselves.

Formation and Change of Philosophy of Life

How is one's POL formulated and changed? The idea of the human as a philosopher is hardly a new one. Kelly's (1955) theory of personal constructs portrays individuals as scientists who formulate and test their own hypotheses in their everyday life. The present model presents humans as philosophers who eventually formulate their own POL based on their personal history and everyday experiences. According to Catlin and Epstein (1992), two kinds of events may have enduring effects on individuals' fundamental beliefs about themselves and the world: everyday life experiences and highly significant life events. Early socialization, especially the interaction of children with their caretakers, gives individuals the earliest sense of what their basic beliefs and values are supposed to be. As many theorists have stated (Bowlby, 1969), the early interactions of individuals with their caretakers shape the patterns of their entire adult life. As individuals mature, their own direct everyday social interactions influence the way they look at the world. Although many of these daily experiences may be of little significance by themselves, together they exert a significant cumulative effect on the individual (and thus on culture and society). Catlin and Epstein (1992) found that reporting of positive interactions with parents as a child was significantly related to positive basic beliefs. A sample report of a positive parental relationship was "When I was a child my mother (father) encouraged me to make my own decisions," and an example of a positive world belief was "By and large, I feel that my personal world is a reasonably safe and secure place" (Catlin & Epstein, 1992, p. 195).

Significant life events and transitions, such as forming a meaningful love relationship, losing someone or something one cares about deeply, or being involved in a serious accident, are also likely to have an impact on one's fundamental beliefs. Posttraumatic stress disorder (PTSD) may be related to the invalidation of one's basic beliefs about the world and the self (Epstein, 1991). The basic beliefs of a group of Vietnam veterans who suffered from PTSD showed more negativity and a greater degree of negative change (compared to control noncombat veterans and nonsymptomatic combat veterans) after their experience in the war than before. Moreover, whereas the other two groups regained their positivity of beliefs a few months after being discharged, the PTSD group continued to show a decline in the favorability of their basic beliefs 15 years after the time of their service. Catlin and Epstein (1992) found that significant life events had "orderly and enduring effects on fundamental attitudes about the self and the world" (p. 204).

Three Important Characteristics of Philosophy of Life

Epstein (1989) contends that the strong and enduring impact of major life events on basic beliefs can be attributed to their significant affective content. As such, Epstein postulates that individuals' theories about self and the world are implicit or subconscious theories, and that individuals will not be able to explain these if they are asked to. This is a main point of difference between the model that I am proposing and Epstein's cognitive–experiential self-theory. Although certain elements of the POL may be unconscious (in particular, those beliefs related to traumatic experiences during childhood), much of the POL is conscious, and people become more aware of their views as they mature and as life circumstances force them to make decisions and select choices.

Delineation of people's basic values on an implicit–explicit continuum is one of the three important characteristics that the present construct and Kluckhohn's conceptualization share. Another characteristic is the portrayal of the processes within the construct as dynamic and as a "system which is constantly in movement through time" (Kluckhohn & Strodtbeck, 1961, p. 7). Individuals continually reshape and modify their POLs as they go through their daily experiences. Because the social world around them is constantly changing, their beliefs and perceptions of this world must change too. For instance, as individuals age, people's behavior toward them may also change. There-fore, it is very likely that the part of Steve's POL pertaining to old age will be different at age 75 from what it is at age 30. Although Steve may not make a decision to change his beliefs about old age or being old, almost certainly he will have to adjust and redefine his POL.

Not only does the content of one's POL constantly change, but the importance that one places on different elements of one's POL also changes through time. For instance, Mary always loved children, but the importance of having children of her own did not become salient to her until she realized that she would not be able to have children with her present husband. Thus, even though the desire to have chil-dren was a part of Mary's POL all along, its importance increased sig-nificantly as the topic became salient to her, in this particular period in her life. Hence, I would like to propose that one's POL is not static, but in a constant process of change and becoming, just as individuals are.

A third important characteristic that the POL model shares with Kluckhohn's conceptualization is that there is a hierarchy in the im-portance that individuals assign to each belief or to each subphilosophy. It is inevitable that some beliefs should be more important to individu-als as a result of their link to the individuals' past experiences, especial-ly if there were some emotional consequences involved. Or perhaps some beliefs become more important as a particular situation arises, or as their significance becomes more salient to an individual at any given time. It is possible that these more important beliefs are more resistant to change as well. According to Epstein (1989), "the greater the number and intensity of the experiences on which [beliefs] are based and the more [beliefs] are interrelated with other beliefs, the more the beliefs are resistant to modification" (p. 7). For instance, beliefs based on a failed marriage that lasted many years are much more resistant to change than those based on a failed relationship that lasted only a few weeks.

In sum, in order to interact effectively with their environment, in-dividuals conceptualize their own philosophies about the world around them and their place in it (i.e., POLs). Their philosophy in regard to any particular concept depends on how three basic questions related to this concept are answered by individuals: What is? What ought to be? And what must be done? On the basis of Kluckhohn's conjecture that individuals' "value orientations" vary across five possible dimen-sions, it is assumed that variations in individuals' POL may also follow the same pattern. Ultimately, what distinguishes one person's POL from another's is the choice of dimension preferred in response to the three basic questions.

The POL construct proposed in this chapter may be distinguished from similar constructs that emphasize the unconscious components of one's basic beliefs. In addition, although early socialization influences the formation of many aspects of one's POL, its internal processes are characterized as dynamic, constantly changing through time. Therefore, the present construct may be distinguished from similar constructs that portray one's basic values as entirely the products of one's personality or traits.

PHILOSOPHY OF LIFE
AND RELATIONSHIP SATISFACTION

The present model submits that the similarity between partners' POLs is the most important determinant of the partners' satisfaction with their relationship. In other words, a greater degree of difference between partners in their POLs translates into lower satisfaction in their relationship. More specifically, individuals who have vastly different POLs will most likely differ greatly from each other in their philosophies of relationships, in their perceptions of their own relationship, and in the attributions they make about aspects of their relationship. Moreover, if the pattern of communication between partners is deficient, they will not be able to come to terms with their differences. The outcome will be lower satisfaction for partners. An example may demonstrate different interrelationships within the present model.

For instance, if one partner's existential belief about financial security is "Financial security for the future is very important" (focus on the future), while the other partner's is "Although financial security for the future is important, we should worry more about now and worry about tomorrow later" (focus on the present), it is likely that they will also differ in their evaluations of how important and desirable it is for their own family to have financial security. In this scenario, it is possible that the first partner may act according to her belief and plan for the future by saving every penny in order to buy a house for the family, whereas the second partner, who is more present-oriented, may prefer to spend the money on a vacation rather than save it for the future. In the absence of adequate communication between the partners about these differences, faulty attributions may result. In this situation, the first partner may view her partner as selfish and as unconcerned about the well-being of their family. The second partner may view his partner as cheap and as overly anxious about the future. Of course, the difference in time orientation may demonstrate itself in other areas of the relationship as well. Depending on the intensity of the differences between the two partners and the salience of these differences, the incompatibility may intensify and turn into a serious conflict. Eventually one or both partners may come to perceive their present relationship as very different from their ideal relationship; if so, the partners' satisfaction with their relationship will inevitably suffer.

Incompatible Philosophies of Life

At what point may differences in partners' POLs begin to cause conflict? First, it is possible for two people to live together for many years before discovering that they have significantly different points of view about life. There are many reasons for this. One possibility is that when partners began their relationship, their POLs were congruent with each other, but as they grew older, their POLs changed in different directions. This may be more typical in cases in which partners marry at an early age (e.g., high school sweethearts marrying in their early 20s), when their POLs still do not contain their adult experiences—that is, the POLs are not completely formed, or the partners are not mature enough to be knowledgeable about them. Second, sometimes significant events in one individual's life may change his or her POL drastically, while the partner is not as much affected; or both partners are affected, but they change in different directions. This may occur in situations in which partners lose a child, or even when one partner experiences a midlife crisis, or growing older changes his or her outlook on life. Third, sometimes partners have different POLs to begin with, yet their initial attraction prevents them from realizing the degree to which they are different. Then, when a situation arises in which a particular conflict becomes salient in their relationship, their differences come to the fore.

For instance, a husband and wife from different religious backgrounds may not consider the difference important until the time comes to select a religion for their child. Then, if it is important for each partner to raise the child in that partner's own religion, a conflict will ensue that can result in lower satisfaction for both partners. Thus, the contribution of any one belief within one's POL (P) to satisfaction depends on the importance of the particular belief to the individual (I) (e.g., raising a Jewish child) and the salience of the belief at the given moment (S) (e.g., having a child). As such, the present model takes into account both personal and situational variables in determining the potential impact of partners' POLs on their relationship satisfaction.

$$P = f(I, S)$$

Measurement of Philosophy of Life

The next important point pertains to the actual differences that may be considered significant in their impact on a couple's level of satisfaction. In other words, how may one measure the POL construct in the context of relationships? The present model considers an individual's philosophy on any given topic as the combination of his or her beliefs on its existential, evaluative, and directive aspects. It will be essential to measure individuals' philosophies on major issues important to couples (e.g., money, in-laws, sex, etc.), and then investigate the difference between partners on their overall POL scores. Partners may differ from each other at several levels. They may be different in the degree to which they adhere to, say, the importance of finances, even though they both may focus on the present in their view of the topic. Or the difference may be in the evaluative aspect of the topic, but not the other two aspects. A more substantial difference may be having a different focus on the topic altogether—for instance, a focus on the future as opposed to the present. Finally, the aggregate total difference may depend on the number of general topics on which the partners vary greatly, and the degree of difference within each topic. Of course, before the differences may be considered, the importance and salience of each topic to each individual should be taken into account.

RESEARCH ON PHILOSOPHY OF LIFE

Researchers of marital conflict have made major contributions to the field by pinpointing how distressed couples may be distinguished from nondistressed ones. One of the important findings in this line of research includes the identification of four dysfunctional interaction patterns related to the deterioration of a relationship: criticism/complaining, contempt, defensiveness (including whining), and stonewalling (withdrawal from interaction) (Gottman, 1994; Gottman & Krokoff, 1989). Gottman (1994) proposes the following as the path to marital dissolution: "Complaining and criticizing leads [sic] to contempt, which leads to defensiveness, which leads to listener withdrawal from interaction (stonewalling)" (p. 110). However, as some researchers have already pointed out (McAllister, 1992), most of the literature on marital interaction and satisfaction seems to have focused on the symptoms of dissatisfaction rather than on its causes. In particular, Levenson, Carstensen, and Gottman (1993) state that the vast majority of this line of research has been and still is concerned with distressed couples and the ways in which their patterns of interaction differ from those of nondistressed couples. The present model attempts to explore why and how relationship conflicts develop in the first place. It is assumed that incompatible cognitions are at the root of distressed relationships:

Simply stated, an individual does not respond to the environment per se; but rather, the individual responds to his or her perceptions and interpretations of the environment. . . . Accordingly, it is not surprising that as researchers in the marital area have become more interested in cognition they have borrowed extensively from the social psychology literature. Indeed, this is a partnership that remains potentially fruitful for the future. (Arias & Beach, 1987, p. 109)

Although research on the role of cognitions in intimate relationships is gaining increasing support, there seems to be a lack of focus and direction in the few studies that have looked at the topic. In particular, Baucom, Epstein, Sayers, and Sher (1989) point to a "dearth of models of marital functioning that incorporate cognitions in a detailed manner" (p. 31). According to Arias and Beach (1987), the application of important topics within the social-cognitive literature to marital satisfaction research has received little attention. So far, research on cognitive factors in marital research has largely focused on the role of causal attribution and unrealistic beliefs about one's relationship, both of which are also a part of the present model and are discussed below. The study of similarity of values and its impact on satisfaction has received even less attention.

Research on Similarity

Research on similarity has been mostly concerned with either similarity of partners in general (e.g., in terms of their socioeconomic background) or their consensus on isolated issues (e.g., political beliefs). Few studies, if any, have dealt with the topic of similarity from a theoretical point of view. Yet similarity was one of the earliest topics of interest in regard to satisfaction in relationships (Gottman, 1994; Kenny & Acitelli, 1994). Many studies have shown that partners who are similar to each other (in terms of important topics in their relationship) have happier relationships than do those who are dissimilar to each other (Allen & Thompson, 1984; Bentler & Newcomb, 1978; Corsini, 1956; Fitzpatrick & Best, 1979; Katz, Glucksberg, & Krauss, 1960; White & Hatcher, 1984). The importance of similarity appears to extend to all phases of a relationship, from early attraction (Berscheid & Walster, 1978) to the later stages, where partners may construct their own new reality (Berger & Kellner, 1964) or, as called here, a shared POL. The areas of similarity have been as diverse as political attitudes (Byrne & Blaylock, 1963), privacy preferences (Craddock, 1994), moral standards and sex (McAllister, 1992), and even food preferences (Ferreira & Winter, 1974).

Similarity of Values or Philosophies of Life

Although I am not aware of any other research to date that has applied the present construct to satisfaction in relationships, Ibrahim and Kahn (1987) developed a scale to assess the "world view" construct, based on the five dimensions of variation in the value orientations proposed by Kluckhohn and Strodtbeck (1961). According to their findings, the scale they developed showed adequate reliability and validity, and the construct proved useful in assessing individuals' world views both within and across cultures. Interestingly, in the context of intermarriages (i.e., marriages between partners from different cultural or ethnic backgrounds), McGoldrick and Preto (1984) considered the extent of partners' differences in their values to be important in their relationship satisfaction. Craddock (1991) found similar attitudes toward marital roles and religious orientation to be related to higher levels of marital satisfaction. He states that homogeneous couples "possess mutual values and role expectations that facilitate their goal setting and goal attainment strategies. In contrast, couples whose attitudes are dissimilar are more likely to struggle with conflicting goals and clashing expectations" (p. 11). It might be asked, however, whether the similarity or dissimilarity of beliefs is always perceived accurately by partners.

Perceptions of Similarity

Interestingly, what seems to have attracted a greater deal of interest among marital satisfaction researchers appears not to be similarity of partners per se, but the partners' perceptions of this similarity. Several investigators have reported that perceptions of similarity between partners are related to their satisfaction; that is, higher perceptions of similarity lead to higher satisfaction (Acitelli, Douvan, & Veroff, 1993; Kenny & Acitelli, 1994). This finding fits the present description of partners who begin their relationship without clear ideas about their points of similarity and difference, and who in fact may be temporarily satisfied with their relationship until specific situations reveal that their perceptions of similarity are incorrect. Therefore, in response to the argument that perhaps the perception of similarity is more consequential than the actual similarity in determining relationship satisfaction, it must be pointed out that perceptions are supposed to reflect the reality that they represent; as such, their accuracy is bound to be compared to reality. The early years of marriage have been found to be crucial to the formation of shared perceptions between partners (Acitelli et al., 1993). Although partners may begin their relationship with widely erroneous perceptions about the similarities of their POLs or values in

life, sooner or later their perceptions will have to be tested in the laboratory of life encounters, and the partners must come to terms with these
differences (i.e., must come to understand that they agree or disagree).
It is my contention that those with different POLs either separate, accept their differences in the form of compromise, or eventually change
their beliefs to resemble their partners' more closely.

In addition, as White (1985) points out, the relationship between
satisfaction and perceptions of similarity may be related to the general
principle of "perceptual congruity" (Heider, 1958; Newcomb, 1961). According to this principle, individuals prefer that people whom they like
agree with their perceptions. In the case of intimate relationships, individuals prefer to perceive their partners as agreeing with them. Yet,
as different situations arise during the course of a relationship in which
one partner's predictions of the other's beliefs turn out to be inaccurate,
"the perceived similarity would become inconsistent in these areas. Assuming that one continues to like one's partner in the face of inconsistency, one can either change one's own attitudes or try to change
the attitude of the spouse to bring about consistency (agreement). Regardless of the strategy, the outcome over time is to increase the accuracy
of both perceived similarity and understanding" (White, 1985, p. 47).

Parallel with Berger and Kellner's (1964) contention that partners'
differences in their perceptions will decrease over time as they build
their own reality together, the present model proposes the following:
In accordance with the delineation of the POL construct as dynamic
and constantly changing, and as a result of the constant interaction
between partners, partners in satisfied relationships, who start their union
with more congruent POLs, will eventually develop a joint POL together.
More congruent POLs may involve similarities in selection of the five
basic dimensions: orientations toward human nature, the human–nature relationship, time, activity, and personal relationships.

As preference for any of these dimensions may be rooted in the
partners' early socialization, a change from one dimension type to another
may prove difficult. However, it may be easier to alter the degree to
which a partner adheres to each dimension. In other words, partners
who begin their life together with preferences for similar types of dimensions (especially in regard to important issues in their relationship), but
who disagree in the degree to which they adhere to each dimension,
may have a high likelihood of reconciling their disparities and perhaps
creating a shared POL together. On the other hand, partners who start
their life together with widely different POLs as a result of disparity
in their choice of dimensions may find it difficult to change their POLs
sufficiently to create a shared one. Of course, effective communication
has a crucial role in the initiation and maintenance of this process.

It might suffice to say at this point that satisfied partners may be those who, through effective communication, have come to share many important values and beliefs about their similarities and differences, such that their perceptions of their relationship have become close to reality.

Individuals' Philosophies in Regard to Close Relationships

An important part of one's POL is the way one thinks about close relationships in general. The existential element of such beliefs denotes how individuals view different aspects of relationships—for instance, their attitudes about gender-related issues (equality of the sexes, etc.). As will be seen later, if these beliefs are irrational, they may have a destructive impact on the functioning of relationships (Eidelson & Epstein, 1982). The evaluative aspect of such a philosophy consists of notions that are related to the ideal kind of relationship as perceived by the individual. For instance, one might fantasize about marrying someone very intelligent, or believe that an ideal wife should have a good job or be highly educated. According to Sternberg and Barnes (1985), one person's feelings toward his or her partner may be mediated by notions about an ideal partner. Baucom et al. (1989) consider two important categories of cognitions as playing important roles in marital adjustment: "assumptions" and "standards." Although differently named, these two concepts are quite similar to the existential and evaluative dimensions as described above. Assumptions are defined as partners' assumptions about the nature of relationships, and standards "involve the characteristics that the individual believes a partner or relationship should have" (p. 32). Finally, the directive dimension of this philosophy is behavior-related and guides individuals' actions in specific situations. For instance, some people may believe that going out with a much older partner is not acceptable, or may add this notion to their POLs after unsuccessful related experiences.

The importance of relationship beliefs has particularly been outlined by gender researchers, who have shown that men and women may differ in their beliefs about love and relationships (Frazier & Esterly, 1990). Jones and Stanton (1988) found that certain relationship beliefs (e.g., thinking in romantic terms about one's relationship) are related to relationship satisfaction for both men and women. In a study by Fitzpatrick and Best (1979), partners who had similar definitions of their relationship were significantly more in agreement about important issues of their relationship and were more cohesive than were partners who did not have similar definitions. Buehlman, Gottman, and Katz (1992) specifically included the variable "philosophy of marriage" in their oral history interviews in order to predict the possibility of future divorce. Included in this procedure was a coding for "marital disappointment/disillusionment," a dimension that assessed the degree to which couples' expectations and ideals about marriage remained unfulfilled, and that proved to be "the most powerful single predictor of divorce" (p. 312).

> In the interview, people who score high in this dimension may say that they do not know what makes a marriage work because all they have seen or experienced are bad ones. Other couples may not be so blunt about their disappointment with marriage but instead will sound disappointed or sad about specific things in their marriage. Couples may mention that they had unrealistic expectations about what marriage would be like or they may give advice to the interviewer about marriage that subtly lets the interviewer know they regret or are displeased with their own. (Buehlman et al., 1992, p. 312)

As Buehlman et al. (1992) report, couples with high scores on this dimension, even when satisfaction at Time 1 was controlled for, were quite likely to have divorced or separated at Time 2 (3 years later).

The role of dysfunctional beliefs and expectations in interfering with the functioning of intimate relationships has received increasing recognition from marital researchers in recent years (Eidelson & Epstein, 1982). Unrealistic relationship beliefs are defined as "the dysfunctional or maladaptive expectations that a person has about close relationships" (Fincham & Bradbury, 1989, p. 71). Jones and Stanton (1988) found that dysfunctional relationship beliefs were more strongly associated with relationship distress than were more general irrational beliefs. In a study by Epstein and Eidelson (1981), measures of partners' specific relationship beliefs were related to measures of marital maladjustment, negative expectations regarding treatment outcome, and overall marital satisfaction. After interviewing marital therapists and reviewing the literature Eidelson and Epstein (1982, p. 715) identified five specific dysfunctional beliefs, including "Disagreement is destructive to relationships" and "Partners who really care should be able to know what their spouses' needs are without overt communication." Irrational beliefs may influence individuals' beliefs about their own relationship in several ways.

Individuals' Beliefs about Their Own Relationship

First, individuals may have incorporated some of their previous negative experiences into their philosophies of relationships. When these general maladaptive beliefs are applied to their specific relationship, the partners' appraisal of each other's behavior may be affected. For instance, a woman's previous negative experience may have included men who were preoccupied with sex. Therefore, her irrational general belief "Men are only interested in sex" may be translated into attributing the cause of her husband's behavior to sexual preoccupation, and thus creating a conflictive situation (Baucom et al., 1989, p. 32). In other words, these irrational beliefs are likely to have a negative impact on attributional processes in relationships (Fincham, 1985). A second way in which irrational beliefs may be problematic is that they may create unrealistic expectations and thus lead to subsequent disappointment. For instance, believing that one's partner should know automatically what one's needs are may result in disappointment once this expectation is unfulfilled, and thus may lead to dissatisfaction with one's relationship. As rational–emotive researchers have stated (Ellis, 1962), the difficulty with irrational beliefs is that they set such high standards and expectations that no real relationship is able to match them (Baucom et al., 1989). Therefore, in a way, by holding such dysfunctional beliefs and expectations, individuals set themselves up for disappointment. According to Fincham and Bradbury (1989), maladaptive expectations influence attributional processes in relationships such that "partner behavior is likely to violate repeatedly unrealistic relationship expectations and thus instigate a causal search to explain the behavior when it occurs" (p. 71). Some of the findings of the attribution theorists indicate, in line with this discussion, that distressed couples may have more unrealistic views of their relationships than nondistressed partners have (Fincham, Fernandes, & Humphreys, 1993), and that higher levels of irrational relationship beliefs predict causal attributions (Fincham & Bradbury, 1989).

Attributions

Studies on attributions in relationships constitute one of the most important lines of research connecting cognitive factors to satisfaction in relationships. The significance of this research may lie partly in its promise of accounting for behavior patterns that distinguish distressed from nondistressed couples (Bradbury & Fincham, 1990). One of the significant findings of attribution studies is that distressed partners are more likely to attribute each other's negative behavior to enduring personality variables, but to attribute each other's positive behavior to situational and temporary variables. On the other hand, research has demonstrated that for partners who are satisfied with their relationship, the opposite pattern appears to be true. In other words, a satisfied partner believes that the other partner's negative behavior (e.g., losing her temper) has a situational explanation ("She is tired" rather than "She has a temper"), whereas the other partner's positive behavior (e.g., giv-ing a hug) has a dispositional cause ("She is warm and caring" rather than "She wants something from me") (Arias & Beach, 1987; Fincham & Bradbury, 1989). In this way, negativity in distressed relationships and positivity in nondistressed relationships are perpetuated.

Several investigators have pointed to the strong causal link between attributional processes and relationship satisfaction (Arias & Beach, 1987; Bradbury & Fincham, 1987, 1990; Fincham & Bradbury, 1993; Karney, Bradbury, Fincham, & Sullivan, 1994; Senchak & Leonard, 1993; Thompson & Snyder, 1986). These findings are consistent with the contention of the present model that attributions are linked directly with satisfaction. However, the literature on attribution has yet to in-vestigate in detail how attributions themselves are originated. Hence the present model may prove useful in both extending the existing research on satisfaction and presenting it within a deeper theoretical level. A closely related issue is the role of communication between part-ners. It is likely that communication patterns may mediate the causal link between relationship attribution and satisfaction. Unfortunately, the investigation of this relationship is beyond the scope of this chap-ter. Future exploration of this topic will certainly enrich the existing body of research on satisfaction.

CONCLUSION

According to the model presented in this chapter, the satisfaction of partners in a close relationship is primarily dependent on the similarity of their basic values and assumptions. As a result of their interaction with the world, and in order to understand their position relative to it, individuals may behave as naive philosophers and develop their own POLs. POL may be defined as the collection of beliefs and assumptions that an individual holds about the world (i.e., nature, society, other people, etc.) and about his or her own place in the world.

Similarity literature dating back to the 1960s has mostly been con-cerned with the role of similarity in attraction rather than satisfaction. No theoretical model has presented an integrated and detailed account of satisfaction based on similarity. Research on similarity and satisfac-tion has been sporadic at best, measuring many diverse points of similarity rather than an underlying construct. Moreover, most of this research has been cross-sectional, and therefore little attention has been paid to the gradual formation or division of similarity and its impact on satis-faction. The present model attempts to offer an account of possible ways in which partners may become more or less similar throughout their relationship, and thus of how each situation may influence their level of satisfaction across different stages of their relationship, not just at any one point in time. In addition, much of the research conducted on this topic considers only the role of internal (e.g., personality) or external (e.g., income) variables in satisfaction. The present model proposes that both internal (i.e., cognitions or philosophies) and external (i.e., salience of the conflict) factors are important determinants of satisfaction and should be taken into account. Another important characteristic of the present model is its portrayal of relationship satisfaction as a dynamic and constantly evolving process, rather than as a static factor limited by partners' personalities or unconscious drives. As such, partners are considered the active creators of a satisfied and fulfilling relationship.

Much of the literature on satisfaction has concentrated on distinguishing satisfied couples from dissatisfied ones on the basis of either their negative patterns of behavior, their attributions, their negative affect, or their faulty patterns of communication. These studies provide us with valuable information in terms of how relationship conflicts may be most effectively characterized and treated. The present model seeks to complement the existing models by offering a social-psychological perspective in an attempt to explain how and why dissatisfaction begins in the first place. It is hoped, however, that the hypotheses put forth in this model may be able to contribute not only to the understanding of relationship dissatisfaction, but also to its prevention. In particular, based on the present model, partners may be able to increase their chances of forming a future satisfied relationship by discussing their POLs early in their relationship. Consideration of similarity of goals and expectations early in the relationship may give the partners more realistic perceptions of the kind of relationship they may have, and therefore may enable them to gauge its success more accurately.

Along with these possible advantages of the proposed model, it is important to consider its shortcomings as well. One possible criticism of the model may be that it does not take into account the unique perspectives of the male and female partners. Yet many studies have shown that female partners' views of their intimate relationships may differ significantly from those of male partners. For instance, is it possible that female partners differ vastly from their male partners in their time orientation (see Chapter 1, this volume) within the context of their close relationships? Providing accurate answers to this and many other important questions may only be possible through empirical testing of the proposed model of satisfaction.

REFERENCES

Acitelli, L. K., Douvan, E., & Veroff, J. (1993). Perceptions of conflict in the first year of marriage: How important are similarity and understanding? *Journal of Social and Personal Relationships, 10,* 5–21.

Allen, A., & Thompson, T. (1984). Agreement, understanding, realization, and feelings understood as predictors of communicative satisfaction in marital dyads. *Journal of Marriage and the Family, 52,* 915–921.

Amato, P. R., & Keith, B. (1991). Consequences of parental divorce for the well-being of children: A meta-analysis. *Psychological Bulletin, 110,* 26–46.

Arias, I., & Beach, R. H. (1987). Assessment of social cognition in the context of marriage. In K. D. O'Leary (Ed.), *Assessment of marital discord: An integration for research and clinical practice* (pp. 109–139). Hillsdale, NJ: Erlbaum.

Baucom, D. H., Epstein, N., Sayers, S., & Sher, T. G. (1989). The role of cognition in marital relationships: Definitional, methodological, and conceptual issues. *Journal of Consulting and Clinical Psychology, 57,* 31–38.

Benesch, K. F., & Ponterotto, J. G. (1989). East and West: Transpersonal psychology and cross-cultural counseling. *Counseling and Values, 33,* 121–131.

Bentler, P. M., & Newcomb, M. D. (1978). Longitudinal study of marital success and failure. *Journal of Consulting and Clinical Psychology, 46,* 1053–1070.

Berger, P., & Kellner, H. (1964). Marriage and the construction of reality. *Diogenes, 46,* 1–24.

Berscheid, E., & Walster, E. (1978). *Interpersonal attraction* (2nd ed.). Reading, MA: Addison-Wesley.

Bloom, B. L., Asher, S. J., & White, S. W. (1978). Marital disruption as a stressor: A review and analysis. *Psychological Bulletin, 85,* 867–894.

Bowlby, J. (1969). *Attachment and loss: Vol. 1. Attachment.* New York: Basic Books.

Bradbury, T. N., & Fincham, F. D. (1987). Affect and cognition in close relationships: Towards an integrative model. *Cognition and Emotion, 1,* 59–87.

Bradbury, T. N., & Fincham, F. D. (1990). Attributions in marriage: Review and critique. *Psychological Bulletin, 107,* 3–33.

Buehlman, K. T., Gottman, J. M., & Katz, L. F. (1992). How a couple views their past predicts their future: Predicting divorce from an oral history interview. *Journal of Family Psychology, 5,* 295–318.

Byrne, D., & Blaylock, B. (1963). Similarity and assumed similarity of attitudes between husbands and wives. *Journal of Abnormal and Social Psychology, 6,* 636–640.

Catlin, G., & Epstein, S. (1992). Unforgettable experiences: The relation of life events to basic beliefs about self and world. *Social Cognition, 10,* 189–209.

Corsini, R. J. (1956). Understanding and similarity in marriage. *Journal of Abnormal and Social Psychology, 52,* 327–332.

Craddock, A. E. (1991). Relationships between attitudinal similarity, couple structure, and couple satisfaction, within married and de facto couples. *Australian Journal of Psychology, 43,* 11–16.

Craddock, A. E. (1994). Relationships between marital satisfaction and privacy preferences. *Journal of Comparative Family Studies, 25,* 371–382.

Dawson, D. A. (1991). Family structure and children's health and well-being: Data from the 1988 National Health Interview Study on Child Health. *Journal of Marriage and the Family, 53,* 573–584.

Eidelson, R. J., & Epstein, N. (1982). Cognition and relationship maladjustment: Development of a measure of dysfunctional relationship beliefs. *Journal of Consulting and Clinical Psychology, 50,* 715–720.

Ellis, A. (1962). *Reason and emotion in psychotherapy.* New York: Lyle Stuart.

Epstein, S. (1977). The ecological study of emotions in humans. In P. Pliner, K. R. Blankstein, & I. M. Spiegel (Eds.), *Advances in the study of communication and affect: Vol. 5. Perception of emotions in self and others* (pp. 47–83). New York: Plenum Press.

Epstein, S. (1989). Values from the perspective of cognitive–experiential self-theory. In N. Eisenberg, J. Reykowski, & E. Staub (Eds.), *Social and moral values: Individual and societal perspectives* (pp. 3–22). Hillsdale, NJ: Erlbaum.

Epstein, S. (1990). Cognitive–experiential self-theory. In L. A. Pervin (Ed.), *Handbook of personality: Theory and research* (pp. 165–192). New York: Guilford Press.

Epstein, S. (1991). The self-concept, the traumatic neurosis, and the structure of personality. In R. Hogan (Series Ed.), D. Ozer, J. Healy, & A. Stewart (Vol. Eds.), *Perspectives in personality: Vol. 3. A research annual, self and emotion* (pp. 63–98). London: Jessica Kingsley.

Epstein, N., & Eidelson, R. J. (1981). Unrealistic beliefs of clinical couples: Their relationship to expectations, goals, and satisfaction. *American Journal of Family Therapy, 9,* 13–22.

Ferreira, A. J., & Winter, W. D. (1974). On the nature of marital relationships: Measurable differences in spontaneous agreement. *Family Process, 13,* 355–370.

Fincham, F. D. (1985). Attributions in close relationships. In J. H. Harvey & G. Weary (Eds.), *Attributions: Basic issues and applications* (pp. 203–234). New York: Academic Press.

Fincham, F. D., & Bradbury, T. N. (1989). The impact of attributions in marriage: An individual difference analysis. *Journal of Social and Personal Relationships, 6,* 69–85.

Fincham, F. D., & Bradbury, T. N. (1993). Marital satisfaction, depression, and attributions: A longitudinal analysis. *Journal of Personality and Social Psychology, 64,* 442–452.

Fincham, F. D., Fernandes, L. O., & Humphreys, K. (1993). *Communicating in relationships: A guide for couples and professionals.* Champaign, IL: Research Press.

Fitzpatrick, M. A., & Best, P. (1979). Dyadic adjustment in relational types: Consensus, cohesion, affectional expression and satisfaction in enduring relationships. *Communication Monographs, 46,* 167–178.

Frazier, P. A., & Esterly, E. (1990). Correlates of relationship beliefs: Gender, relationship experience and relationship satisfaction. *Journal of Social and Personal Relationships, 7,* 331–352.

Gottman, J. M. (1994). *What predicts divorce?: The relationship between marital processes and marital outcomes.* Hillsdale, NJ: Erlbaum.

Gottman, J. M., & Krokoff, L. J. (1989). Marital interaction and satisfaction: A longitudinal view. *Journal of Consulting and Clinical Psychology, 57*, 47–52.

Heider, F. (1958). *The psychology of interpersonal relations.* New York: Wiley.

Hong, G. K. (1989). Application of cultural and environmental issues in family therapy with immigrant Chinese Americans. *Journal of Strategic and Systemic Therapies, 8*, 14–21.

Ibrahim, F. A. (1985). Effective cross-cultural counseling and psychotherapy: A framework. *The Counseling Psychologist, 13*, 625–638.

Ibrahim, F. A., & Kahn, H. (1987). Assessment of world views. *Psychological Reports, 60*, 163–176.

Janoff-Bulman, R. (1991). Understanding people in terms of their assumptive worlds. In R. Hogan (Series Ed.), D. J. Ozer, J. M. Healy, & A. J. Stewart (Vol. Eds.), *Perspectives in personality: Vol. 3. A research annual, self and emotion* (pp. 99–116). London: Jessica Kingsley.

Jones, M. E., & Stanton, A. L. (1988). Dysfunctional beliefs, belief similarity, and marital distress: A comparison of models. *Journal of Social and Clinical Psychology, 7*, 1–14.

Karney, B. R., Bradbury, T. N., Fincham, F. D., & Sullivan, K. T. (1994). The role of negative affectivity in the association between attributions and marital satisfaction. *Journal of Personality and Social Psychology, 66*, 413–424.

Katz, I., Glucksberg, S., & Krauss, R. (1960). Need satisfaction and Edwards PPS scores in married couples. *Journal of Consulting Psychology, 24*, 205–208.

Kelly, G. A. (1955). *The psychology of personal constructs.* New York: Norton.

Kenny, D. A., & Acitelli, L. K. (1994). Measuring similarity in couples. *Journal of Family Psychology, 8*, 417–431.

Kluckhohn, C. (1951). Values and value orientations in the theory of action. In T. Parsons & E. A. Shields (Eds.), *Toward a general theory of action* (pp. 388–433). Cambridge, MA: Harvard University Press.

Kluckhohn, F. R., & Strodtbeck, F. L. (1961). *Variations in value orientations.* Evanston, IL: Row, Peterson.

Kluckhohn, F. R., & Strodtbeck, F. L. (1973). *Variations in value orientations* (2nd ed.). Westport, CT: Greenwood Press.

Koltko-Rivera, M. E. (1995). *The psychology of world views.* Manuscript submitted for publication.

Levenson, R. W., Carstensen, L. L., & Gottman, J. M. (1993). Long-term marriage: Age, gender, and satisfaction. *Psychology and Aging, 8*, 301–313.

Markus, H. R., & Kitayama, S. (1991). Culture and the self: Implications for cognition, emotion, and motivation. *Psychological Review, 98*, 224–253.

Marsella, A. J. (1993). Counseling and psychotherapy with Japanese Americans: Cross-cultural considerations. *American Journal of Orthopsychiatry, 63*, 200–208.

Martin, T., & Bumpass, L. (1989). Recent trends in marital disruption. *Demography, 26*, 37–52.

McAllister, I. (1992). Marital satisfaction in Australia: A path model. *Australian Journal of Sex, Marriage and Family, 7*, 199–206.

McGoldrick, M., & Preto, N. (1984). Ethnic intermarriage: Implications for therapy. *Family Process, 23,* 347–364.

McGuire, W. (1980). W. McGuire. In R. I. Evans (Ed.), *The making of social psychology: Discussions with creative contributors* (pp. 171–187). New York: Gardner/Wiley.

McKay, M., Rogers, P. D., Blades, J., & Gosse, R. (1984). *The divorce book.* Oakland, CA: New Harbinger.

Newcomb, T. M. (1961). *The acquaintance process.* New York: Holt, Rinehart & Winston.

Parkes, C. M. (1975). What becomes of redundant world models? A contribution to the study of adaptation to change. *British Journal of Medical Psychology, 48,* 131–137.

Rokeach, M. (1973). *The nature of human values.* New York: Free Press.

Rotter, J. (1954). *Social learning and clinical psychology.* Englewood Cliffs, NJ: Prentice-Hall.

Rotter, J. (1975). Some problems and misconceptions related to the construct of internal versus external control of reinforcement. *Journal of Consulting and Clinical Psychology, 43,* 56–67.

Senchak, M., & Leonard, K. E. (1993). The role of spouses' depression and anger in the attribution–marital satisfaction relation. *Cognitive Therapy and Research, 17,* 397–408.

Sternberg, R. J., & Barnes, M. L. (1985). Real and ideal others in romantic relationships: Is four a crowd? *Journal of Personality and Social Psychology, 49,* 1586–1608.

Sue, D. W. (1978). World views and counseling. *Personnel and Guidance Journal, 56,* 458–462.

Sue, D. W., & Sue, D. (1990). *Counseling the culturally different: Theory and practice* (2nd ed.). New York: Wiley.

Terman, L. M., Buttenwieser, P., Ferguson, L. W., Johnson, W. B., & Wilson, D. P. (1938). *Psychological factors in marital happiness.* New York: McGraw-Hill.

Terman, L. M., & Wallin, P. (1949). The validity of marriage prediction and marital adjustment tests. *American Sociological Review, 14,* 497–504.

Thompson, J. S., & Snyder, D. K. (1986). Attribution theory in intimate relationships: A methodological review. *American Journal of Family Therapy, 14,* 123–138.

White, J. M. (1985). Perceived similarity and understanding in married couples. *Journal of Social and Personal Relationships, 2,* 45–57.

White, S. G., & Hatcher, C. (1984). Couple complementarity and similarity: A review of the literature. *American Journal of Family Therapy, 12,* 15–25.

Yum, J. O. (1988). The impact of Confucianism on interpersonal relationships and communication patterns in East Asia. *Communication Monographs, 55,* 374–388.

Zavalloni, M. (1980). Values. In H. C. Triandis & R. W. Brislin (Eds.), *Handbook of cross-cultural psychology: Vol. 5. Social psychology* (pp. 73–120). Boston: Allyn & Bacon.

Zimbardo, P. G. (1980). P. G. Zimbardo. In R. I. Evans (Ed.), *The making of social psychology: Discussions with creative contributors* (pp. 199–214). New York: Gardner/Wiley.

PART 2

*SATISFACTION
OVER THE COURSE
OF CLOSE RELATIONSHIPS*

CHAPTER 6

———•◆•———

A Temporal Model
of Relationship Satisfaction
and Stability

ELLEN BERSCHEID
JASON LOPES

Happy people tend to be those who are satisfied with their close personal relationships. Freedman (1978), for example, concluded: "There is no simple recipe for producing happiness, but all of the research indicates that for almost everyone, one necessary ingredient is some kind of satisfying, intimate relationship" (p. 48). If so, many people are destined to experience disappointment in their pursuit of happiness. Some demographers project that two out of three first marriages are likely to fail (e.g., Martin & Bumpass, 1989), and married individuals also seem to be less happy than they once were, at least when their happiness is contrasted with that of their never-married counterparts (e.g., Glenn & Weaver, 1988; Lee, Seccombe, & Shehan, 1991). But, illustrating what Samuel Johnson called "the triumph of hope over experience," most of the disenchanted and disillusioned will try again. And again. And in some cases, yet again. Clearly, many people could use some help.

The experts have been trying to help. But their quest to find the determinants of relationship satisfaction has not been as successful as they had hoped. After reviewing the quantitative research on marital quality conducted in the 1980s, Glenn (1990) concluded that this research "produced only a modest increment in understanding of the causes and consequences of marital success" (p. 818), with "success" viewed as satisfaction in an intact marriage. The determinants of relationship satisfaction are important in themselves, of course, but interest in their identification has been heightened by their presumed association with relationship stability. The popular answer to the question "Why do some relationships endure and others dissolve?" is this: "If people are satisfied with their relationship, they maintain it; if they become dissatisfied, they end it." This is a simple answer, but perhaps too simple; it is surprisingly difficult to find hard empirical evidence to support this seemingly obvious assumption, at least with respect to marital relationships (e.g., White, 1990).

In this chapter we examine the assumption that satisfaction with a relationship determines its stability. Neither we nor anyone else believes that this is always true (see Heaton & Albrecht, 1991, for a discussion of unhappy but stable marriages), but consideration of when it is true and when it is not illuminates many important relationship dynamics. We begin our discussion of the satisfaction–stability association by briefly describing the theoretical perspective from which it most often has been viewed—the social exchange perspective (see Karney & Bradbury, 1995, for a review of other theoretical perspectives).

SOCIAL EXCHANGE THEORIES

The fundamental assumption underlying the social exchange theories is that people's exchange of rewards and punishments is the essence of social interaction and constitutes the important underlying dynamic of all relationships. Most exchange theories predict that rewarding and satisfying interactions will be repeated and dissatisfying interactions will not; thus, they link relationship satisfaction with stability.

Unlike other exchange theories, however, Thibaut and Kelley's social interdependence theory (Thibaut & Kelley, 1959; Kelley & Thibaut, 1978) theoretically decouples satisfaction from stability. Interdependence theory recognizes that many relationships are "nonvoluntary," in that individuals sometimes feel compelled to maintain unsatisfying relationships, although they would prefer to end them. To account for involuntary relationships, Thibaut and Kelley introduced the concept of "comparison level," or "the standard against which the member [of the relationship] evaluates the 'attractiveness' of the relationship or how satisfactory it is" (1959, p. 21), and the concept of "comparison level for alternatives," or "the standard the member uses in deciding whether to remain in or to leave the relationship" (1959, p. 21). In distinguishing between these two standards, Thibaut and Kelley argue that although satisfaction and stability are often positively associated, they need not be. Each standard—one for satisfaction with the relationship, and the other for deciding to maintain or dissolve the relationship—is theorized to derive from two different sources. Comparison level, formed from the outcomes the individual has experienced or observed in similar relationships, is the level of outcomes the individual feels he or she deserves from the relationship. Comparison level for alternatives, on the other hand, derives from "the quality of the best of the member's available alternatives, that is, the reward–cost positions experienced or believed to exist in the most satisfactory of the other available relationships" (1959, p. 22).

Interdependence theory thus predicts that a person will sometimes dissolve a satisfying relationship simply because he or she believes that an alternative relationship will be even more satisfying. It also predicts that a person often remains in an unsatisfying relationship because the best alternative relationship is even more unattractive. If the theory is correct, some of the inferences we commonly make about relationships are false; it is not always true, for example, that a dissolved relationship must have been an unsatisfying relationship, or that a stable relationship is satisfying.

Interdependence theory predicts that an individual's behavior in a relationship is a function not simply of the goodness of outcomes associated with that individual's *own* behavioral options, but rather is determined by the configuration presented by the individual's and the partner's *joint* outcome matrix. Later revisions of interdependence theory (Kelley, 1979; Kelley & Thibaut, 1978) extended its relational theme by emphasizing that in choosing among behavioral options, not only does an individual take into consideration the goodness of outcomes that both the individual and the partner will receive if a particular behavioral option is exercised; the individual also often makes agreements with the partner about how both will exercise their behavioral options in the future. Such agreements override the influence that each individual's personal outcomes would otherwise exert on his or her behavioral choices. For example, an individual who voices the traditional marriage vow is promising the partner to maintain the relationship "until death do us part" even if the partner should become sick or poor. Such a vow represents the individual's personal commitment to continuing the relationship even if circumstances should arise where abandoning the relationship might prove more rewarding to the individual.

The concept of "commitment," usually viewed as an individual's subjectively felt intention to continue a relationship, has come to play a central role in much current theorizing about the determinants of relationship stability. Rusbult's (1983, 1991) investment model, one of several theoretical elaborations of interdependence theory, proposes that an individual will feel more satisfied with a relationship to the degree that numerous rewards are derived from the partner and the relationship, few costs are suffered, and each partner has a lower rather than a higher comparison level. It predicts that a person should be committed to a relationship to the extent that he or she is satisfied with it. Satisfaction is viewed as only one of three aspects of commitment, however. The quality of the individual's alternatives to the present relationship and the individual's "investment" in the relationship (e.g., time, money, and the development of activities, friends, and possessions uniquely associated with the relationship) are also theorized to contribute to commitment. Changes in feelings of commitment are hypothesized to mediate an individual's decision to continue or leave the relationship. As Rusbult (1991) puts it, "Importantly, it is *increasing satisfaction*, the perception that one's alternatives are *becoming less and less attractive*, and the recognition of *increasingly great investment* that leads to increased commitment" (p. 160), which in turn is theorized to be associated with stability.

Kelley (1983) takes a somewhat different view of commitment and the prediction of stability. To understand and predict stability, Kelley points out that one must identify (1) the conditions that keep a person in a relationship—that is, the conditions responsible for the positive aspects of the relationship, as well as the costs that would be incurred upon leaving the relationship—which he calls the "pros" of the relationship; and (2) those that act to push or draw the individual out of the relationship, which he terms the "cons" of the relationship. Kelley theorizes that the key feature of these conditions for the prediction of stability is the "consistency with which, over time and situations, the pros outweigh the cons" (p. 289) for each person in the relationship: "If membership is to be stable, the average degree to which the pros outweigh the cons must be large relative to the variability in this difference" (p. 289). If there is a large difference in favor of the pros, then there can be a great deal of fluctuation in the level of the pros and cons over time without affecting the stability of the relationship, because the pros are likely to continue to outweigh the cons even if they fluctuate markedly. If, however, there is little difference in the level of the pros and cons, then it is important that they stay at a relatively constant level, because even a slight fluctuation may result in the cons overwhelming the pros and thus endangering the relationship.

Because the conditions associated with commitment often fluctuate over time, stability forecasters not only need to identify the conditions influencing the relationship at the present time, but also must predict how each of these forces is likely to fluctuate in the future. Because it takes two people to maintain a relationship but only one to dissolve it, this theoretical view also implies that a separate forecast must be made for each partner; if even one partner's pros dip below the cons, the relationship may be in trouble. In short, Kelley's theoretical view of commitment differentiates between two outwardly similar relationships in which the two sets of relationship partners may feel equally committed to continuing their relationships at the present time. An analysis of the stability of the forces underlying the partners' present feelings of commitment may reveal that one of these relationships is like a great ocean liner capable of riding out violent storms, while the other is a fragile canoe that will capsize in a single gust of wind. Thus Kelley's theoretical perspective suggests that simply asking people how committed they are at present to their relationships may give a misleading forecast of the relationships' future stability.

Yet another view of relationship stability, Levinger's (1965, 1976, in press) cohesiveness model, was originally developed to integrate the fragmented literature on divorce. Levinger drew upon interdependence theory as well as on Lewin's (1951) field theory, which proposes that certain forces either attract a person to, or repel him or her from, a particular region of the person's life space or "field" (e.g., to or from a specific relationship). Levinger calls these attracting and repelling forces "attraction forces," and he links them with the individual's satisfaction with the relationship. In addition, Levinger posits "barrier forces" that restrain a person from leaving a relationship; these forces represent the costs associated with leaving the relationship should it become dissatisfying and should a better alternative arise. The barriers that may act to contain an individual within a relationship are theorized to be factors that lead the individual to anticipate sustaining costs (e.g., financial, social, psychological, emotional) should he or she voluntarily terminate the relationship. Levinger (1991) theorizes that "barriers only influence one's decision to continue in a relationship if one begins to contemplate exit" (p. 148).

Levinger's concept of barriers is somewhat similar to the concept of "structural commitment" in Michael Johnson's theoretical framework. The basic assumption of Johnson's (1982, 1991a) commitment theory is that an individual's decision to continue a relationship is a function of three distinct subjective experiences of commitment: (1) personal commitment, or the individual's feeling that he or she *wants* to continue the relationship; (2) moral commitment, or the individual's feeling that he or she *ought* to continue it; and (3) structural commitment, or the individual's feeling that he or she *must* continue it. In contrast to personal and moral commitment (which Johnson theorizes to be experienced by individuals as having originated within themselves), "structural commitments are experienced as external and constraining factors in one's environment that make it costly or difficult to leave a relationship, whatever one's own personal or moral commitment to it may be" (Johnson, 1991a, p. 119). Structural commitments are viewed as including irretrievable investments in the relationship, social reaction, the difficulty of termination procedures (e.g., the procedures of obtaining a legal divorce), and the availability of acceptable alternatives. In sum, Johnson theorizes that an individual's experiences associated with the three types of commitment jointly determine the individual's motivation to maintain or dissolve the relationship.

Berscheid and Campbell (1981) have used Levinger's cohesiveness model to analyze the causes of "the changing longevity of heterosexual close relationships" (p. 209). Endorsing the view of many family researchers that "a shift in the lifetime divorce probability from 10% to well over 50% cannot be explained at the micro level" (White, 1990, p. 904)—for example, the partners' satisfaction with the microevents of their personal interactions—Berscheid and Campbell review the many macro-level changes in societal conditions that coincided with the sharp upward turn of the divorce rate that occurred around 1960, and contend that most represented a dramatic reduction in the barriers that previously had contained people in their marital relationships. (See Attridge & Berscheid, 1994, for a more recent review of current societal conditions that indicate further weakening of barriers to marital dissolution.) In their analysis, Berscheid and Campbell illustrate not only how changes in macro-level societal conditions influence the likelihood of relationship dissolution *directly* through the presence or absence of barriers to dissolution, but also how barriers *indirectly* influence dissolution through their influence on the partners' satisfaction with the relationship. They argue that as the external barriers to marital dissolution have weakened, "the burden of purpose and justification for maintaining the relationship has increasingly fallen on the 'sweetness' of its contents" (1981, p. 222).

When the burden of justifying a relationship is placed on satisfaction with its internal contents, or the rewards and costs arising from microevents in the partners' interaction, Berscheid and Campbell predict that the contents themselves are more likely to turn sour than if they did not bear the burden of providing the sole *raison d'être* of the relationship. When there are few barriers to leaving a relationship, for example, an individual must choose to continue the relationship with the partner and forsake all others not once, but again and again. The freedom of perpetual choice means that the individual must continually expend time and energy to reevaluate the wisdom of the previous choice through monitoring his or her satisfaction with the relationship, the quality of the available alternatives, and the depth of his or her investments. Moreover, the individual must perform this decision analysis not only for himself or herself but for the partner as well, in order to arrive at a probability estimate of the partner's leaving the relationship. If this latter analysis reveals that the partner, like the individual, has few barriers to dissolution, then the costs of insecurity and anxiety are added to other costs the individual is currently experiencing in the relationship. These added costs should reduce satisfaction with the relationship. In sum, Berscheid and Campbell argue that few barriers to relationship dissolution often signal that both partners must spend much time and energy "taking the pulse" of the relationship and attending to even the slightest symptom of malaise, for fear that it ultimately will prove fatal to the relationship.

OVERVIEW OF THE TEMPORAL MODEL

The conceptual framework we sketch in the remainder of this chapter is intended to build on the contributions that the theories we have outlined have made to our understanding of relationship satisfaction and stability. Our analysis focuses on the temporal interaction between satisfaction with the relationship and changes in the relationship's environment.

An important difference between our approach and those we have just described is that we do not incorporate the concept of psychological commitment; that is, we do not treat in any way the individual's commitment to the relationship, if commitment is defined (as it usually is) as the individual's subjective wish or intent to continue the relationship. Rather, taking our cue from Kelley (1983), we focus on the forces associated with stability, particularly environmental forces, and their likely effect on satisfaction with the relationship. Thus, we extend the line of reasoning begun in Berscheid and Campbell (1981) to achieve a better understanding of the interplay over time between the internal dynamics of the relationship and its external context. Moreover, in our emphasis on environmental conditions associated with stability, we highlight the partners' attempts to manipulate these forces with the intent of preserving or destroying their relationship. Our approach, then, is not phenomenological. Whether, how, and when partners become aware of the environmental forces affecting their relationship and deliberately attempt to manipulate them encompass a set of important empirical questions that have not captured the attention they deserve.

Our emphasis on the environmental forces associated with relationship stability and the need to forecast how these are likely to change in the future is similar to the view often taken by older and wiser observers of young couples about to launch their relationships on their voyage through time. Although noting the couples' vows of personal commitment never to abandon their ships, these observers often look to the horizon. There, for some couples, they see only a calm and benevolent sea ahead; for other couples, however, they see on the horizon a tsunami rolling toward the relationship. We begin our analysis of the influence of environmental factors on relationship stability by discussing the essence of a relationship—the partners' interaction with each other.

THE RELATIONSHIP ORGANISM: INTERACTION

A relationship between two people resides in neither of the partners, but rather in the interaction that takes place between them. That interaction can be viewed as constituting the living organism, or dynamic system, we call an interpersonal "relationship." Put another way, relationship researchers generally view the interaction that takes place between an individual and his or her partner as the living tissue of the relationship. If an individual and his or her partner never interact, there is no relationship. If they seldom interact, there is not likely to be much of a relationship between them. If they do interact frequently, it is the recurrent pattern of their interaction that relationship researchers seek to understand.

To understand the interaction pattern characteristic of any relationship, researchers try to identify the relatively stable conditions that are responsible for that pattern, as well as such outcomes of the interaction as the partners' satisfaction with the relationship. Attempts by the partners or by a relationship therapist to change the nature of the relationship, as well as forecasts of the likelihood that the relationship will spontaneously change, depend on the identification of these conditions. The conditions that influence the interaction between an individual and his or her partner have been classified as "personal" and "environmental" (see Kelley et al., 1983), with the attributes of the person, the attributes of the partner, and the interaction between them constituting "personal" causal conditions, and the physical and social contexts of their interaction constituting "environmental" causal conditions.

Considerable effort has been devoted to identifying the personal conditions that influence interaction and the satisfaction or dissatisfaction that results from it. For example, the personality trait of "neuroticism" is one personal condition that has frequently been examined. Not surprisingly, many studies find that possession of this personality trait bodes ill for marital satisfaction and stability (e.g., Kelly & Conley, 1987; Kurdek, 1993). The answer such studies give to the question "How can I find a satisfying relationship?", then, is "First, you have to be the right person [e.g., one who is not neurotic]." This answer contrasts with the assumption that is usually made in a quest for a satisfying relationship. Rather than *being* the right person, an individual assumes that he or she must *find* the right person, who possesses the personal attributes the individual believes conducive to a satisfying relationship. To aid in this search for the right person, an individual often spends a good deal of time making up a shopping list of desirable attributes a partner should possess (e.g., see Buss & Barnes, 1986). Researchers also have examined how the fit between an individual's attributes and his or her partner's attributes influence relationship satisfaction and stability. One of the most important of these for relationship satisfaction is the similarity of the partners (see Berscheid & Reis, in press). Studies showing that the fit between the partners' attributes influences satisfaction suggest that to develop a satisfying relationship "you have to find the right person for *you*," and this is not going to be the right person for everyone.

In contrast to personal forces influencing partners' satisfaction with their interaction, the influence of environmental forces—the relationship's social and physical contexts—has been relatively ignored. The aspect of the social environment that represents the availability of attractive alternatives to the relationship is an exception (e.g., Udry, 1981; and see Berscheid & Reis, in press), thanks largely to the emphasis interdependence theory places on the role of comparison level for alternatives in decisions to maintain or terminate a relationship. Levinger (1994) has discussed the tendency for relationship researchers to focus on the relationship partners themselves and the microevents occurring in their interaction, and to neglect the relationship's environmental context (but see Brown, Werner, & Altman, 1994, for an interesting exception). Johnson (1991a), too, has observed: "Work on relationship stability has long been hampered by an American 'free-will' bias that has led social scientists to focus almost entirely on forms of commitment I have identified as personal. Most research and theory on marital dissolution, for example, have emphasized 'marital satisfaction' or 'dyadic adjustment' or 'relationship quality' " (pp. 128–129). As a consequence, little is known about how relationships are affected by dramatic and widespread changes in the sociocultural context in which they are embedded.

RELATIONSHIP STABILITY:
THE CONTINUANCE OF INTERACTION

If the essence of a relationship is interaction, then relationship stability can be viewed as the continuance of the partners' interaction with each other. But what *kind* of relationship it is, and whether it is that kind or another kind of relationship that is continued, poses important questions not often discussed. One of these questions concerns the kind of relationship the partners have in mind when they say they are committed to their relationship. In his discussion of psychological commitment, Johnson (1991a) pauses to discuss the question "Commitment to what?" He observes: "When one asks a married respondent if she is committed to the maintenance of her relationship with her husband, she responds in terms of her understanding of the meaning of marriage . . . [and] would probably not count 'getting divorced but continuing to see each other because of the children' as maintaining the relationship" (1991a, p. 120). An external observer, however, might say that these ex-spouses clearly do have a relationship with each other, as they still interact and are interdependent. However, the *kind* of relationship they have has changed from a marital relationship to some other type.

In addition to the difficulty of interpreting people's answers to questionnaire items assessing their commitment to their relationships, there is also the problem of interpreting their responses to items assessing their satisfaction with their relationships. Johnson (1991a), for example, defines "personal commitment," or the sense of wanting to continue a relationship, as being a function of several components, two of which figure in almost all theories of commitment: (1) the individual's attitude toward the relationship, and (2) the individual's attitude toward the partner. The critical question is whether an individual who answers relationship satisfaction queries is expressing satisfaction with the relationship but not necessarily the partner, satisfaction with the partner but not necessarily the relationship, or some combination of both.

These problems of interpreting the meaning of an individual's subjective responses to commitment and satisfaction measures may be bypassed, at least theoretically, by defining a relationship as existing when the partners have some impact on each other. This implies that there has been interaction of some kind. But it is not clear how much interaction—or impact or interdependence—is necessary before we can say that two people are in a relationship with each other. Researchers have attempted to define a "close" relationship (e.g., Aron, Aron, & Smollan, 1992; Kelley et al., 1983), an "intimate" relationship (e.g., Reis & Shaver, 1988), and relationships of other kinds, but the elemental question of when two people are or are not in a relationship with each other is not frequently considered.

Theorists of relationship development are an exception to the rule, for they must identify the "beginning" of a relationship to study its development. Several of these theorists view the relationship as beginning the first time one person has some impact on another (e.g., Berscheid & Graziano, 1979; Levinger, 1974). Others, however, do not agree that one such interaction, or even a good deal more such interactions, necessarily qualify as a relationship (e.g., Homans, 1979). The question of how much interaction and interdependence constitute a relationship is similar to the question of when a human becomes a human. At the moment of conception (or the first impact)? At the point of the fetus's viability (or when the relationship is able to continue in circumstances other than when interaction first occurred)? After birth (or after the relationship is fully formed along certain specified dimensions)? Obtaining agreement on the answer to the question of when interactions become a relationship is likely to be as difficult as agreement on the answer to the question of when a fetus becomes a human.

Avoiding all of these thorny issues, we view relationship stability as the continuance of interaction. Thus, we assume that understanding stability requires an identification of the forces that compel people to continue, or repel them from continuing, to interact with each other. We take it as a given that relationships often change in kind over time (e.g., from a coworker relationship to a friendship to a romantic relationship to a marital relationship) and recognize that a consideration of changes in the attributes of the partners (e.g., from child to adult), changes in the nature of their interaction (e.g., from frequent to seldom), and changes in the relationship's environmental context (e.g., from voluntary to involuntary) may lead observers to conclude that the type of relationship we are observing has changed over time.

THE "VOLUNTARINESS" OF INTERACTION

All theories of commitment, satisfaction, and stability attempt to identify the forces that compel people to continue to interact with each other. Perhaps the simplest view is offered by Murstein (1970) in his stimulus–value–role theory of marital choice. Murstein's interest in the forces under which an individual will attempt to interact with another for the first time led him to distinguish between interactions that take place in an "open field" as opposed to a "closed field." Murstein defines a closed field as one "in which both [individuals] . . . are forced to interact by reason of the environmental setting in which they find themselves.

. . . Examples of such situations might be that of students in a small seminar in a college, members in a law firm, and workers in complementary professions such as doctor–nurse and 'boss'–secretary" (1970, p. 466). In a closed field situation, the compelling forces responsible for the interaction are usually located in the relationship's physical and social environments rather than in personal conditions. In contrast, an "open field" situation "refers to a situation in which the [individuals] . . . do not as yet know each other. . . . Examples of such 'open field' situations are 'mixers,' presence in a large school class at the beginning of a semester, and brief contact in the office. The fact that the field is 'open' indicates that either [individual] . . . is free to start the relationship or to abstain from initiating it, as they wish" (1970, p. 466). As Murstein suggests, if the individual does initiate interaction in an open field situation, it is likely to be the result of a personal condition (e.g., the partner's physical attractiveness).

The closed field versus open field distinction refers to the "voluntariness" of the interaction that takes place between two people. All of the theories we have discussed imply such a dimension. Thibaut and Kelley (1959) address nonvoluntary relationships, as previously noted. Johnson's concept of structural commitment, defined as the feeling that one must continue (or, presumably, initiate) a relationship, is said to derive "from factors that are experienced as external to the individual and constraining" (1991a, p. 122). And Levinger's barriers are clearly conceptualized as forces that keep the individual in the relationship involuntarily.

Nevertheless, the idea that every human relationship can be placed on a dimension of voluntariness, anchored at one end with total freedom to interact or not to interact with another (i.e., with no negative consequences suffered as a consequence of the failure to interact) and anchored at the other end with the most severe consequences resulting from a failure to interact with the partner, is rarely discussed (but see Rusbult's [1991] and Johnson's [1991b] debate on this issue). This neglect of the voluntariness dimension underlying relationships can probably be attributed to the same forces that have been responsible for the neglect of the influence of environmental conditions on relationships in favor of examining the influence of personal conditions. Not only do people like to think that whether and with whom they have relationships are matters of personal choice and volition, but relationship researchers, especially social psychologists, have preferred to study types of relationships that are usually voluntary in nature (e.g., romantic relationships). Whatever the reason for the neglect, we believe that voluntariness of interaction is a fundamental dimension underlying all relationships, and that many relationship phenomena cannot be well understood without explicitly considering this aspect of relationships.

External forces that compel an individual to interact with a specific other involuntarily (i.e., the individual would not choose to interact with the other if those forces were not present) constitute only one side of the coin. To understand and predict when an individual will or will not interact with a specific other, one also needs to identify the forces that repel the individual from interacting with the other (i.e., the individual would choose to interact with the other if those repelling forces were not present). Again, all the theories we have discussed assume such a dimension. For example, the concept of barriers implies that in addition to strong forces compelling interaction, there exist strong forces repelling interaction. The compelling forces are perceived as "barriers" to the termination of interaction with the partner only because such repelling forces are present.

CONDITIONS INFLUENCING INTERACTION PROBABILITY

We conclude, then, that if the essence of a relationship lies in the partners' interaction with each other, the question of relationship stability—or why one relationship endures and another dissolves—can be rephrased as follows: "What forces compel an individual to interact (or continue to interact) with a specific other, resulting in a stable relationship with that person, and what forces repel the individual from interacting, resulting either in no relationship or in termination of a once viable relationship?" The central question we address, then, is this: "What is the probability that an individual will attempt to interact with his or her partner at any given time?" The answer we give to this question is the following: "The probability of an individual's attempt to interact with his or her partner at any given time is a function of a set of personal and environmental causal conditions, some of which are exogenous to the relationship and some of which are endogenous to it." (For convenience in the discussion below, we shall assume that both partners are simultaneously subject to the same conditions and to the same degree, although this is probably never true.)

Personal Exogenous Forces

Some of the forces that compel or repel interaction are "exogenous" to a relationship, in that they are introduced from or produced outside the organism or system. Thus, exogenous forces that facilitate or inhibit an individual's interaction with his or her partner are external to the interaction pattern, content, and outcomes. Such exogenous forces may be personal. Personal exogenous forces compelling interaction with a partner may include an individual's loneliness, or an individual's strong affiliative need and extraverted personality, or an individual's uncertainty about the correctness of his or her attitude or opinion (e.g., Festinger, 1954). Exogenous personal forces repelling interaction may include an individual's chronic shyness, introverted personality, fatigue and poor health, or lack of time because of demands elsewhere.

Personal Endogenous Forces

Some of the forces that compel or repel an individual to interact with his or her partner are "endogenous" to the relationship, in that they are produced within the organism or system. Endogenous forces that influence the probability of interaction are thus those conditions that are "produced by," or are "a result of," or "emerge from" the microevent of interaction. Love, trust, intimacy, and many of the other variables of traditional interest to relationship researchers are of this nature. Relationship satisfaction is an endogenous force, in that it is usually viewed as emerging from the partners' interaction and as representing a relatively stable force that compels continued interaction. (It should be noted that there is some empirical evidence that an individual's satisfaction with a relationship is best viewed as emerging from the interaction between the two partners rather than as a personal trait; Johnson, Amoloza & Booth, 1992.[1]) As we have discussed, all social exchange theories view satisfaction as primarily the result of the partners' exchange of rewards and punishments in interaction.

In addition to satisfaction, of course, many agreements and understandings often emerge from the partners' interaction. These often achieve enough stability and force that they come to represent important endogenous personal conditions that influence subsequent interaction. Many such agreements represent conditions that regulate both the frequency of interaction and the environment in which it will take place. For example, friends may agree that every Friday night is reserved for each other and that they will meet at the bowling alley, or ex-spouses may agree that they will avoid certain locations so as to avoid any circumstances under which they might be compelled to interact. Also, as we have discussed, marriage vows and other such joint relationship resolutions are promises that each partner will continue to interact with the other, regardless of strong repelling forces that might arise.

In sum, the personal exogenous and endogenous forces that will influence the partners' probability of continued interaction can be placed on a continuum ranging from positive (compelling interaction) to negative (repelling interaction). If an initial interaction is ever to occur, there must be at least one positive exogenous force impinging on an individual and/or his or her partner. To forecast the probability of continued interaction, then, it is necessary to assess the relationship's present location along this continuum, and to forecast how these personal forces are likely to change over time and thus to change the relationship's location on the compelling–repelling dimension.

Environmental Exogenous and Endogenous Forces

Environmental forces may also be exogenous or endogenous. Exogenous environmental forces that compel or repel interaction may include physical environmental forces (e.g., the close physical proximity of an individual and his or her partner has been demonstrated to compel interaction), as well as social environmental forces (e.g., an individual's friends may either facilitate or hinder interaction with his or her partner). Environmental exogenous conditions are viewed as representing rewards and costs that are incurred by the individual as a result of his or her interaction with the partner (or failure to interact), but whose source is an agent other than the partners.

Those who wish to predict the stability of a relationship must forecast the appearance and disappearance over time of exogenous environmental conditions (e.g., an economic downturn, or an AIDS epidemic that decimates an individual's social network) that compel or repel interaction. These changes in the exogenous environmental context of the relationship often arise from events of which the partners may not be aware; even if they are aware of them, they may have no control over them. Nevertheless, they help form the environmental context in which the relationship is embedded, and, from the point of view of the relationship forecaster, they may contain the vital clue to the relationship's future—a future the forecaster may predict more accurately than the partners themselves, who may tend to focus on the micro-events of their interaction with each other and on the goodness of outcomes they are presently receiving in that interaction and their satisfaction with these. (See Fletcher & Kininmonth, 1992, for some tangential empirical support for the proposition that partners typically accord environmental conditions little importance in the fate of their relationship.)

In addition to forecasting the appearance and disappearance of exogenous environmental conditions over time, to predict relationship stability it is also necessary to forecast the appearance or disappearance of endogenous forces, or how the partners themselves will attempt to change the environmental conditions that are currently facilitating or inhibiting their interaction. For example, depending on the first interaction (e.g., it is rewarding or it is punishing), partners may subsequently act to change the environmental conditions surrounding their relationship. If the interaction has been rewarding, for example, they may increase their physical proximity by moving into the same neighborhood. If so, the stable and compelling environmental condition of physical proximity has become a new environmental force that will influence the relationship. It is an endogenous force because it has emerged from the relationship.

Although environmental forces are often created in the partners' interaction, they may thereafter achieve independence from the partners' future interactions and may not be affected by those interactions (e.g., by momentary fluctuations in the partners' satisfaction with subsequent interactions). In some cases, for example, the endogenous personal or environmental force that has emerged from previous interactions may be immutable or difficult to change (e.g., an individual has undergone surgical removal of a segment of the intestine in an effort to lose weight and improve his or her appearance, or has renounced his or her national citizenship to adopt the partner's). Some endogenous environmental conditions, then, assume a life of their own—a life that later may be regarded by the relationship partners in the same way that Dr. Frankenstein came to view the life of the monster he had created. More often, perhaps, their very immutability and stability may lead the partners to forget the existence of that environmental force, their active role in creating it, and its continued effect on their interaction.

The question of the partners' awareness of the environmental forces influencing their interactions has not yet received direct empirical investigation. It should be noted, however, that the partners need not be aware of the existence of such conditions for those conditions to affect the relationship. To take the example of social reaction to the relationship, theorized by Johnson (1991a) to be one source of structural commitment, people in the partners' social environment who approve of the relationship may surreptitiously devise circumstances that increase the probability of the partners' interaction (as matchmakers often do); those who disapprove may secretly create a host of obstacles that make it difficult or impossible for the partners to interact. The partners are likely to be subject to these effects whether they are aware of them or not. If they are aware that their social environment compels continued interaction, such awareness may contribute to their subjective feeling of structural commitment.

The question of when partners are likely to be aware of environmental forces influencing their relationship is important for several reasons. For example, if one thinks of the partners' relationship as a ship sailing through time in environmental waters that either facilitate or inhibit continued interaction, then it can be seen that whether the partners recognize the role that these environmental forces play in their relationship—and how successful they are in eliminating repelling environmental forces and constructing compelling ones—will determine whether they subsequently become the captains of their relationship or whether they, and the relationship, may become just the victims of what the partners later describe as "fate" or "bad luck."

On the whole, however, one can guess that people generally are not attuned to situational or contextual conditions that influence their own or their partners' interaction behavior. As Heider (1958) put it long ago, and as much social psychological research has confirmed, "behavior engulfs the field"—the "field" in this case being the environmental context of the partners' interaction. Far more salient factors to the partners are likely to be their own and their partner's behaviors in their current interactions and the goodness of outcomes they receive directly from those interactions. Thus, when the partners are dissatisfied with their interaction outcomes, it seems more likely that they will attempt to change personal forces (e.g., each partner may attempt to increase his or her own or the other's communication skills, love, trust, etc.) than to attempt to change environmental forces. Again, however, this is an empirical question. It might be noted that relationship therapists, too, seem to focus on personal forces in their attempt to remedy relationship dissatisfaction (e.g., by changing the partners' expectations, attributions, and conflict resolution skills) and only rarely practice what we would term "environmental therapy" (see Berscheid, in press). Nevertheless, it is clear that partners are sometimes aware of compelling and/or repelling environmental forces, that these forces are sometimes modifiable, and that sometimes the partners do attempt to change them. At other times, however, despite awareness of their influence, these conditions may be beyond the power of the partners to change.

SATISFACTION AND THE PARTNERS' MANIPULATION OF ENVIRONMENTAL FORCES

To predict relationship stability, it would be useful to know when partners are likely to attempt to change the environmental forces in which the relationship is embedded. High satisfaction with the goodness of outcomes received in interaction with another should be one circumstance that leads an individual to attempt to construct stable personal and environmental conditions that will increase the probability of future interaction, thus helping to ensure that the individual will continue to receive the rewards the interaction presently offers. We have

noted that such manipulations often are directed toward the modification of personal conditions that increase interaction probability. Here,
however, we shall focus on how successful manipulations of compelling or repelling environmental forces are likely to affect relationship
satisfaction and, in turn, the stability of the relationship. To do so, we
return to the romantic relationship scenario discussed by Berscheid and
Campbell (1981).

To illustrate how macrosocietal conditions may influence the microevents of interaction and, through them, relationship satisfaction and
stability, Berscheid and Campbell (1981) examine a relationship in which
the partners find their interaction rewarding (and thus, presumably, are
highly satisfied with the quality of their relationship) and presently experience no barriers to relationship termination. Figure 6.1 depicts the
location of that relationship (at Time$_1$) on a grid defined by two
dimensions: (1) the quality,[2] positive or negative, of the interaction,
or the degree to which the rewards and costs of the interaction together
contribute to feelings of relationship satisfaction and constitute a compelling or repelling force for future interaction; and (2) the environmental forces surrounding the relationship, which together represent
forces compelling or repelling future interaction.

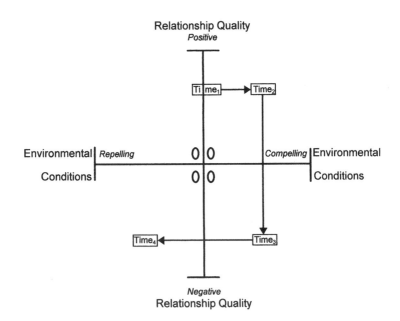

FIGURE 6.1. The development of a romantic relationship (described in Berscheid
& Campbell, 1981) as plotted on the Q-E grid.

The location of this particular relationship on the "quality–environment" (Q-E) grid depicts the fact that currently there are no environmental forces present that compel or repel future interaction; that is, the social and physical environments of this relationship are providing no facilitative or hindering forces, and both partners are free to terminate their interaction without incurring costs from agents outside the relationship. Rather, the "fuel" that is propelling this relationship through time is wholly personal and endogenous. As Berscheid and Campbell discuss, the absence of compelling environmental forces ought to increase insecurity about the future of the relationship and anxiety about the continuation of interaction rewards, thereby reducing the degree of satisfaction the partners would otherwise enjoy.

THE TEMPORAL COURSE
OF A ROMANTIC RELATIONSHIP
ON THE QUALITY-ENVIRONMENT GRID

We pick up here where Berscheid and Campbell (1981) left off and predict that under such circumstances, the partners will take actions to assure the relationship's future. These actions may include personal vows of commitment to continue the relationship. However, most people are aware that, as one sage put it, oral vows are worth the paper they're not written on. As a consequence, the partners may attempt to put a stronger shell around the interaction tissue of their relationship by constructing compelling environmental forces that help guarantee the continuance of their satisfying interaction. The literature on the development of romantic relationships describes the nature of some of these endogenous environmental forces the partners may construct. For example, the partners often move their residences or jobs to be in closer proximity, sign legal contracts together (including the marital contract), and eliminate interfering friends from their social network. Recent evidence suggests that in addition to actual changes, some environmental changes the partners make are perceptual. For example, the appearance in the social environment of attractive and available alternative partners seems to lead individuals who are highly committed to a relationship to devalue the attractiveness of those alternative partners (Johnson & Rusbult, 1989; Simpson, Gangestad, & Lerma, 1990).

As a result of the successful construction of these endogenous and compelling environmental forces, this relationship will move to a new location on the Q-E grid (see Figure 6.1, Time$_2$). The relationship's new location on the grid reflects both its high interaction quality and the existence of new compelling environmental forces. One presumes that many newlywed relationships are located in this quadrant of the Q-E grid, but so too are many employee–employer relationships in which the partners have been so satisfied with their interaction that, to guarantee its future, they have signed a long-term contract with high penalties for its abrogation. Similarly, friends, in an effort to preserve their satisfying relationship, may decide to attend the same college and join the same fraternity or sorority in order to be roommates; they thus may also be located in this Q-E quadrant.

The question of interest now becomes how the creation of these endogenous compelling environmental forces, intended to increase the likelihood of the continuance of the relationship and the receipt of its satisfying benefits, is likely to influence satisfaction and relationship stability. In other words, is the relationship likely to remain in its new location, and, if not, to what location on the Q-E grid is it likely to move next (i.e., at Time$_3$)? If the relationship is a newlywed relationship, there is a great deal of research that indicates where it will move. A decrease in marital satisfaction over time is one of the most frequently documented findings in the marital literature (Glenn, 1990; Karney & Bradbury, 1995). Along with a decrease in satisfaction over time, there also appears to be a decrease in the amount of interaction between the partners (e.g., Johnson et al., 1992), or a shrinking of the vital interaction tissue of the relationship, just as one might expect if interaction has become less satisfying. Although a "decrease" in satisfaction must be viewed in the light of the fact that, on an absolute basis, most people are satisfied with their marriages,[3] for illustrative purposes we shall assume that in this particular relationship the decrease has been severe enough that the partners are now dissatisfied with it.

It is this decrease over time in marital satisfaction that many researchers have been trying to understand, but with limited success. Has the partners' active construction of compelling environmental conditions to assure their continual interaction paradoxically played a role in decreasing their satisfaction with the relationship? Probably. But how? To consider this question, we return to the motivation that partners often have for constructing these conditions in the first place—insecurity about the continuance of the relationship. With respect to the marital relationship, for example, although young, never-married adults appear to worry about whether a marriage will be able to meet their needs for personal fulfillment, security also appears to be in the forefront of their concerns (see Attridge & Berscheid, 1994, for a discussion, and Zimmer, 1986, for evidence relevant to this point). Nock's (1995) recent finding that the perceived commitment of the spouse to the relationship strongly influences the individual's own degree of commitment is also congruent with security being a major concern of individuals in this type of relationship.

Feelings of insecurity about the relationship's continuance should diminish after the partners construct compelling (and after they banish repelling) environmental conditions to protect their relationship's future. They can relax. There is no longer any need for either partner to monitor his or her own or the other's moment-to-moment interaction outcomes or alternatives. They can get about their other business. And they can revert to old, comfortable habits without worrying about whether those behaviors will immediately threaten the relationship. As often observed anecdotally, that polite and considerate prince of a suitor becomes the toad of a husband who leaves the sugar bowl empty and often forgets to shave. That attractive and vivacious fiancée becomes the phlegmatic wife who gobbles Oreos by the dozen and finds that resumption of her Zen meditations leaves her no time to watch all those football games she previously professed to enjoy.

As a result of the partners' construction of strong compelling environmental forces, more subtle cognitive effects may be taking place as well. For example, extending research on the effects of the "overjustification" attribution effect to the relationship arena, Seligman, Fazio, and Zanna (1980) induced dating couples to adopt either an "intrinsic" cognitive set, in which each individual was encouraged to think about the partners' enjoyment of each other as motivations to continue the relationship, or an "extrinsic" set, in which the external reasons and potential pressures to continue the relationship were emphasized. These investigators found that, as contrasted to the condition in which intrinsic conditions were made salient, individuals who were made acutely aware of their extrinsic reasons for continuing the relationship viewed the probability of marrying their partners as significantly lower (and lower than that of a control group as well); they also reported less love (but not less liking) for their partners. Similarly, in a correlational study, Fletcher, Fincham, Cramer, and Heron (1987) found that individuals who gave more external reasons for the maintenance of their relationships and described them in fewer interpersonal terms also reported lower levels of commitment, happiness, and love for their partners. Other theorists have highlighted the partners' subjective perceptions of their intrinsic and extrinsic motivations in continuing the relationship as factors influencing each individual's trust and satisfaction with the relationship[4] (e.g., Blais, Sabourin, Boucher, & Vallerand, 1990; Rempel, Holmes, & Zanna, 1985).

If satisfaction with the interaction decreases enough, we can predict that the partners will further decrease their interaction, and yet maintain the relationship if there are sufficient compelling reasons to do so. A prospective correlational study of married individuals reported by White and Booth (1991) indicates that when there are compelling environmental reasons to continue a marriage (e.g., lower perceived remarriage prospects, home ownership), great unhappiness with the partner[5] seems to be required before the relationship is dissolved. Some marital relationships, then, will move over time from their former location on the Q-E grid, where they enjoyed both high interaction quality and security in the form of environmental forces compelling the continuance of the relationship, to a new location that reflects compelling environmental reasons for maintaining the relationship but lower quality (see Figure 6.1, Time$_3$).

Should the compelling environmental forces present at Time$_3$ disappear (e.g., an individual achieves economic independence from his or her partner), one can predict that the relationship will eventually (for one must assume some inertia) move once again. It will move to that location on the Q-E grid that represents the "boneyard" of once vital relationships (see Figure 6.1, Time$_4$). "What happened?" friends ask. "We became dissatisfied with the relationship," the partners say, "and so we ended it." Their simple answer is true enough, but it can be seen that the process by which they became dissatisfied was complex.

The path that relationships take over time is usually even more complicated of course. In Figure 6.2, we depict a hypothetical romantic relationship between Mary and John, who met in the course of their work. Originally (at Time$_1$), their only contact occurred as one of them waited for the other to finish using the copy machine, and as neither was patient, their interaction was dissatisfying. Few other environmental forces compelled their interaction (e.g., their offices were on different floors). One day, however, their supervisor assigned Mary and John to a work team to develop a marketing campaign for a new product, thus creating a strong exogenous environmental force compelling Mary and John to interact frequently (see Figure 6.2, Time$_2$); their failure to do so would, in fact, cost them their jobs. As their interaction increased, Mary and John found that they shared many attitudes and values. As a result, the quality of their interaction grew increasingly positive (see Figure 6.2, Time$_3$), and thus a new—and endogenous—compelling force was born.

After several months the work team dissolved and, with it, the exogenous environmental force that initially compelled Mary and John to interact frequently (see Figure 6.2, Time$_4$). However, the endogenous compelling force that had emerged in the meantime, the positive quality of their interaction, continued to motivate Mary and John to interact. Their relationship was now similar to the relationship Berscheid and Campbell (1981) focused on in their illustration; that is, the only force compelling Mary and John's interaction was its positive quality. After a time of increasing anxiety about the future of their relationship, Mary and John decided to marry. Marriage, of course, created many

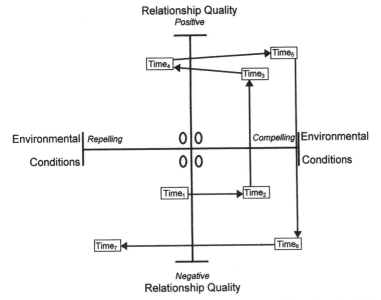

FIGURE 6.2. The development of an office romance as plotted on the Q-E grid.

environmental forces that compelled Mary and John to maintain their interaction, and it also eliminated several repelling environmental forces (e.g., John's former girlfriend stopped calling him; see Figure 6.2, Time$_5$).

After a few years of happy married life, Art was named the new supervisor of Mary's sales department. Art made Mary his star protégée, and as a consequence, Mary found interaction with Art extremely rewarding. She gradually devoted more and more of her time to her work and less to interacting with John. Moreover, when did she interact with John, she was often tired and distracted. Thus, the quality of her interaction with John, as well as its frequency, decreased (see Figure 6.2, Time$_6$). Disgusted and frustrated, John decided to move out and file for divorce, even though many environmental forces continued to compel him to interact with Mary (e.g., the health problems of their beloved dog). Believing that their relationship could not be revived, John decided to destroy what little relationship was left by accepting a transfer to a distant city, thereby setting in place an environmental force that strongly repelled continued interaction with Mary (see Figure 6.2, Time$_7$). One fortunate result for John was that his new geographical relocation increased his prospects for remarriage, for that city had one of the most favorable sex ratios for single men in the country; the plenitude of opposite-sex persons constitutes an exogenous environmental force facilitating the formation of new romantic relationships.

ASYMMETRY OF PARTNERS
ON THE QUALITY-ENVIRONMENT GRID

For the sake of convenience, we have assumed that both partners experience the same degree of satisfaction in the relationship and that both are subject to the same environmental conditions compelling or repelling their interaction, although, as we have noted, this is probably never true. Because it takes two people to maintain a relationship and only one to dissolve it, we have stated that forecasts of stability need to locate both partners on the Q-E grid to identify the partner who constitutes the relationship's "weak link," or the partner who is more likely to dissolve the relationship (see Attridge, Berscheid, & Simpson, 1995, for a discussion of this point and some supporting empirical evidence). Such information may also facilitate the prediction of which partner is likely to be motivated to construct environmental forces that compel or repel continued interaction.

Many familiar types of relationships are characterized by one of the two partners occupying different locations on the Q-E grid, and some of these appear to move systematically to different grid locations over time. A parent–child relationship, for example, is asymmetrical for much of the life of the relationship. The child's developmental changes alone will change the location of the relationship on the Q-E grid, as any parent can testify. As the child ages, for example, environmental forces compelling interaction will probably decrease for the child, and environmental forces repelling interaction (e.g., the adolescent's peer network) may increase.

Assessing the partners' locations on the environmental dimension of the Q-E grid is difficult at present. Although many instruments are available to assess the quality of the partners' interaction, both partners' subjective perceptions of its quality, and observers' evaluation of its quality, there are few means of measuring the compelling–repelling nature of the environmental conditions in which a relationship is embedded. This makes it difficult to investigate the temporal interplay of personal and environmental causal forces, whether endogenous and exogenous, and their effect upon satisfaction and stability. One exception is an inventory developed by Stanley and Markman (1992), who, inspired by Johnson's (1982) theory of commitment, attempted to assess "constraint commitment," or the "forces that constrain individuals to maintain relationships regardless of their personal dedication to them"

(Stanley & Markman, 1992, pp. 595–596) in marital and dating relationships. Three of their constraint commitment subscales appear to assess environmental conditions that compel or repel continued interaction. More efforts to develop inventories assessing a relationship's environmental conditions are needed. Such inventories (1) should be applicable to all types of relationships, not only romantic or marital relationships; and (2) should require respondents to report only on whether certain specified conditions do or do not exist, rather than to report their subjective views of whether these conditions constitute forces that are influencing their personal decisions to continue the relationship. The latter requirement is a consequence of our suspicion that many of the conditions that relationship stability forecasters would consider compelling or repelling environmental conditions are not presently recognized as such by the partners.

SUMMARY

In their review of theory, method, and research on the longitudinal course of marital quality and stability, Karney and Bradbury (1995) conclude that the need for theory is especially acute in the study of marriage, because "much of the longitudinal work has not been explicitly theoretical in orientation and because subsequent progress in understanding how marriages change is likely to depend heavily on the quality of available models" (p. 4). These authors evaluate the available theories against three criteria: (1) whether the theory encompasses a full range of possible predictors of marital outcome and provides links between different levels of analysis (e.g., the theory specifies how macro-level variables such as cultural norms are linked to micro-level variables such as interaction events); (2) whether mechanisms of change within marriage are specified (e.g., the theory explains, not simply predicts, how marriages achieve different outcomes); and (3) whether the theory accounts for variability in marital outcomes both between couples and within couples (e.g., the theory explains why some marriages persist despite dissatisfaction and others dissolve). Karney and Bradbury conclude that all available theories are deficient with respect to one or more of these criteria.

The positive features of a perspective based on social exchange theories, as characterized by Karney and Bradbury, include the facts that many types of variables can be incorporated into this conceptual framework and that it distinguishes between marital satisfaction and marital stability. These critics observe, however, that social exchange theories "[do] not address how change in marriage comes about" (p. 5), and that "a temporal perspective is also lacking from conceptualizations of attractions and barriers" (p. 5). The temporal model of satisfaction and stability we have sketched in this chapter is an attempt to address some of these limitations. We now summarize the model's features.

First, it departs from the customary focus on psychological commitment, or an individual's subjectively experienced motivation to continue the relationship, and simply posits that two people are in a relationship with each other if they interact and thus show at least some interdependence in their behavioral activities. The question of predicting relationship stability then becomes one of predicting the continuance of interaction. The model assumes that to predict whether interaction will continue, it is necessary to identify the relatively stable personal and environmental causal conditions that currently compel and repel interaction, and to forecast how these conditions are likely to change over time.

Second, the model adopts the social exchange perspective, which assumes that the prime internal dynamic of social interaction is the partners' exchange of rewards and punishments, and that relationship satisfaction results from the positive and negative outcomes the partners experience in interaction with each other. It views relationship satisfaction as an endogenous personal condition; it is endogenous because it emerges from the interaction, it is personal because it is an attribute of the individual, and it constitutes a condition because it is relatively stable. Relationship researchers agree that relationship satisfaction, or dissatisfaction, is an important condition that compels, or repels, continued interaction.

Third, the model highlights environmental conditions that compel or repel continued interaction because, in comparison to personal conditions, these have been neglected in relationship research (see Berscheid, 1994). It emphasizes the need to identify how the environmental context of a relationship may change in systematic ways over time, and it distinguishes changes in environmental conditions that are endogenous to the relationship from those that are exogenous. Endogenous changes in the environmental context of the relationship emerge from the interaction and are made by the partners themselves. Other compelling and repelling environmental forces influencing the relationship are exogenous to it; they originate outside the relationship, and the rewards and costs such conditions produce for the partners as a result of their interaction are delivered by outside agents.

Fourth, and most importantly, the model attempts to show how relationship satisfaction and the environmental context of the relationship may interact with each other over time to determine the fate of the relationship. A "quality–environment" grid is used to plot progressions over time. The Q-E grid represents the positive or negative quality of the partners' interaction (or whether that interaction represents a compelling or a repelling force for future interaction) on the Q dimension, and the compelling and/or repelling nature of the relationship's environment on the E dimension.

Finally, the model suggests that further research is needed (1) to investigate the extent to which partners are aware of the impact of the environment on their relationship; (2) to identify the conditions under which, and the means by which, people manipulate the environment in which the relationship is embedded, in order to strengthen or weaken their relationship; and (3) to develop instruments to measure the degree to which a relationship's current environment compels or repels continued interaction.

ACKNOWLEDGMENT

We wish to thank George Levinger, University of Massachusetts at Amherst, for his helpful comments on an earlier draft.

NOTES

1. It might be noted that although psychological commitment, or subjective intent to continue a relationship, is usually viewed as emerging from interaction with another and probably usually does, it need not. That is, in some circumstances the individual may vow to make the *next* relationship endure (whether with a romantic partner, an employer or employee, or some other person) "no matter what!" In such cases, commitment is an exogenous variable, an individual condition, that has not emerged from the interaction with the partner and does not depend on the partner's qualities or on the nature of the interaction that subsequently ensues.

2. We label this dimension of the grid relationship "quality," rather than relationship satisfaction, because it is not yet clear how relationship quality might be most usefully assessed and how its putative dimensions (e.g., satisfaction, intimacy, commitment, etc.) might be most usefully conceptualized (see, e.g., Kurdek, 1996, for a recent discussion). Attridge, Berscheid, and Simpson (1995) have found evidence that self-reports of multiple relationship dimensions appear to reflect a global latent factor of positive–negative sentiment, as has Kurdek (1996). Thus we simply use the term "quality," rather than satisfaction, as a general label for the subjective affective character of the relationship; we hold in abeyance the question of what factors contribute to that positive or negative affect and how it is most reliably assessed.

3. In a longitudinal study of marital satisfaction of newlyweds over a 9-year period, Lindahl, Clements, and Markman (in press), for example, found that scores on the Marital Adjustment Test (Locke & Wallace, 1959) declined over

the early years of the relationship, together with other marital satisfaction findings; however, after 3¼ years, these scores seemed to stabilize. The investigators, so far, have observed no further significant declines over time. This pattern was not true for all couples, of course, as approximately 20% of their sample had decided to divorce or separate by the 9-year date.

4. It should be noted that the question of whether answers to satisfaction items on questionnaires represent satisfaction with the *relationship* or satisfaction with the *partner* (or some varying combination of the two) arises in this context. That is, one wonders whether individuals who experience strong compelling environmental forces to continue a relationship are often satisfied with their relationships but not necessarily with their partners. Compelling environmental forces usually represent rewards received from the social and physical environment contingent on maintaining interaction with the partner, regardless of the nature of the interaction and its direct outcomes. The Internal Revenue Service, for example, allows parents to take tax deductions even if their interactions with their children are unrewarding, and permits married people to file joint returns whether or not they love their partners. One can speculate, then, that "satisfaction with the partner" may translate quickly into satisfaction with the quality of the interaction, whereas "satisfaction with the relationship" may be more highly correlated with the existence of strong compelling reasons to continue a relationship of this type. Again, this issue is in need of empirical investigation.

5. Of the 11 items on White and Booth's (1991) "marital happiness" scale, 8 assessed happiness with the partner, while only 3 had to do with the happiness of the marriage itself; this suggests that the scale may essentially may be a "happiness with partner" scale.

REFERENCES

Aron, A., Aron, E. N., & Smollan, D. (1992). Inclusion of Other in the Self Scale and the structure of interpersonal closeness. *Journal of Personality and Social Psychology, 63*, 596–612.

Attridge, M., & Berscheid, E. (1994). Entitlement in romantic relationships in the United States: A social-exchange perspective. In M. J. Lerner & G. Mikula (Eds.), *Entitlement and the affectional bond* (pp. 117–147). New York: Plenum Press.

Attridge, M., Berscheid, E., & Simpson, J. A. (1995). Predicting relationship stability from both partners versus one. *Journal of Personality and Social Psychology, 69*, 254–268.

Berscheid, E. (1994). Interpersonal relationships. *Annual Review of Psychology, 45*, 79–129.

Berscheid, E. (in press). A social psychological view of marital dysfunction and stability. In T. N. Bradbury (Ed.), *The developmental course of marital dysfunction.* New York: Cambridge University Press.

Berscheid, E., & Campbell, B. (1981). The changing longevity of heterosexual close relationships: A commentary and forecast. In M. J. Lerner &

S. C. Lerner (Eds.), *The justice motive in social behavior* (pp. 209–234). New York: Plenum Press.

Berscheid, E., & Graziano, W. (1979). The initiation of social relationships and interpersonal attraction. In R. L. Burgess & T. L. Huston (Eds.), *Social exchange in developing relationships* (pp. 31–60). New York: Academic Press.

Berscheid, E., & Reis, H. T. (in press). Attraction and close relationships. In S. Fiske, D. Gilbert, & G. Lindzey (Eds.), *Handbook of social psychology* (4th ed.). New York: McGraw-Hill.

Blais, M. R., Sabourin, S., Boucher, C., & Vallerand, R. J. (1990). Toward a motivational model of couple happiness. *Journal of Personality and Social Psychology, 59,* 1021–1031.

Brown, B. B., Werner, C. M., & Altman, I. (1994). Close relationships in environmental context. In A. L. Werner & J. H. Harvey (Eds.), *Perspectives on close relationships* (pp. 340–358). Needham Heights, MA: Allyn & Bacon.

Buss, D. M., & Barnes, M. (1986). Preferences in human mate selection. *Journal of Personality and Social Psychology, 50,* 559–570.

Festinger, L. (1954). A theory of social comparison processes. *Human Relations, 7,* 117–140.

Fletcher, G. J. O., Fincham, F. D., Cramer, L., & Heron, N. (1987). The role of attributions in the development of dating relationships. *Journal of Personality and Social Psychology, 53,* 481–489.

Fletcher, G. J. O., & Kininmonth, L. A. (1992). Measuring relationship beliefs: An individual differences scale. *Journal of Research in Personality, 26,* 371–397.

Freedman, J. (1978). *Happy people: What happiness is, who has it, and why.* New York: Harcourt Brace Jovanovich.

Glenn, N. D. (1990). Quantitative research on marital quality in the 1980's: A critical review. *Journal of Marriage and the Family, 52,* 818–831.

Glenn, N. D., & Weaver, C. N. (1988). The changing relationship of marital status to reported happiness. *Journal of Marriage and the Family, 50,* 317–324.

Heaton, T. B., & Albrecht, S. L. (1991). Stable unhappy marriages. *Journal of Marriage and the Family, 50,* 747–758.

Heider, F. (1958). *The psychology of interpersonal relations.* New York: Wiley.

Homans, G. (1979). Foreword. In R. L. Burgess & T. L. Huston (Eds.), *Social exchange in developing relationships* (pp. xv–xxii). New York: Academic Press.

Johnson, D. J., & Rusbult, C. E. (1989). Resisting temptation: Devaluation of alternative partners as a means of maintaining commitment in close relationships. *Journal of Personality and Social Psychology, 57,* 967–980.

Johnson, D. R., Amoloza, T. O., & Booth, A. (1992). Stability and developmental change in marital quality: A three-wave panel analysis. *Journal of Marriage and the Family, 54,* 582–594.

Johnson, M. P. (1982). Social and cognitive features of the dissolution of commitment to relationships. In S. Duck (Ed.), *Personal relationships 4: Dissolving personal relationships* (pp. 51–73). New York: Academic Press.

Johnson, M. P. (1991a). Commitment to personal relationships. In W. H. Jones

& D. Perlman (Eds.), *Advances in personal relationships* (Vol. 3, pp. 117–143). London: Jessica Kingsley.

Johnson, M. P. (1991b). Reply to Levinger and Rusbult. In W. H. Jones & D. Perlman (Eds.), *Advances in personal relationships* (Vol. 3, pp. 171–176). London: Jessica Kingsley.

Karney, B. R., & Bradbury, T. N. (1995). The longitudinal course of marital quality and stability: A review of theory, method, and research. *Psychological Bulletin, 118*, 3–34.

Kelley, H. H. (1979). *Personal relationships: Their structures and processes.* New York: Wiley.

Kelley, H. H. (1983). Love and commitment. In H. H. Kelley, E. Berscheid, A. Christensen, J. H. Harvey, T. L. Huston, G. Levinger, E. McClintock, L. A. Peplau, & D. L. Peterson, *Close relationships* (pp. 265–314). New York: Freeman.

Kelley, H. H., Berscheid, E., Christensen, A., Harvey, J. H., Huston, T. L., Levinger, G., McClintock, E., Peplau, L. A., & Peterson, D. L. (1983). *Close relationships.* New York: Freeman.

Kelley, H. H., & Thibaut, J. W. (1978). *Interpersonal relations: A theory of interdependence.* New York: Wiley.

Kelly, E. L., & Conley, J. J. (1987). Personality and compatibility: A prospective analysis of marital stability and marital satisfaction. *Journal of Personality and Social Psychology, 52*, 27–40.

Kurdek, L. A. (1993). Predicting marital dissolution: A 5-year prospective longitudinal study of newlywed couples. *Journal of Personality and Social Psychology, 64*, 221–242.

Kurdek, L. A. (1996). The deterioration of relationship quality for gay and lesbian cohabiting couples: A five year prospective longitudinal study. *Personal Relationships, 3*, 417–442.

Lee, G. R., Seccombe, K., & Shehan, C. L. (1991). Marital status and personal happiness: An analysis of trend data. *Journal of Marriage and the Family, 53*, 839–844.

Levinger, G. (1965). A social psychological perspective on marital dissolution: An integrative review. *Journal of Marriage and the Family, 27*, 19–29.

Levinger, G. (1974). A three-level approach to attraction: Toward an understanding of pair relatedness. In T. L. Huston (Ed.), *Foundations of interpersonal attraction* (pp. 100–120). New York: Academic Press.

Levinger, G. (1976). A social psychological perspective on marital dissolution. *Journal of Social Issues, 32*(1), 21–47.

Levinger, G. (1991). Commitment vs. cohesiveness: Two complementary perspectives. In W. H. Jones & D. Perlman (Eds.), *Advances in personal relationships* (Vol. 3, pp. 145–150). London: Jessica Kingsley.

Levinger, G. (1994). Figure versus ground: Micro- and macroperspectives on the social psychology of personal relationships. In R. Erber & R. Gilmour (Eds.), *Theoretical frameworks for personal relationships* (pp. 1–28). Hillsdale, NJ: Erlbaum.

Levinger, G. (in press). Duty toward whom? Reconsidering attractions, barriers, and commitment in a relationship. In W. H. Jones & J. M. Adams

(Eds.), *Handbook of interpersonal commitment and relationship stability*. New York: Plenum Press.

Lewin, K. (1951). *Field theory in social science*. New York: Harper.

Lindahl, K., Clements. M., & Markman, H. (in press). The development of marriage: A nine-year perspective. In T. Bradbury (Ed.), *The developmental course of marital dysfunction*. New York: Cambridge University Press.

Locke, H. J., & Wallace, K. M. (1959). Short marital adjustment and prediction tests: Their reliability and validity. *Marriage and Family Living, 21,* 251–255.

Martin, T., & Bumpass, L. (1989). Recent trends in marital disruption. *Demography, 26,* 37–52.

Murstein, B. (1970). Stimulus–value–role: A theory of marital choice. *Journal of Marriage and the Family, 32,* 465–481.

Nock, S. L. (1995). Commitment and dependency in marriage. *Journal of Marriage and the Family, 57,* 503–514.

Reis, H. T., & Shaver, P. (1988). Intimacy as an interpersonal process. In S. W. Duck (Ed.), *Handbook of personal relationships* (pp. 367–389). Chichester, England: Wiley.

Rempel, J. K., Holmes, J. G., & Zanna, M. P. (1985). Trust in close relationships. *Journal of Personality and Social Psychology, 49,* 95–112.

Rusbult, C. E. (1983). A longitudinal test of the investment model: The development (and deterioration) of satisfaction and commitment in heterosexual involvements. *Journal of Personality and Social Psychology, 45,* 101–117.

Rusbult, C. E. (1991). Commentary on Johnson's "Commitment to personal relationships": What's interesting, and what's new? In W. H. Jones & D. Perlman (Eds.), *Advances in personal relationships* (Vol. 3, pp. 151–169). London: Jessica Kingsley.

Seligman, C., Fazio, R. H., & Zanna, M. P. (1980). Effects of salience of extrinsic rewards on liking and loving. *Journal of Personality and Social Psychology, 38,* 453–460.

Simpson, J. A., Gangestad, S. W., & Lerma, M. (1990). Perception of physical attractiveness: Mechanisms involved in the maintenance of romantic relationships. *Journal of Personality and Social Psychology, 59,* 1192–1201.

Stanley, S. M., & Markman, H. J. (1992). Assessing commitment in personal relationships. *Journal of Marriage and the Family, 54,* 595–608.

Thibaut, J. W., & Kelley, H. H. (1959). *The social psychology of groups*. New York: Wiley.

Udry, J. R. (1981). Marital alternatives and marital disruption. *Journal of Marriage and the Family, 43,* 889–897.

White, L. K. (1990). Determinants of divorce: A review of research in the eighties. *Journal of Marriage and the Family, 52,* 904–912.

White, L. K., & Booth, A. (1991). Divorce over the life course: The role of marital happiness. *Journal of Family Issues, 12*(1), 5–21.

Zimmer, T. A. (1986). Premarital anxieties. *Journal of Social and Personal Relationships, 3,* 149–160.

CHAPTER 7

Marital Satisfaction and Spousal Interaction

JUDITH A. FEENEY
PATRICIA NOLLER
CARLA WARD

THE CHANGING MARRIAGE

What makes for a happy marriage? In the past, marital researchers tended to rely on demographic variables (e.g., education, income) to predict marital success. However, changes in the functions and goals of marriage have resulted in less emphasis on demographic predictors. Whereas marriage was previously seen as a union of economy, designed to reinforce and strengthen social class lines (Duby, 1983), romantic love and attraction have since become important parts of the marital equation. Accordingly, patterns of interaction between spouses are now regarded as key predictors of marital satisfaction. In these days of growing divorce rates, it would seem imperative to understand the forces that can bind a relationship together or, alternatively, encourage its dissolution. Research into marital satisfaction has been prolific; theory construction, however, has been less common. A notable exception has been the work of Lewis and Spanier (1979).

LEWIS AND SPANIER'S MODEL
OF MARITAL QUALITY

Lewis and Spanier (1979; Spanier & Lewis, 1980) extensively reviewed the literature on marital satisfaction, quality, and happiness (terms that tend to be used interchangeably). The focus of their review was on trying to "better understand the complex interrelationship between the host of variables which are purported to be related to the quality and stability of marriage" (p. 268). Based on this review, Lewis and Spanier developed a model of marital quality that emphasized three main sets of variables as predictors of marital quality: (1) social and personal resources (the resources that each individual brings into the marriage, such as self-esteem, mental and physical health, and abilities); (2) satisfaction with lifestyle (including household composition, satisfaction with wife's working, and extent of support from friends, relatives, and the community); and (3) rewards from spousal interaction (including role fit, communication effectiveness, and amount of interaction). These sets of variables, and their proposed relation to marital quality, are summarized in Figure 7.1.

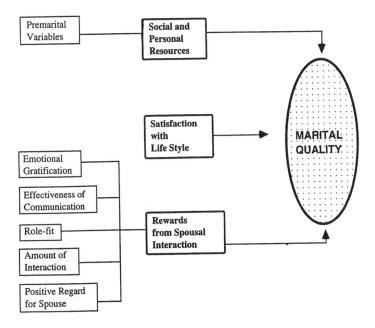

FIGURE 7.1. A model of marital quality (Lewis & Spanier, 1979).

In this chapter, we focus on the third set of variables—that is, rewards from spousal interaction. As Figure 7.1 shows, Lewis and Spanier discuss five dimensions of such rewards: positive regard for spouse (including perceived similarity, attractiveness, ease of communication), emotional gratification (expressions of love and affection, emotional interdependence), communication effectiveness (self-disclosure, empathy, accuracy of nonverbal communication), role fit (role sharing, role complementarity), and amount of interaction (shared activities, effective problem solving). We chose to focus on these proposed rewards from spousal interaction, because interactions between spouses are particularly central to the marital relationship. Such interactions both reflect and shape the day-to-day functioning of a couple, and are an appropriate focus for increasing our understanding of marital quality. Also, as we have noted above, the "romantic" view of marriage highlights the importance of issues concerning spousal interaction.

In this chapter, we discuss research in which our primary goals were (1) to see whether married couples describe their marital interactions in terms of the five dimensions proposed by Lewis and Spanier; (2) to check whether these five dimensions are relevant to marital satisfaction in the 1990s; and (3) to see whether some or all of these dimensions help to explain the frequently reported finding that marital quality tends to change over the lifespan (Lerner & Spanier, 1979; Olson, McCubbin, Larsen, Muxen, & Wilson, 1983).

WHAT ARE THE IMPORTANT DIMENSIONS OF MARITAL QUALITY?

Again, Lewis and Spanier's (1979) model was based on a review of the research on predictors of marital quality. From this review, a set of 38 propositions was generated concerning the relations between marital quality and specific aspects of marital interaction—for example, having mutual respect, having similar personalities, having a mutually pleasurable sexual relationship, being good companions, and having a deep love for each other. These propositions were then grouped together, according to the major themes that they seemed to represent; these themes are the five dimensions of rewards from spousal interaction shown in Figure 7.1. An important goal of our research was to see whether married couples perceive their interactions in terms of these five dimensions—a task that, to our knowledge, has not previously been undertaken.

Although no previous research has looked specifically at the five dimensions proposed by Lewis and Spanier, the question of which dimensions underlie marital quality has been addressed more generally by a considerable body of research. Much of this research has reported two main dimensions of marital quality, which seem to be largely independent of each other: one that includes sources of satisfaction from the relationship, such as shared activities, warmth, understanding and involvement, and one that includes sources of dissatisfaction from the relationship, such as indifference, lack of involvement, quarreling and arguments (Gilford & Bengtson, 1979; Marini, 1976; Orden & Bradburn, 1968). In a similar way, Argyle and Furnham (1983) explored the dimensions of relationships at a more general level (including relationships between neighbors, friends, and spouses), and found evidence for both positive dimensions (instrumental reward, emotional support, and shared interests) and negative dimensions (emotional conflict and criticism). Despite the considerable support for positive and negative factors as separate aspects of marital quality, the focus in Lewis and Spanier's (1979) work on rewards from spousal interaction is more clearly on the positive aspects of the marital relationship.

ASSESSING MARITAL QUALITY

What kind of items are best suited to assessing marital quality? There has been considerable debate about whether measures of marital quality should include evaluative items, descriptive items, or both (e.g., Norton, 1983). "Evaluative" items are those that ask the individual to make a global evaluation of his or her marriage (e.g., "I have a good marriage"), whereas "descriptive" items assess specific marital behaviors (e.g., the extent to which spouses engage in joint activities, the way they make decisions, etc.).

Two main arguments have been made against the use of descriptive items (Norton, 1983). The first argument is that these items presuppose particular models of marriage; for example, it is assumed that leaving the house after a fight is always negative. On the other hand, it should be noted that if the models of marriage underlying descriptive items are soundly based in empirical research, then such items are likely to be valuable indices of marital quality. The second argument against descriptive measures of marital quality is that the behaviors described in these items are often similar to other variables that researchers wish to study (e.g., communication, decision making; Norton, 1983). In other words, if marital quality is assessed by means of descriptive items, relations between marital quality and some other variables may be overestimated because of the partial overlap in item content. Given that the 38 propositions of Lewis and Spanier (1979) are descriptive in nature, a secondary goal of our research was to look at the relations between these variables and previous measures of marital quality, both evaluative and descriptive.

STAGE OF THE LIFE CYCLE AND MARITAL QUALITY

There is evidence that couples' reports of marital quality vary across the life cycle (Gilford & Bengtson, 1979; Lerner & Spanier, 1979; Olson et al., 1983). However, studies in this area have produced contradictory findings concerning the *nature* of these changes (Finkel & Hansen, 1992). Some studies have shown a relatively steady increase in quality over the course of marriage (e.g., Gilford, 1986), whereas others have found that marital quality tends to decline after the early years of marriage (Blood & Wolfe, 1960; Paris & Luckey, 1966). A third group of researchers has reported a more complex curvilinear pattern, in which marital quality increases over the early years of marriage, declines during the child-rearing and middle years, and increases again in the later years (Anderson, Russell, & Schumm, 1983; Rollins & Cannon, 1974; Rollins & Feldman, 1970).

Vaillant and Vaillant (1993) examined trends in marital satisfaction over the course of 40 years of marriage. As couples progressed through the marital life cycle, their satisfaction remained relatively stable, particularly in the middle and later years. On the other hand, when couples were asked to think back over their marriages and to rate their satisfaction at various points, there was some evidence of curvilinear patterns. Similarly, it has been argued that patterns of change in marital quality may depend on the methods used by the researchers: The curvilinear pattern seems to be more common in cross-sectional studies (which compare groups differing in length of marriage) than in longitudinal studies (which follow one group of couples over time). Some researchers have queried cross-sectional reports of an increase in satisfaction late in the life cycle; it is possible, for example, that this apparent increase partly reflects the loss of the most unhappy couples from "long-term married" groups because of divorce. Other researchers, however, have shown that cross-sectional reports of increased satisfaction in later life do not stem from other confounding variables, such as growing financial security (Anderson et al., 1983).

It also seems that different dimensions of marital quality may show different patterns of change over time. Gilford and Bengtson (1979) found that young couples were generally high on both positive and negative aspects of marital quality (sources of satisfaction and dissatisfaction), whereas older couples were moderately high on the positive aspects, but low on the negative aspects. Similarly, Argyle and Furnham (1983) found that young couples had lower levels of satisfaction and higher levels of conflict than older couples. These results suggest that the various dimensions of marital quality may show different patterns over the life cycle.

Given the conflicting findings in this area, a further goal of our research was to look at the effects of life cycle stage and the presence-absence of children on the different dimensions of marital quality. The effects of life cycle stages were assessed cross-sectionally, with subjects at different stages of the marital life cycle reporting on the current state of their relationships. For this reason, we expected to find curvilinear patterns for at least some of the factors being measured.

REWARDS FROM SPOUSAL INTERACTION: A PRELIMINARY TEST OF THE MODEL

To explore spouses' perceptions of their marital interactions, we first developed a 38-item questionnaire, based on the 38 propositions contained in the "rewards from spousal interaction" section of Lewis and Spanier's (1979) model (again, see Figure 7.1). As we explain in more detail later, each of the 38 items consisted of two parts: one in which subjects were asked to rate the extent to which a particular aspect of marital quality (e.g., having a mutually pleasurable sexual relationship, being good companions) characterized their current marital relationship, and a second in which they were asked to rate the importance of that particular characteristic to marriage in general.

We included the two sets of ratings because we wanted to assess subjects' perceptions not only of their own marriages, but also of the factors important to the quality of marriage *in general*. We expected that previous measures of marital quality would be less strongly related to dimensions based on the ratings of general importance than to those based on ratings of the current relationship; spouses may consider a particular aspect of marriage to be important, regardless of whether that aspect is present in their own marriage, and regardless of their overall perceptions of their own marital quality. In fact, it could be argued that spouses may sometimes see certain aspects of marriage as important precisely *because* those aspects are lacking in their own relationship.

As already indicated, our research questions focused on the major dimensions of marital interaction, on the links between these dimensions of marital interaction and previous measures of marital quality, and on changes in the dimensions of marital interaction across the life cycle. We expected that when the 38 items were rated in terms of individuals' own marriages, the dimensions derived from the items would be closely related to global evaluations of the quality of those marriages. We expected weaker relations between the importance dimensions and global evaluations of marital quality. We also expected the dimensions of marital interaction (rated in terms of individuals' own marriages) to vary with life cycle stage; in particular, we expected these dimensions generally to follow the curvilinear pattern described earlier, although we were open to the possibility that this pattern might not occur for all dimensions.

In a preliminary test of the theoretical model, 355 married people (170 husbands and 185 wives) completed a set of questionnaires, described below. The participants were recruited from the general community by students enrolled in a course on the family, as part of their required classwork. Each pair of students recruited six subjects—one male and one female in each of three categories of years married: 10 years or less, 11–20 years, and more than 20 years. Completed questionnaires were sealed for confidentiality, and were returned to us via the recruiting students. Participants were urged to fill in the questionnaires without consulting their partners, and only one member of any couple completed the questionnaires.

The length of participants' marriages ranged from 1 year to 52 years, with an average of about 16 years. Participants had an average of 1.97 children, a figure approximately equal to the national average for Australia; the number of children ranged from zero to six, and the number of children living at home ranged from zero to five. Of the total sample, 131 participants had no children living at home, and 89 had never had children. The sample represented a broad range of educational and occupational levels. One hundred and three subjects reported that they were not at all religious, 168 described themselves as somewhat religious, and 74 characterized themselves as very religious.

The main components of the set of questionnaires consisted of the items written to test the 38 propositions concerning rewards from spousal interaction (Lewis & Spanier, 1979). Two items were written to correspond with each proposition: one that assessed spouses' perceptions of the particular aspect of marital interaction within their own relationship, and one that assessed perceptions of the importance of that aspect of interaction to marriage in general. These two sets of 38 items are referred to here as the Quality of Dyadic Interaction Scale and the Importance of Dyadic Interaction Scale (or, for short, the Quality items and the Importance items), respectively. Each set of items was rated on a 6-point scale, from 1 = "totally disagree" to 6 = "totally agree." Table 7.1 shows sample Quality and Importance items for each of the five dimensions of rewards from spousal interaction described by Lewis and Spanier.

TABLE 7.1. Sample Items for the Five Dimensions of Rewards from Spousal Interaction Proposed by Lewis and Spanier

Dimension	Items from Quality of Dyadic Interaction Scale	Items from Importance of Dyadic Interaction Scale
Positive regard for spouse	My partner and I are similar in lots of ways.	It is important for partners to be similar to one another.
	My partner and I agree in our basic values.	It is important for partners to agree about basic values.
Emotional gratification	My partner and I are very affectionate to one another.	It is important for partners to be very affectionate to one another.
	My partner and I have a great deal of respect for one another.	It is important for partners to respect one another.
Communication effectiveness	My partner and I agree in our views of one another.	It is important for partners to agree in their views of one another.
	My partner and I are very understanding of each other.	It is important for partners to be understanding of one another.
Role fit	My partner and I are very compatible sexually.	It is important for partners to be sexually compatible.
	My partner and I are able to meet each other's needs.	It is important for partners to be able to meet each other's needs.
Amount of interaction	My partner and I are good companions to one another.	It is important for partners to be good companions to one another.
	My partner and I share a lot of activities.	It is important for partners to share a lot of activities.

In addition to the items based on Lewis and Spanier's model, spouses completed the Quality Marriage Index (QMI; Norton, 1983), which is a six-item measure of marital quality that uses only evaluative items. As already noted, Norton argued that evaluative items offer the advantage of avoiding overlap between the measure of marital quality and other variables of potential interest to researchers (such as communication). Five of the six QMI items were rated on a 7-point scale, from 1 = "not at all true" to 7 = "very true." The other item asked subjects to rate their marriages on a 7-point scale, from 1 = "extremely unhappy" to 7 = "perfectly happy." Scores on the QMI for the present sample ranged from 7 to 42, with a mean of 34.95. These figures show that the average level of reported marital happiness was quite high, but that the sample nevertheless spanned the full range from extremely unhappy to extremely happy.

Finally, spouses answered some background questions concerning their level of education (year 10 or 11, year 12, some tertiary education, university degree), religiosity (not at all religious, somewhat religious, very religious), length of marriage, number of children, and number of children currently living at home.

Major Dimensions of the Quality of Dyadic Interaction Scale

A prinicipal-component factor analysis was carried out on the items assessing spouses' perceptions of their current marital relationships. The purpose of this statistical technique is to find a limited set of factors (or dimensions) that describe the relationships among a larger set of variables (in this case, the 38 aspects of marital interaction). Those variables that are strongly interrelated tend to correlate with (or "load on") the same factor, and the factors are interpreted and labeled in terms of the variables that load highly on them.

Given that Lewis and Spanier (1979) described the rewards from spousal interaction in terms of five dimensions (positive regard for spouse, emotional gratification, communication effectiveness, role fit, and amount of interaction), we first tested whether the five-factor solution provided a good description of the data. Only one of our five factors corresponded to any of the five factors discussed by Lewis and Spanier. The first factor contained all nine items reflecting the effectiveness of communication, as described by Lewis and Spanier, but also contained four other items about communication and about meeting needs and expectations. Other factors included one predominantly about physical intimacy, one about respect and equality, and one about similarity and involvement. The final factor could not be interpreted with confidence, because it contained a single item about regular church attendance as a couple. Because of the lack of correspondence with Lewis and Spanier's proposed structure, together with the fact that one factor was defined by only a single item, the five-factor solution was not considered to describe the data adequately.

The most readily interpretable solution comprised three factors. The first factor was defined by 13 items; the items that loaded most highly on it were about the quality of the sexual relationship, expression of feelings, love, affection, attraction, and companionship. Based on the content of these items, this factor was labeled Intimacy. The second factor was defined by eight items, which focused on respect, consideration, equality, encouraging growth, and flexibility. This factor was labeled Respect. The third factor contained nine items, which were about having similar personalities, having similar views of the world and of each other, and meeting one another's expectations. This factor was labeled Consensus. Scales corresponding to each of the three factors were formed by summing participants' ratings on the relevant items. Each of the three scales showed high reliability (alpha coefficients ranged from .87 to .93).

Major Dimensions of the Importance of Dyadic Interaction Scale

The items in which spouses rated the importance of each aspect of marital interaction to marriage in general were analyzed in a similar way, and the analysis showed that these items were best described by two factors. The first factor was defined by 24 items; those with the highest loadings were about showing each other respect, communicating successfully, being good companions, and being understanding of each other. This factor was labeled Importance of Communication. The second factor contained 14 items, which focused on having similar personalities, seeing the world in similar ways, agreeing in views of each other, and fitting each other's ideal. This factor was labeled Importance of Consensus. Scores were again calculated for each of the two scales, which showed high reliability (alpha coefficients ranged from .82 to .92).

Relations between Quality and Importance Factors and Marital Quality

Mean scores on the Quality factors were relatively high. For example, the mean score for Intimacy was 61.75, with the possible range of scores being from 13 to 78. This result shows that, on average, participants saw their marriages as quite high in Intimacy, and also as high in Respect and Consensus. This finding is not surprising; in studies of marriage, community-based samples usually contain a large proportion of individuals who report high marital quality. (The high mean scores on the Quality factors are also consistent, of course, with the high mean score on the QMI.) Similarly, mean scores on the Importance factors tended to be high, indicating that most of the aspects of spousal interaction described by Lewis and Spanier (1979) were generally seen as quite important to marriage. For all five scales, however, there were substantial individual differences, with scores spanning almost the full possible range.

Correlations were calculated between the Quality and Importance factors and the QMI. For all three Quality factors, the correlations were greater than .65. This result suggests that the major dimensions of spousal interaction are indeed closely linked with spouses' global evaluations of their marriages. In other words, spouses who describe their marital interactions as high in Intimacy, Respect, and Consensus, as indicated by ratings of specific behaviors, tend to see their marriages as strong and stable.

Correlations between the Importance factors and the QMI were not nearly as strong (although these correlations were statistically significant, ranging from .19 to .36). This result was as expected; as noted earlier, spouses may see a particular aspect of marriage as important, regardless of whether that aspect is present in their own marriage, and regardless of their overall perceptions of their own marital quality.

Education, Religiosity, and Marital Quality

How do the background variables of education and religiosity relate to marital quality? At the start of this chapter, we have noted that research into marital quality has placed increasing emphasis on patterns of communication and interaction between spouses, rather than on demographic predictors of marital success. The background variables that we measured in this sample provided rather mixed findings with regard to the importance of demographic predictors of marital quality.

Educational level was related only to ratings of the Importance of Consensus. Specifically, those with higher levels of education rated consensus as less important to marriage than those with lower levels of education rated it. These more educated individuals seem to take the position that agreeing may not be the crucial issue in relationships, given that differences between spouses can often be accepted and/or resolved.

In contrast, religiosity was related to all three Quality factors, but not to the Importance factors. Higher levels of religiosity were associated with higher ratings of Intimacy, Respect, and Consensus. These results are consistent with a number of studies indicating that religiosity is predictive of marital adjustment, and suggesting more generally that religion provides a belief system that supports positive family life and constructive family behavior (see Thomas & Cornwall, 1990, for a review).

Gender and Marital Quality

Although some researchers have found that men tend to describe their relationships more positively than women do, results from this sample showed no gender differences in ratings of the three Quality factors.

Gender was related to the Importance of Communication scale, however, with women emphasizing the importance of communication to a much greater extent than men.

This finding fits with some of the claims of Tannen (1986, 1990), who discusses the different approaches of males and females to communication. She argues that females tend to see communication about relationship problems as providing opportunities for closeness, whereas men are more likely to be anxious about the outcome of such communication (see also Noller, 1993; Guthrie & Noller, 1988).

Length of Marriage, Number of Children, and Marital Quality

We have noted earlier that couples' reports of marital quality may vary across the life cycle: Researchers have variously reported that satisfaction increases over the course of marriage, declines over time, or shows a curvilinear pattern (increasing over the early years, declining during the middle years, and increasing again in the later years). In this sample, we tested for these various effects of length of marriage on marital quality. That is, we tested whether length of marriage has a simple relation with marital quality (with quality tending to increase or to decrease over the course of marriage), and we also tested for the more complex, or curvilinear, pattern.[1]

These analyses provided very little evidence of a simple relation between length of marriage and marital quality. By contrast, four of the five dimensions of marital quality showed a curvilinear link with length of marriage. Specifically, for all three Quality factors (Intimacy, Respect, and Consensus), higher marital satisfaction was reported by those in both early and late stages of their marriages than by those in the middle years. A similar curvilinear pattern was found for the Importance of Communication factor. The Importance of Consensus factor was not related to length of marriage, in terms of either the simple or the curvilinear pattern. The curvilinear patterns that we observed in this sample fit with the patterns found in other studies, such as those of Lerner and Spanier (1979) and Olson et al. (1983).

The most frequent explanation for the curvilinear relation between length of marriage and marital quality centers on the presence of children in the middle stages (Olson et al., 1983). Given this explanation, we were interested in comparing the levels of marital quality reported by three groups within our sample: those who had never had children, those who had children who were no longer living at home, and those who still had children living at home. The extent to which spouses endorsed the Importance of Consensus factor did not differ across these three groups (note that this factor was also unrelated to length of marriage). The remaining four factors, however, did differ across the three groups. Those who had never had children reported the highest levels of Intimacy in their own marriages, and also reported higher levels of Respect than those who had children living at home. Those who had children living at home reported the lowest levels of Consensus in their marriages. Those who had never had children endorsed the Importance of Communication factor to a greater extent than either of the other groups did.

Although these findings suggest that the presence of children has a negative impact on marital happiness, it is important to note that presence of children is likely to be confounded with length of marriage; in other words, groups that differ in terms of the presence–absence of children are likely to differ also in length of marriage. In order to separate out these two variables, we compared the marital quality reported by the three groups, after controlling for length of marriage; all the group differences described above remained significant. This finding suggests that the greater marital quality reported by those without children cannot be explained simply in terms of their having been married for a shorter length of time.

When we carried out additional analyses that focused on the effects of the actual *number* of children, we found that the number of children respondents had was related only to reports of Intimacy in the current marriage: Those who had more children reported less Intimacy in their spousal interactions. The number of children *currently living at home* was related primarily to perceptions of Consensus: Those who had more children living at home reported less Consensus in their marriages, and also assigned lower ratings to the Importance of Consensus.

REWARDS FROM SPOUSAL INTERACTION: A FURTHER TEST OF THE MODEL

The results that we have described so far support the argument that aspects of spousal interaction are very important to individuals' perceptions of marital quality. At the same time, it is not at all clear that the five dimensions of rewards from spousal interaction discussed by Lewis and Spanier provide the best description of patterns of marital interaction. For this reason, we decided to extend our research in several ways that would allow for a more powerful test of Lewis and Spanier's model.

In designing the next stage of the research, we wanted to overcome some limitations of the earlier work. First, all of the items we had developed for that work were worded positively—that is, in terms of favorable patterns of interaction between spouses. This form of wording is consistent with the way in which Lewis and Spanier's propositions were originally phrased, but may have precluded the possibility of finding separate factors related to sources of satisfaction and dissatisfaction, as obtained by some other researchers. That is, the wording of our items may have influenced the nature of the three Quality factors reported above, which focus on the more positive aspects of marriage, at the expense of negative aspects.

Second, and again with regard to the wording of the items, it should be noted that we wrote only one item to represent each of Lewis and Spanier's propositions. Unfortunately, a few of these propositions were double-barreled, and hence the corresponding items addressed more than one issue. For example, the item "My partner is very attractive to me both physically and mentally" contains two distinct ideas (physical attractiveness and mental attractiveness), which may have made it more difficult for spouses to give a reliable answer. There were also some items that included references to the behavior of both marital partners, and such items may also have been difficult to answer; for example, responding to the item "My partner and I are very affectionate to one another" may have been difficult for individuals who see their marriage as rather one-sided in terms of the giving of affection.

Finally, we wanted to study married *couples*, rather than married individuals. In the first stage of our research, our decision to use married individuals was primarily a pragmatic one; this procedure meant that the students who were recruiting subjects would need to get the cooperation of only one member of a couple, rather than both, and would not be so limited in the subjects available to them. By obtaining a sample of intact couples, however, researchers can look at the extent of agreement (i.e., the correlation) between spouses in their perceptions of their relationships. Couple data also provide a strong test of gender differences in marital quality: Because the husbands and wives in such a sample are describing the same marriages, any systematic difference between their reported levels of marital quality should reflect real differences in perception, rather than sampling artifacts.

In order to extend and strengthen the research, we collected data from a second sample. Before doing so, we made fairly substantial changes to the Quality of Dyadic Interaction Scale, as detailed below. A further change from the earlier work was that we recruited both members of couples, so that we could look at levels of agreement between partners. We also included an established measure of marital satisfaction that consisted of both evaluative and descriptive items, so that we could relate the Quality and the Importance factors to both types of items.

Finally, we were interested in the discrepancies between subjects' perceptions of the interactions in their *own* marriages, and their perceptions of the *ideal* marriage; for this reason, we calculated a "dissonance" score for each item, by subtracting the rating of the current relationship from the corresponding importance rating. In particular, we were interested in the relation between the dissonance scores and previous measures of marital satisfaction (both evaluative and descriptive).

We expected that the major dimensions of the Quality items would be generally similar to those found with the first sample (although the substantial number of additional items might produce a slightly different set of findings). As before, we also expected that the dimensions based on the Quality items would be closely related to the spouses' subjective assessments of the quality of their marriages. Once again, we expected weaker relations between the Importance dimensions and marital quality. In addition, we expected the dissonance scores to be closely related to measures of marital satisfaction. In line with the findings from the first sample, we expected that the dimensions of marital quality would vary with life cycle stage, and that they would generally follow a curvilinear pattern. We also expected the dimensions of marital quality to be related to the presence of children, with marital quality generally being higher where there were no children in the family.

For this stage of the research, we sampled 84 married couples. Some participants (but usually not their partners) came from a pool of introductory psychology students, and the rest were recruited from the general community. All participants were asked to complete the questionnaires without discussing the items with their spouses, to place each questionnaire in a separate envelope, and to return these two envelopes together to us.

Participants had been married for an average of approximately 12 years (with a range from 1 year to 46 years). The average number of children was 1.54; the number of children ranged from zero to six, and the number of children living at home also ranged from zero to six. Thirty-seven couples had no children living at home, and 29 couples had never had children. Educational levels again varied widely, from not completing high school to tertiary education. Sixty-nine subjects described themselves as not at all religious, 82 as somewhat religious, and 16 as very religious.

As before, the questionnaire package completed by spouses included the Quality of Dyadic Interaction Scale, the Importance of Dyadic Interaction Scale, an established measure of marital satisfaction, and demographic questions. The Quality and Importance measures were modified in terms of item format (as described below), but the items were rated on the same 6-point scale used in the original versions.

The Quality of Dyadic Interaction Scale was again based on Lewis and Spanier's 38 propositions concerning the rewards from spousal interaction. Some items were modified, however, to deal with the limitations of the earlier version. First, items that referred to more than one marital behavior, or to the behavior of more than one spouse, were rewritten. (Items that referred to similarity, compatibility, or communication between partners were kept as single items.) This change resulted in an expanded set of 58 items. For example, the proposition "The greater the expression of affection between spouses, the greater the marital quality" was represented in the earlier version by the item "My partner and I are very affectionate to one another"; the revised version used two items, "I am very affectionate towards my partner" and "My partner is very affectionate towards me." Second, in order to minimize response bias, half of the items were reworded in a negative direction. For example, the item "My partner and I are very compatible sexually" became "My partner and I are not very compatible sexually."

The only change to the Importance of Dyadic Interaction Scale involved the item referring to mental and physical attractiveness; this item was rewritten as two separate items, so that the importance of these two aspects of attractiveness could be rated separately. Thus the revised scale included 39 items.

The established measure of marital satisfaction completed by this sample was a short version of Snyder's (1979) Marital Satisfaction Inventory (MSI), a measure consisting of 280 items in a true–false format, forming 11 scales. We chose four scales that have proved particularly useful in distinguishing between happy and unhappy spouses; within each scale, items were chosen that loaded most highly on that particular factor of the MSI. The scales used were an evaluative scale, Global Distress (e.g., "My marriage has been disappointing in several ways"); two descriptive scales, Problem-Solving Communication (e.g., "Our arguments often end with an exchange of insults") and Affective Communication (e.g., "There is a great deal of love and affection expressed in our marriage"); and a scale assessing Conventionalization, or the tendency to portray one's marriage in a very favorable light (e.g., "My spouse has all of the qualities I have ever wanted in a mate"). As in the earlier sample, participants also answered background questions assessing educational level, religiosity, length of marriage, number of children, and number of children currently living at home.

Major Dimensions of the Revised Quality Scale

Because of the changes made to the items and to the sampling procedure, we conducted new principal-component factor analyses separately for the Quality and Importance items. The best solution for the 58 Quality items involved five factors. The factors were labeled Communication (10 items), Compatibility (6 items), Attraction (6 items), Respect (6 items), and Intimacy (5 items).

The items loading most highly on the Communication factor were about the partner's being very understanding and being able to relate to one's thoughts and feelings, and about successful communication between the spouses (see Table 7.2 for sample items). The highest-loading items on the Compatibility factor were about being understanding of the partner, being a good companion to the partner, and fitting the partner's ideal. Items loading highest on the Attraction factor were about sexual pleasure and compatibility, physical attraction, and having a deep love for the partner. Items loading highest on the Respect factor were about respecting the partner as a separate and unique person, the partner's having a deep love for the spouse, and the partner's being helpful and considerate toward the spouse. The highest-loading items on the Intimacy factor were about being highly emotionally involved in the partner's life, being able to express feelings and attitudes to the partner, and sharing deepest feelings with the partner. All five scales were highly reliable (alpha coefficients ranged from .74 to .87). Correlations between the factors were also high, ranging from .58 to .72.

TABLE 7.2. Sample Items for the Five Dimensions Obtained from the Quality of Dyadic Interaction Scale (Revised)

Dimension	Items
Communication	*My partner is unable to relate to my thoughts and feelings.
	My partner and I are able to communicate successfully with one another.
Compatibility	I am a very good companion to my partner.
	*I do not completely fit my partner's picture of an ideal partner.
Attraction	*My partner and I are not very compatible sexually.
	My partner is highly physically attractive to me.
Respect	I respect my partner as a separate and unique person.
	My partner is always considerate and helpful towards me.
Intimacy	*I am not highly emotionally involved in my partner's life.
	*I do not share my deepest feelings with my partner.

Note. Items preceded by an asterisk (*) loaded negatively on the associated factor, and were reverse-scored.

It is important to note that although the five Quality factors could be easily interpreted, they did *not* correspond to the five dimensions of rewards from spousal interaction described by Lewis and Spanier (1979). We come back to this point later (see "General Discussion" below). In that section, we also compare these Quality factors with those found in the first sample.

Major Dimensions of the Revised Importance Scale

The 39 items of the revised Importance of Dyadic Interaction Scale produced two factors that were readily interpretable. The pattern of correlations between the items and the two factors was very similar to that obtained with the first sample, and the two factors were again labeled Importance of Communication (13 items) and Importance of Consensus (6 items). The highest-loading items on the Importance of Communication factor were about spouses' respecting each other, being considerate and helpful, and communicating successfully and easily. The highest-loading items on the Importance of Consensus factor were about spouses' fitting each other's ideal, sharing spaces in the home, having similar personalities, and agreeing in views of each other. Reliability estimates were high (alpha coefficients ranged from .79 to .94), and the two factors were moderately intercorrelated ($r = .38$).

As before, mean scores for the five Quality factors and for the two Importance factors were toward the high end of possible scores. In other words, spouses in this sample tended to report positive patterns of marital interaction, and also perceived the various aspects of interaction as important to marriage in general. Again, however, there was substantial range on all of the factors.

Agreement between Spouses for Quality and Importance Factors

As we have noted earlier, studying married couples allows researchers to assess the extent to which husbands and wives agree in their perceptions of their relationships. To address this issue, we calculated correlations between husbands' and wives' scores for each factor (see Table 7.3). Agreement between husbands and wives was generally moderate to low. The level of agreement reached significance for Compatibility, Attraction, Respect, Intimacy, and Importance of Consensus; even for these factors, however, the amount of variance shared between husbands' and wives' reports was quite small, varying from only 5% to about 25%.

Interestingly, there was no significant agreement between husbands

TABLE 7.3. Agreement between Husbands
and Wives on Quality and Importance Factors

Factor	Extent of spousal agreement
Communication	.21
Compatibility	.23*
Attraction	.41***
Respect	.47***
Intimacy	.28**
Importance of Communication	− .11
Importance of Consensus	.41***

Note. *$p < .05$. **$p < .01$. ***$p < .001$.

and wives in scores either on the Communication or the Importance of Communication factors. One reason for this result may have been the restricted range of scores on the scales assessing communication. The Importance of Communication scale was particularly problematic in this regard, with spouses' mean score being 72.47, and the highest possible score being 78. In other words, most participants saw communication as extremely important to marriage, and this fact may have tended to mask any link between the responses of husbands and wives.

Relations between the Quality and Importance Factors and the Marital Satisfaction Inventory Scales

Correlations were calculated between the five Quality and two Importance factors and the four scales of the MSI (Global Distress, Problem-Solving Communication, Affective Communication, and Conventionalization). Significant relations with the MSI scales were restricted almost completely to the Quality factors. Each of the five Quality factors showed significant correlations with each of the MSI scales; most of these correlations were about .50. By contrast, the Importance factors were only weakly related to the MSI scales. This result replicates the earlier finding that spouses may rate a given aspect of marriage as important, regardless of whether that aspect is seen as present in their own relationship.

Given that the MSI scales are well-established measures of marital satisfaction, the strong correlations between these scales and the five Quality factors suggest that the latter are valid indices of marital quality. These correlations also make sense intuitively; they show, for example, that spouses who rate their interactions with their partners as high in Respect also tend to rate their marriages as high in Affective and Problem-Solving Communication, and low in Global Distress.

At the same time, it is possible that the strong links between the Quality factors and the MSI scales might be attributable to a form of response bias, whereby some subjects consistently try to portray their relationships in a favorable light. To check this possibility, we conducted hierarchical multiple-regression analyses to predict each of the three major MSI scales (Global Distress, Problem-Solving Communication, Affective Communication) from the five Quality factors, controlling for the degree of marital conventionalization. The results showed that even after the MSI Conventionalization scores were controlled for, the Quality factors were closely related to the other three MSI scales.

"Dissonance" between Perceptions of the Current Relationship and of the Ideal Marriage

We have mentioned above that we were also interested in the discrepancies between subjects' perceptions of their own marital interactions, and their perceptions of the ideal marriage. As a measure of these discrepancies, "dissonance" scores were computed. These scores were defined by subtracting ratings of items on a particular Quality factor (e.g., Compatibility) from ratings of the corresponding Importance items. In this calculation, Quality items were reverse-scored where appropriate. In this way, five dissonance scores were obtained for each spouse (one for each Quality factor).

The five dissonance scores all correlated positively with MSI Global Distress. That is, spouses who saw their own marital interactions as falling short of the ideal were likely to rate their marriages as generally disappointing and unhappy. Similarly, those spouses who saw their marital interactions as falling short rated their marital communication (both Affective and Problem-Solving Communication on the MSI) as poor, and were less likely to describe their marriages in highly favorable ways.

Education, Religiosity, and Marital Quality

Again, we were interested in how the background variables of education and religiosity related to reports of marital quality. The only significant effect of education was for the Intimacy scale: Spouses with higher levels of education reported more Intimacy in their marriages. In contrast to findings from the previous sample, religiosity did not significantly predict any of the factors. This result may be attributable to differences between the two samples of subjects, with only a small minority of the second sample describing themselves as very religious.

Gender and Marital Quality

Gender was related to reports of Intimacy and Respect in participants' current relationships. Although, as noted earlier, some researchers have found that men describe their relationships more positively than women do, wives in this sample reported higher levels of Respect and Intimacy than husbands did. As in the previous sample, gender was also related to the Importance of Communication, with wives emphasizing the Importance of Communication to a much greater extent than husbands.

Length of Marriage, Number of Children, and Marital Quality

As in the previous sample, we tested for the effects of length of marriage on marital quality. Specifically, we tested whether length of marriage shows a simple relation with marital quality (i.e., increasing or decreasing quality over the course of marriage), and we also tested for curvilinear patterns over time.

There was again very little evidence of a simple relation between length of marriage and marital quality. In contrast, five of the seven scales showed a curvilinear link with length of marriage. Specifically, higher marital satisfaction was reported by those in both early and late stages of marriage for four of the five Quality factors: Compatibility, Attraction, Respect, and Intimacy. A similar pattern was found for the Importance of Consensus. Neither the Communication factor nor the Importance of Communication factor was reliably predicted from length of marriage, in terms of either simple or complex relations. Again, the curvilinear patterns observed in this research are consistent with previous research.

Given the earlier results suggesting that the presence of children may have a negative impact on marital happiness, the effects of presence of children were again assessed by comparing the marital quality reported by three groups of couples: those that had children still living at home, those that had children no longer at home, and those that had not had children. These analyses revealed significant differences among the three groups for all of the Quality factors, but not for the Importance factors. The strongest findings were that childless couples reported greater Compatibility, Respect, and Intimacy than those with children still living at home.

In discussing these results from the first sample, we have pointed out that the presence of children is likely to be confounded with length of marriage. To try to separate these effects, we again compared these three groups (those with children still at home, those with children no longer at home, and those without children), while controlling for length of marriage. The differences among the three groups were retained for all the Quality factors, but were reduced in size. These results suggest that the lower marital quality reported by those with children is partly a function of their greater length of marriage, and partly a function of the actual presence of children.

The total number of children in the family did not significantly predict any of the Quality or Importance factors. The number of children at home, however, was inversely related to Communication, Compatibility, Respect, and Intimacy. In other words, couples with more children living at home saw their marriages as characterized by fewer of these aspects of relationship quality.

GENERAL DISCUSSION

The Quality factors from the revised instrument only partially replicated those from the original version. This result is not surprising, given the substantial changes in item format across the two samples. Specifically, 20 new Quality items were added, because a number of items in the original set referred to more than one behavior or to more than one partner. In addition, for the revised instrument, half of the items were reworded in a negative direction.

Despite these substantial changes in item format, it is interesting to note that there were points of correspondence in the Quality factors across the two samples. When the major items defining the factors are examined, it seems that the Respect factor was relatively stable across the two versions; this result suggests that Respect is a very important and robust dimension of marital interaction. The Intimacy factor from the first sample divided into two factors in the expanded version: Attraction (with a focus on sexual compatibility, sexual satisfaction, and deep love) and Intimacy (with a focus on sharing of attitudes, feelings, and ideas). The Consensus factor also split into two factors: Compatibility (with an emphasis on meeting each other's expectations, seeing the world in similar ways, and understanding each other), and Communication (with an emphasis on partners' understanding, communicating successfully, and agreeing in views of each other).

Although the five-factor solution from our revised instrument provided the best description of the data, it did not replicate the five hypothetical dimensions discussed by Lewis and Spanier (1979). For example, the Compatibility factor from our second sample cut across Lewis and Spanier's dimensions; it included items from four of their five dimensions, with no more than two items coming from any one of them.

In attempting to explain the poor correspondence between the present dimensions and those advanced by these theorists, it is useful to examine the original classification of their propositions. Although their items were based on an extensive review of empirical studies, their decisions about how to *group* the items were conceptually driven. More importantly, it appears to us that at least some of the items do not have high face validity for the category in which they were placed. For example, the item pertaining to sharing deepest feelings seems to involve the quality or effectiveness of communication (or intimacy), rather than the amount of interaction. Similarly, the item about communicating easily seems to involve the quality or effectiveness of communication, rather than positive regard for spouse. There also seems to be no compelling reason for including the item about seeing each other as equals within the category of emotional gratification (which centers on the expression of affection between spouses).

An interesting issue addressed by this research is whether the behaviors suggested by Lewis and Spanier as predictive of marital quality are as important in the 1990s as in the '60s and '70s. The results we have presented suggest that most of the specific behaviors (e.g., aspects of communication, respect for spouse) included in their model are still relevant today. However, as we have noted above, the broad categories that are defined by these behaviors (see Figure 7.2) do not conform closely to those proposed by Lewis and Spanier (Figure 7.1).

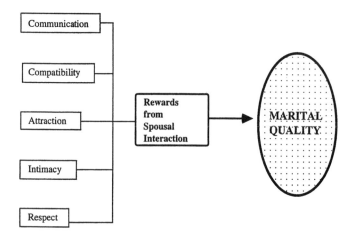

FIGURE 7.2. Dimensions of rewards from spousal interaction found in the present research.

Despite the fact that most of the specific behaviors discussed by Lewis and Spanier appear to be relevant today, issues concerning role fit (or the absence of role conflict) did *not* emerge as important in the current research. Most of the items reflecting the role fit category did not load on any of the five Quality factors. The only exception was the item concerning sexual compatibility, which loaded on the Attraction factor in the present research. It would seem that our subjects saw the question of sexual compatibility as part of the broader issue of love, sex, and attraction, rather than in terms of role fit or role conflict.

The Quality dimensions found in the present research show only limited overlap with those from previous studies of marital satisfaction. There is some agreement between the present factor structure and that reported by Spanier and Cole (1974); in particular, the Attraction factor in the present study is similar to the factor that they labeled Affection. In addition, the basic themes in the present Compatibility and Intimacy factors show partial overlap with Spanier and Cole's Consensus and Cohesion factors, respectively.

In contrast to the work of Argyle and Furnham (1983) and Gilford and Bengtson (1979), however, all of our Quality factors reflected positive aspects of marital interaction. Perhaps the presence of only positive factors is related to the way in which Lewis and Spanier set up their model, which focused on positive aspects of marital interaction. Note that even though half of the items were worded negatively in the revised instrument, still only positive factors emerged. Perhaps it is necessary to include items that explicitly deal with conflict, arguments, and disagreements, in order to obtain negative factors.

Unlike the Quality factors, the Importance factors were replicated quite closely across our two samples. In fact, all of the items that loaded on either of the Importance factors in Sample 1 also loaded on the same factor in Sample 2. In Sample 1, however, each factor was defined by more items; this may have been so because the larger sample in Study 1 provided a somewhat stronger picture of the dimensions underlying the item set. The fact that the structure of the Importance items was relatively stable suggests that the two factors that were obtained reflect major issues that couples see as critical aspects of marital quality. This stability may also be explained, at least in part, by the fact that only a single item was added to the Importance set for the second sample.

It is interesting to note that, as with the Quality factors, the Importance factors contained very few items from Lewis and Spanier's role fit category. Indeed, no item from this category loaded consistently on either Importance factor across the two samples. It seems that issues concerning role expectations and role performances are not generally seen as central to marriage today, possibly because changing patterns of participation in the work force have resulted in more varied and more flexible ways of managing the demands of work and family.

As we have noted above, the stability of the two Importance factors suggests that these factors reflect issues that are central to marital quality. In fact, it is possible to see the two Importance factors as defining two different models of marital quality. The first model involves an emphasis on the importance of communication as the process by which relationships are built and maintained. Via communication, differences between spouses can be resolved and issues dealt with, even when there are not high levels of consensus initially. The second model involves an emphasis on the importance of similarity, agreement and compatibility; there seems to be an implication that communication is not nearly so important in relationships where there are high levels of agreement, and similarity. Because there was a low to moderate correlation between the two factors, it is clearly possible for couples to endorse both models to some extent. It is interesting to note that in the first sample, those with higher levels of education were less likely to endorse the compatibility model.

The Quality factors from the current research related strongly to an evaluative measure of marital quality in the first sample, and to both evaluative (MSI Global Distress) and descriptive (MSI Affective Communication and Problem-Solving Communication) scales in the second sample. We also found that the dissonance scores, which reflect the difference between perceptions of real and ideal marriages, were highly correlated with both evaluative and descriptive measures of marital quality. Although the Quality factors and the dissonance scores were strongly related to previous measures of satisfaction and to MSI Conventionalization, it would seem clear that these results cannot be explained simply in terms of a global response bias: The Quality factors were only weakly related to the Importance factors, and responses to the Importance factors were not reliably related to previous measures of marital quality.

We would also argue that the fact that the MSI Conventionalization scale was quite strongly related to the Quality factors and the dissonance scores is not necessarily problematic. If one's marriage is perceived to be close to the ideal, then it is possible that very high scores on all these measures reflect honest reporting. That is, people may report high levels of satisfaction because they are indeed, satisfied with their marriages. The generally accepted assumption seems to be that marital quality and marital conventionalization are highly correlated because marital quality measures are contaminated by a social desirability artifact. However, research consistently shows that a substantial proportion of respondents see their marriages as very successful (Edmonds, 1967; Russell & Wells, 1992); this finding is likely to reflect respondents' genuine positivity about their relationships, as well as a tendency to present them in a favorable light. The results of the present study suggest that dissonance scores may also be effective as an index of marital satisfaction, because they focus on the extent to which one's actual marriage differs from one's ideal marriage.

The extent of agreement between husbands and wives was significant for four of the five Quality factors (Compatibility, Attraction, Respect, and Intimacy), as well as for the Importance of Consensus factor. Although the agreement was far from perfect, and the correlations did not explain a large percentage of the variance, this relatively low level of agreement between partners is not unusual in research in the marital area. Bernard (1964) argued that some spouses see their relationships so differently that it is possible to think in terms of "his marriage" and "her marriage." The fact that the extent of agreement between spouses did not reach significance for either the Communication factor or the Importance of Communication factor is in keeping with the claims made by Tannen (1990), who addresses the different communication styles of men and women. She argues for a cultural explanation of these differences, and suggests that whereas women see talk as strengthening relationships, men tend to see talk as indicative of problems and as likely to weaken relationships.

We found that length of marriage had a curvilinear relation with four of the five Quality factors: Compatibility, Attraction, Respect, and Intimacy. In other words, those in the middle years of marriage tend to report lower marital quality than those in either the early or the later years. It is important to keep in mind, however, that, as in the present research, this issue has generally been addressed with cross-sectional rather than longitudinal data. A detailed study of 17 long-term marriages (using retrospective data) found that although the curvilinear pattern was the most common, there were also small groups of couples whose members were stable in their evaluations of their relationships, whether those evaluations were positive, negative, or neutral (Weishaus & Field, 1988).

There was no relation between length of marriage and the quality of communication, either simple or curvilinear. This finding supports previous research (e.g., Noller, Feeney, Bonnell, & Callan, 1994) in suggesting that spouses are either good communicators or poor ones. That is, communication patterns are likely to be relatively stable over time, unless some intervention takes place.

The findings with regard to the presence of children were similar to those for length of marriage, suggesting that the curvilinear relation between length of marriage and marital quality may be attributable, at least in part, to the presence of children in the family during the middle years. In considering the effects of children on marital happiness, it is interesting to note that the highest ratings of Intimacy and Respect in the current relationship were made by those who had never had children. These couples also gave the Importance of Communication very high ratings. Together, these findings may reflect the greater opportunities for intimacy among these couples; in addition, childless couples may have fewer issues about which to disagree. This interpretation is supported by the finding that couples with children living at home reported lower Consensus in their relationships than other couples did.

The research described here has two main limitations. The first limitation is the cross-sectional nature of the design, with comparisons being made across the stages of marriage, rather than within subjects. It is possible that different results may have been obtained had subjects' relationships been assessed longitudinally. The second limitation concerns the factor analysis of the Quality items in the second sample: Given the large number of items in the expanded questionnaire, the sample size was smaller than optimal. This limitation was offset by the recruiting of couples, rather than just married individuals. Having to obtain the cooperation of both members of a couple tends to make the recruitment of subjects more difficult, although additional research questions can be addressed.

SUMMARY

In this chapter, we have reported on research that provides a partial test of Lewis and Spanier's (1979) model of marital quality, focusing on their proposed "rewards from spousal interaction." We initially developed a questionnaire that was derived from the 38 propositions contained in Lewis and Spanier's model, and that assessed both the quality of the subject's own relationship and the perceived importance of each behavior to marriage. Factor analyses revealed three Quality factors (Intimacy, Respect, and Consensus) and two Importance factors (Importance of Communication and Importance of Consensus).

In extending this research, we recruited a sample of married couples, expanded the set of items, and included a measure of social desirability (conventionalization) and more detailed measures of marital satisfaction. Factor analysis of the Quality of Dyadic Interaction Scales yielded five factors, similar in many ways to the three found with the previous sample. For the Importance items, the same two factors were found as in the first sample. The five Quality factors were related to previous measures of marital satisfaction, and to variables such as years married and presence of children.

Together, these two studies have enabled us to test the validity of Lewis and Spanier's (1979) model, which proposes that rewards from spousal interaction constitute an important aspect of marital quality. Certainly it seems that many of Lewis and Spanier's propositions are still strongly related to marital quality in the 1990s, although the factors found in this research are different in a number of respects from those of Lewis and Spanier. These differences may stem in part from changes in ideas about what makes a marital relationship satisfying. Communication was generally seen as a particularly crucial aspect of marital relationships. Differences in results for the Quality factors and the Importance factors suggest that subjects were able to discriminate clearly between the state of their own relationships and the importance of various behaviors to marriage in general.

ACKNOWLEDGMENT

An earlier version of this chapter was presented at the National Council on Family Relations Conference, Baltimore, Maryland, November 1993.

NOTE

1. These tests were made by means of regression analysis, in which the aim is to predict scores on some criterion variable (in this case, marital quality) from other relevant variables—in this case, both the simple scores and the "quadratic term" for length of marriage, with the quadratic term providing a test of the curvilinear relation.

REFERENCES

Anderson, S., Russell, C., & Schumm, W. (1983). Perceived marital quality and family life-cycle categories: A further analysis. *Journal of Marriage and the Family, 45*, 127–139.

Argyle, M., & Furnham, A. (1983). Sources of satisfaction and conflict in long-term relationships. *Journal of Marriage and the Family, 45*, 481–492.

Bernard, J. (1964). The adjustment of married mates. In H. T. Christensen (Ed.), *Handbook of marriage and the family* (pp. 675–739). Chicago: Rand McNally.

Blood, R. O., & Wolfe, D. M. (1960). *Husbands and wives: The dynamics of married living.* Glencoe, IL: Free Press.

Duby, G. (1983). *The knight, the lady and the priest: The making of a modern marriage in medieval France.* New York: Pantheon.

Edmonds, V. H. (1967). Marital conventionalization: Definition and measurement. *Journal of Marriage and the Family, 29,* 681–688.

Finkel, J. S., & Hansen, F. J. (1992). Correlates of retrospective marital satisfaction in long-lived marriages: A social constructivist perspective. *Family Therapy, 19,* 1–16.

Gilford, R. (1986). Marriages in later life. *Generations, 10,* 16–20.

Gilford, R., & Bengtson, V. L. (1979). Measuring marital satisfaction in three generations: Positive and negative dimensions. *Journal of Marriage and the Family, 41,* 387–398.

Guthrie, D. M., & Noller, P. (1988). Spouses' perceptions of one another in emotional situations. In P. Noller & M. A. Fitzpatrick (Eds.), *Monographs in social psychology of language: No. 1. Perspectives on marital interaction* (pp. 153–181). Clevedon, England: Multilingual Matters.

Lerner, R. M., & Spanier, G. B. (1979). *Child influences on marital and family interaction: A lifespan perspective.* New York: Academic Press.

Lewis, R. A., & Spanier, G. B. (1979). Theorizing about the quality and stability of marriage. In W. R. Burr, R. Hill, F. I. Nye, & I. L. Reiss (Eds.), *Contemporary theories about the family* (Vol. 1, pp. 268–294). New York: Free Press.

Marini, M. (1976). Dimensions of marriage happiness: A research note. *Journal of Marriage and the Family, 38,* 443–448.

Noller, P. (1993). Gender and emotional communication in marriage: Different cultures or differential social power. *Journal of Language and Social Psychology, 12,* 92–102.

Noller, P., Feeney, J. A., Bonnell, D., & Callan, V. J. (1994). A longitudinal study of conflict in early marriage. *Journal of Social and Personal Relationships, 11,* 233–252.

Norton, R. (1983). Measuring marital quality: A critical look at the dependent variable. *Journal of Marriage and the Family, 45,* 141–151.

Olson, D. H., McCubbin, H. I., Larsen, H. L., Muxen, M. J., & Wilson, M. A. (1983). *Families: What makes them work?* Beverly Hills, CA: Sage.

Orden, S. R., & Bradburn, N. M. (1968). Dimensions of marriage happiness. *American Journal of Sociology, 73,* 715–731.

Paris, B. L., & Luckey, E. B. (1966). A longitudinal study in marital satisfaction. *Sociology and Social Research, 50,* 212–222.

Rollins, B. C., & Cannon, K. (1974). Marital satisfaction over the life-cycle: A reevaluation. *Journal of Marriage and the Family, 36,* 271–292.

Rollins, B. C., & Feldman, H. (1970). Marital satisfaction over the family life-cycle. *Journal of Marriage and the Family, 32,* 20–28.

Russell, R. J., & Wells, P. A. (1992). Social desirability and quality of marriage. *Personality and Individual Differences, 13,* 787–791.

Snyder, D. K. (1979). Multidimensional assessment of marital satisfaction. *Journal of Marriage and the Family, 41,* 813–823.

Spanier, G. B., & Cole, C. (1974). Toward clarification and investigation of marital adjustment. *International Journal of Sociology of the Family, 6,* 121–146.

Spanier, G. B., & Lewis, R. A. (1980). Marital quality: A review of the seventies. *Journal of Marriage and the Family, 42,* 825–839.

Tannen, D. (1986). *That's not what I meant: How conversational styles make or break relationships.* New York: Ballantine Books.

Tannen, D. (1990). *You just don't understand.* New York: Ballantine Books.

Thomas, D. L., & Cornwall, M. (1990). Religion and family in the 1980s: Discovery and development. *Journal of Marriage and the Family, 52,* 983–992.

Vaillant, C. O., & Vaillant, G. E. (1993). Is the U-curve of marital satisfaction an illusion? A 40-year study of marriage. *Journal of Marriage and the Family, 55,* 230–239.

Weishaus, S., & Field, D. (1988). A half-century of marriage: Continuity or change? *Journal of Marriage and the Family, 50,* 763–774.

CHAPTER 8

---·---

Rethinking Satisfaction in Personal Relationships from a Dialectical Perspective

LARRY A. ERBERT
STEVE W. DUCK

An attempt to summarize the literature on satisfaction in personal relationships is complicated not only by the considerable amount of research generated on the topic, but by conceptual and definitional ambiguity (see Glenn, 1990, for discussion). Measures of satisfaction are often used as barometers for, or are correlated with measures of, the quality of relational interaction (Fincham & Bradbury, 1987; Glenn, 1990; Johnson, Amoloza, & Booth, 1992), adjustment in marriage (Long & Andrews, 1990; Long, 1993), marital functioning (Honeycutt, 1986), and communicative effectiveness in marriage (e.g., Noller & Fitzpatrick, 1990). It is difficult to ascertain precisely what scholars have learned about what it means to "be in" or "maintain" a satisfying relationship. Although it may be safe to conclude that people who consistently engage in negative, destructive, conflictual interaction will report higher levels of relational dissatisfaction (resulting in the increased likelihood of relational dissolution; see Gottman, 1994), this generalization does not begin to reflect the complexity and variability in interaction that characterize most relationships (Duck, 1994).

The intent of rethinking satisfaction in close relationships from a dialectical perspective is not to supplant current conceptualizations of the construct, but to suggest a complementary view, an expansion of what it means to examine satisfaction in human interaction. What is missing theoretically and empirically from the literature in relational satisfaction (and/or quality) is a discussion of the dilemmas or contradictions faced by people in everyday life (Duck, 1994), especially those that affect the determination of satisfaction. Although relational theorists are embracing a dialectical perspective with increasing frequency, scholars writing about satisfaction issues have rarely used this lens from which to theorize about or reconceptualize "relationship satisfaction" as a consequence of the practical management of dilemmas and contradictions. While the matters of variability, stability, change, and variance in relationship experience may be seen from different perspectives as an inherent part of relational experience (Duck, 1994), the present chapter explores one particularly well-developed theoretical framework for looking at these phenomena—namely, dialectical theory (Baxter & Montgomery, 1996).

UNDERSTANDING CONTEMPORARY DIALECTICAL THEORY

Dialectical theory, as it is conceptualized here, is based on the scholarship of Mikhail Bakhtin (Bakhtin, 1981, 1986; Baxter, 1994; Holquist, 1983; Morson & Emerson, 1990), a Russian theorist, who wrote about the open-ended complexity of social life. In any relationship or interaction, self and other are involved in a dance of open-endedness that is perpetually indeterminate and subject to changing social and environmental conditions. Indeed, as Holquist (1983) noted, "It was his sense of the world's overwhelming multiplicity that impelled Bakhtin to rethink strategies by which heterogeneity had traditionally been disguised as unity" (p. 307). The primal forces underlying Bakhtin's philosophy of social life are evident in the oppositional nature of the "centripetal–centrifugal" dynamic (Baxter, 1994; Baxter & Montgomery, 1996). That is, centripetal forces (those that create a sense of togetherness and unification) are in a dynamic and oppositional relationship with centrifugal forces (those that separate and divide). For example, coordinating relational actions for enjoyable activity sharing requires cooperation and unity, yet also requires individual expression of the differences or preferences for certain activities. Centripetal–centrifugal forces represent, at least for Bakhtin, the "deep structure of all social experience" (Baxter, 1994, p. 25). It is important to recognize that for Bakhtin, structure is not a closed, determinate system, but instead represents a dynamism where indeterminacy and fluidity dominate so-cial interaction (see Baxter, 1994, and Volosinov/Bakhtin, 1973, for further discussion). To explain the handling of such indeterminism, Bakhtin focused on the role of dialogue (see below, and Billig, 1987; Duck, 1994).

As Baxter and Montgomery (1996) have argued, dialectics is not a theory in the traditional sense, where a set of formal propositions or axiomatic arguments are laid forth; instead, a dialectical viewpoint represents a metaperspective that is held together by a number of com-mon assumptions. Baxter and Montgomery's version of dialectical the-ory, referred to as "relational dialectics," embraces dialogic processes as central to all types of interactions. Although universal agreement may not exist with regard to these assumptions, the four defining con-cepts of a dialectical perspective are "contradiction," "change," "praxis," and "totality."

First, "contradiction" is defined as the "dynamic interplay between unified opposition" (Baxter & Montgomery, 1996, p. 8). For example, relational partners strive to cope with ongoing tension between oppo-site needs, such as autonomy and connection. A contradiction represents not only such opposites, but the interplay *and* unity of the opposites (Baxter & Montgomery, 1996; Goldsmith, 1990). Temporarily fulfill-ing connection needs with a partner—through intimacy and activity sharing, for example—can lead to an increased desire for fulfilling au-tonomy needs. Not only is there interplay between oppositions, but Alt-man, Vinsel, and Brown (1981), addressing social-psychological issues, have asserted that oppositions assist in defining one another: "The idea of harmony in social relationships helps define and is partly defined by the idea of conflict, and the idea of interpersonal closeness con-tributes to our understanding of openness and vice versa" (p. 118). Ac-cording to this view, contradictions not only are important to examine in social interaction, but also constitute important metaphysical (Corn-forth, 1968) and ideological (Volosinov/Bakhtin, 1973) foundations of social experience. Individuals and couples are constantly faced with choices over competing demands within a larger social milieu. When contradictions are apparent, individuals will not necessarily resolve these contradictions through a synthesis of the two competing needs or de-mands (as in the Hegelian notion of a dialectic).

Second, the focus on "change" represents a concern for develop-ment and interaction over time (Goldsmith, 1990; Werner & Baxter, 1994). To study change in personal relationships means that scholars examine both linear (or one-time) change and cyclical change (see Wern-er & Baxter, 1994). Although operationalizing "change" in dialectical research is difficult, and often differs among leading dialectical scholars (see Altman et al., 1981; Baxter & Wilmot, 1983; Conville, 1983, 1988), change is not generally regarded as a dysfunction in a system or a disturbance that needs to be corrected (Altman et al., 1981). Even though change in dialectical theory has typically been conceived of in terms of the Hegelian "thesis–antithesis–synthesis" dynamic (see Baxter, 1994, and Rychlak, 1976, for discussion), some recent dialectical theorists object to the limitations of this tripartite scheme. In discussing Bakhtin's conception of dialogism, for example, Baxter (1994) argued that

> dialogism [which constitutes the foundation of Baxter and Montgomery's relational dialectics] does not presuppose a systematic, evolutionary process of change that culminates in a state of transcendence or synthesis to some higher order of development; rather, dialogism conceives of change as a perpetual ongoingness of centrifugal–centripetal forces that are manifested in multitudinous ways as relationships change through time. (p. 32)

Hence, change does not necessarily or generally follow stable or predictable patterns. Change is a product of the ongoing dialogue between self and other, which is sustained through the use of the "utterance" within the context of everyday interaction (see Bakhtin, 1986). Even amidst the variety of conceptualizations of change, it is regarded as critical for understanding the nature of human interaction.

The third concept necessary for understanding dialectical theory is "praxis." Praxis is defined as the quality that designates people as both actors and objects of their actions.

> People function as proactive actors who make communicative choices in how to function in their social world. Simultaneously, however, they become reactive objects, because their actions become reified in a variety of normative and institutionalized practices that establish the boundaries of subsequent communicative moves. (Baxter & Montgomery, 1996, p. 13)

The central feature of praxis is the consideration of the concrete, specific actions taken by people in everyday interaction, and of the ways in which those practices serve both to free and to constrain future interaction. Scholars, then, are concerned with the nature of symbolic contradictions, as opposed to materialistic contradictions (as in Marxist dialectics), which surface in the interaction of relational parties.

Fourth, "totality" refers to making connections among a number of related phenomena, in order to comprehend a more holistic view of such phenomena. At least two ways of dividing the conceptual territory for "totality" exist. In the first, totality reflects a multitude of social and cultural factors that affect the functioning of relationships. This perspective on relationships suggests that a holistic view of human interaction is necessary for examining not only psychological processes, but temporal qualities, cultural conditions, and physical and social contexts (see Altman, 1993; Altman et al., 1981; Werner, Altman, & Brown, 1992; Werner, Altman, Brown, & Ginat, 1993; Rawlins, 1983, 1992). The environments in which interaction take place are multifaceted and are not easily reducible to individual construction of relational experiences. The aim in this research is to understand personal relationships as holistic experiences affected by numerous personal and social circumstances.

A second view of totality refers to the basic interrelatedness of contradictions. Baxter and Montgomery (1996) have asserted that totality implicates three essential features of contradictions: (1) the location of contradictions—that is, the location is within the interpersonal relationship and not a product of an individual; (2) interdependencies among contradictions—which include primary and secondary contradictions, internal and external contradictions, or a "knot" of contradictions (see also Cornforth, 1968); and (3) the contextual factors that influence the interplay of contradictions. Taken together, these two broad descriptions of totality require scholars to recognize what Bakhtin (1981) has referred to as the "chronotopic conditions of human interaction." That is, "chronotope" refers to those conditions of time and space in which interaction occurs; all interaction, and the multiplicity of contradictions that surround interaction, can be placed within a specific sociohistorical context.

These four dialectical components provide a larger perspective or philosophy from which to explore the nature of satisfaction and dissatisfaction in personal relationships. It is with this lens that we begin to question some of the underlying assumptions within the literature on relationship satisfaction, and explore ways in which a dialectical theory can improve the kinds of questions that scholars and researchers ask.

DEFINING RELATIONSHIP SATISFACTION

"Relationship satisfaction" is defined in a variety of ways, but it is generally regarded as a subjective evaluation by each relational partner of the quality, or happiness level, within an intimate relationship (see Huston & Vangelisti, 1991). Satisfaction measures are not designed as objective assessments of relational interaction, but as measures of the attitudes and feelings of relational partners. "Satisfaction" is often used as equivalent to other terms, such as relational or marital "quality" (Fincham & Bradbury, 1987; Johnson et al., 1992), "adjustment" (Long & Andrews, 1990), "well-being" (Acitelli, 1992), "functioning" (Honeycutt, 1986), or "success" (Glenn, 1990). Sabatelli (1988), however, when comparing assessments of satisfaction and adjustment, maintained that whereas measures of *satisfaction* assess the individual, subjective attitudes of relational partners, measures of *adjustment* are objective in nature because the latter do not include judgments of interactions. Quality, for Sabatelli (1988), either may be a hybrid of adjustment and satisfaction, or may function as a global indicator of the state of the relationship. In this interpretation of relational quality, both subjective and objective assessments of the state of the relationship are considered.

Although (as noted above) the term "satisfaction" is often used synonymously with other related concepts, which may result in obscurity or other definitional and conceptual problems (see Fincham & Bradbury, 1987, for discussion), the purpose here is not to provide a definitive solution to the problem of definitional ambiguity. Instead, it is to recognize the need to understand how people manage to nurture and maintain relationships that are enjoyable (and perhaps unenjoyable or challenging) and that may or may not endure over time. There is probably general agreement, even within this volume, about the need to examine the conditions that are conducive to pleasurable and positive feelings, attitudes, and interactions. However, "satisfaction" as the term is currently used may speak more to an unattainable ideal than to the actual experiences of people in everyday life. It is not that people don't want or shouldn't seek to "feel" satisfied, but real-life satisfaction depends on more of the variances in the relational landscape than researchers typically consider.

More importantly, however, when global assessments of quality or satisfaction are determined, the nature of the relationship between everyday, specific interaction and global assessments may remain vague. Behaviorally oriented scholars have attempted to examine "specific categories of behavior that give rise to reports of satisfaction in marriage" (see Fincham & Bradbury, 1987, p. 800) for the purpose of determining overall satisfaction. However, the way in which specific behaviors relate to overall satisfaction is unknown, except that they permit generalizations to be made about happy versus unhappy couples. Gottman and Levenson (1992), for example, argued that placing couples within dichotomous categories of "happy" versus "unhappy" would aid in predicting marital dissolution. One of their goals was to develop a parsimonious model for understanding marital processes that would lead to the prediction of marital *outcomes*. Even so, determining happiness or satisfaction at one point in time does not necessarily predict future satisfaction (e.g., Gottman & Krokoff, 1989). In addition, Huston and Van-gelisti (1991) have asserted: "Although a number of correlational studies support these propositions [that more satisfied spouses express more warmth and less hostility than dissatisfied spouses], such studies fail to establish whether the patterns of positive and negative behavior pre-cede the development of satisfaction and dissatisfaction, whether they reflect prior or current satisfaction, or both" (p. 721). Certainly there remains a need to clarify the nature of the relationship between the particular and the global, *and* the dynamic interplay between satisfac-tion and dissatisfaction over time. Dialectical theory can help us bet-ter understand the nature of ongoing contradictions in personal relationships by embracing the indeterminacy and variability inherent in the interactions that people experience in their real lives.

DIALECTICAL THEORY AND RELATIONSHIP SATISFACTION

Dialectical theory makes an assumption that social experience is or-ganized around tensions or contradictory forces that are inherent in relat-ing (Montgomery, 1993). Clearly, relationships are not unitary, invariable states; they consist instead of various experiences, different moods, plea-sures, and pains, and plenty of "for better, for worse" (Duck, 1994; Duck & Wood, 1995). Therefore, it stands to reason that examining satisfac-tion in personal relationships should lead to questions that seek to de-termine whether and/or how varied experiences—understood as dialectical contradictions—are related not only to the global assessment of satisfaction, but also to the everyday types of experiences that lead people to view their general experiences as satisfying and/or dissatisfy-ing. In this section, we identify a number of emphases in the satisfac-tion literature, and we explore how each of the four dialectical concepts (contradiction, change, praxis, and totality) can help scholars under-stand the interrelationship of both positive and negative, satisfying and dissatisfying dimensions of interaction (Duck & Wood, 1995)

Contradiction and Relationship Satisfaction

Within a dialectical frame, it is impossible to examine relational satis-faction without also considering its opposite, dissatisfaction. Research-ers tend to construe satisfaction and dissatisfaction as a duality, rather than an as interconnected interplay of opposites (Duck & Wood, 1995). The implications for viewing satisfaction as part of a larger process in which both satisfaction and dissatisfaction are integral, undeniable elements of relational interaction needs to be considered more fully. If contradiction and oppositions are part of the "deep" structure of relating, then satisfaction is intimately connected to and never far away from dissatisfaction. As Altman et al. (1981) have noted, one term helps to define and is defined by its opposite; therefore, understanding satisfaction requires an examination of dissatisfaction, as well as of all other functional oppositions that may be relevant to relational satisfaction (Duck, 1994; Duck & Wood, 1995).

Opposition is central to dialectical theory and is an important feature in understanding relational contradictions. In this section, we argue that many constructions of relationship satisfaction are based on dualities, which are characterized by either–or thinking. A dualistic construction of opposition does not seek to understand the dynamic *interplay* of two or more oppositions, or how one side of an opposition feeds into the other, both in theory and in practice. The implications of examining satisfaction as a dualistic compared with a dialectic construction are both practical and ideological. Therefore, two emphases and possible limitations that spring from a dualistic construction of satisfaction in close relationships merit further consideration.

The Emphasis on the Ideal Relationship

Since satisfaction is generally studied in marital relationships more than in other types of relationships, an implicit ideological construction of the ideal type of marriage—and, indeed, the ideal type of intimate relationship—is based on a premise of closeness, bonding, and togetherness. In essence, researchers categorize couples as belonging to one of two groups: either "satisfied" *or* "dissatisfied," "distressed" *or* "nondistressed" (Levenson & Gottman, 1983), "regulated" *or* "nonregulated" (Gottman & Levenson, 1992), and so forth. One purpose of such classifications, of course, is to determine which couples are in need of counseling (or which couples may benefit from some type of intervention, such as communication and conflict management training; see Markman, Renick, Floyd, Stanely, & Clements, 1993). Another purpose may reside in an inherent desire to understand issues of stability (Heaton & Albrecht, 1991), longevity, and/or divorce (e.g., Gottman, 1994) in marital relationships. Those couples in the satisfied, regulated, and nondistressed groups are somehow "doing it right," compared to those in whose relationships negativity, conflict, and dissatisfaction abound. Even so, membership in either of the two categories is argued to represent or be the product of the overall patterns of interaction, and those patterns are labeled as either positive or negative. All of this is predicated on an underlying belief of an ideal relational type that values intimacy over

closedness, togetherness over individuality, and disclosure over privacy. For example, Zuo (1992) has identified past research in which marital couples' time together is basically theorized to be correlated with
greater marital happiness. In addition, Sabatelli (1988), in a review of
marital survey instruments, noted that past conceptualizations of a "well-
adjusted" marriage—as measured by the Locke and Wallace (1959) instrument, for example—may no longer apply to marital interaction today. For example, couples who scored high on marital adjustment
engaged "in *all* outside interests together . . . generally preferred to 'stay
at home' rather than be on the go" (Sabatelli, 1988, p. 896). These approaches are consistent with exchange theories of marital interaction,
and to some extent represent a type of "quid pro quo" thinking about
marital relationships.

Alternative conceptions of couple types, which go beyond dualistic constructions, have been proposed. Fitzpatrick (1988) has classified
couples as (1) "traditionals," characterized by a high degree of connection and by endorsement of stereotypical gender roles; (2) "indepen-
dents," characterized by a strong commitment to individual autonomy
and independence; and (3) "separates," characterized by emotional distance and little intimate interaction. In addition, Gottman (1993) has
proposed five different couple types, but classifies three couple types
within this category scheme as "stable" and two as "unstable." Within
the stable category, which Gottman argues roughly parallel the types
identified by Fitzpatrick, couples are classified as "validators," "volatiles,"
and "avoiders." Although Gottman (1993) has discovered that stability
is somewhat correlated with satisfaction (a correlation of .20; Gottman
& Levenson, 1992), he speculates about the costs and benefits of each
of the three stable relational types, arguing that each has potential for
positive and/or negative interaction. However, the bias of the ideal relationship creeps to the surface of Gottman's (1993) description of the
different types:

> The volatile marriage tends to be quite romantic and passionate, but
> it has the risk of dissolving into endless bickering. The validating
> marriage (which is consistent with current models of marital thera-
> py) is calmer and intimate; these couples appear to value a compan-
> ionate marriage and shared experiences, not individuality. The risk
> may be that romance will disappear over time, and partners will be-
> come merely close friends. The third type avoids the pain of con-
> frontation and conflict, but the risk may be emotional distance and
> loneliness. (p. 13)

If one is forced to choose among endless bickering, emotional distance
and loneliness, and merely being close friends, the selection seems ob-

vious. Even when the ideal type is deconstructed, a bias is still evident in the choice among the least of three evils—in this case, settling on close friendship. Gottman's overall purpose in this research, however, is to argue for a balance between positive and negative interaction episodes, although in this case "balance" is constructed as a ratio of approximately five positive interaction episodes to one negative episode.

The Emphasis on Positivity as the Relational Goal

When the ideal relational type is embraced—one in which intimacy is preferred over detachment—positive interaction becomes teleologically important. According to the extant literature, the way to satisfaction is through a preponderance of positive interaction episodes. "Positive" interaction is argued to occur when people are agreeable, avoid conflict, and seek togetherness and unity. Gottman (1993, 1994) and his colleagues (e.g., Levenson & Gottman, 1983) appear to be among the few who argue that instances of negative interaction, such as the expression of anger and disagreement (see Gottman & Krokoff, 1989) or conflict between partners, can serve a long-term positive function in intimate relationships. However, when considering issues of marital stability, Gottman (1993) has noted that too much expression of negative affect and behavior appears to be corrosive to the long-term stability of marriage. Gottman (1993) recognizes the interplay between positive and negative interaction, and argues that negative interaction is as necessary as positive interaction for desirable marriages. Even so, the simple recognition of the importance of negative interaction episodes does not do justice to the potential interplay and interdependency with positive interaction episodes. Viewing opposition without interdependency is a dualistic construction of interaction episodes. For example, how often can interaction episodes be construed by relational partners as both positive and negative? Or in what ways do couples cycle between periods of satisfying interaction and dissatisfying interaction? When couples report satisfaction scores of 5 or 6 on a 7-point Likert scale (e.g., Quality of Marriage Index; Norton, 1983), doesn't this suggest that some dissatisfaction exists simultaneously in the global assessment? It may be that tensions and contradictions constitute a significant structural basis for the simultaneous existence of satisfaction and dissatisfaction. More importantly, we need to explore how the dialectical issues of contradiction and opposition can help researchers move beyond the simple dichotomies. Before answering these inquiries, we should determine how the emphasis on the relational ideal and on the positivity as the relational goal limits theoretical and empirical investigation of satisfaction in close relationships.

The Ideal Relationship and the Goal of Positivity as Limitations

First, if the basic ideological foundations of each partner in an intimate relationship are predicated on the ideal relationship, attaining that ideal becomes an almost impossible task. On the one hand, people may use the ideal as a cornerstone for their personal belief systems and subsequent behavior in relational interaction, which can serve a relationship well, up to a point (McCall, 1988; Simmel, 1950). On the other hand, the inability to attain perpetual states of satisfaction and to exclude negative episodes may create dissonance within the relationship and/or the individual(s), leading to the denial of important oppositions. Unfortunately, the ideal relational type implies that couples should function in a state of happiness and satisfaction. Furthermore, if both partners explicitly or implicitly "agree" on working toward the ideal satisfying relationship, it is hard to imagine that tensions and contradictions will not emerge between what Rawlins (1983) has described as the dialectic of the ideal and the real.

In a critique of empirical and theoretical notions of the ideal relationship, Marks (1989) has argued that the intrinsic style of marriage, which is an ideal type (similar to Fitzpatrick's traditional and Gottman's validating types), limits conceptions of styles or types of high-quality marriages. That is, no longer should people be trapped by a marital type in which the ideal of "near-perfect companion" or making heroic sacrifices for the relationship is the dominant mode. If unity or togetherness themes dominate conceptions of the marital ideal, a rigid structural prison that serves to limit the validation of other types of relationships is constructed. However, Marks (1989) noted that since dilemmas emerge in relational interaction, balancing competing needs (e.g., autonomy and jointness) is the solution to relational contradictions. Clearly, a closer examination of relational types indicates a need to explore the ideological foundations of what constitutes an intimate and/or marital relationship. Classification of intimate or marital types of relationships into even two or three categories may tend to limit our conceptualization of what constitutes a "workable" relationship (Duck & Wood, 1995).

Second, when positive interaction becomes the goal of relational interaction, partners may purposefully eliminate any perceived negative interaction, which includes episodes of conflict. Perhaps a dualistic construction of any relational ideal perpetuates cycles in which people fail miserably to attain the ideal, but in which they also fail to embrace anything that is perceived as leading to or resulting in negativity, distance, or dissatisfaction. Admittedly, there are many situations where the reduction of negative episodes is critical for relational survival—for example, when highly distressed couples come in for counseling and therapy (see Markman et al., 1993), or when violence is the outcome of out-of-control conflictual interaction. However, for couples that are not identified as extremely dissatisfied and/or in need of intervention, the reduction of interaction that the partners perceive as negative may serve to produce and reproduce patterns of unnecessary and damaging avoidance and accommodation behaviors (Duck & Wood, 1995). Scholars have long advocated the positive, beneficial functions of conflictual interaction (Deutsch, 1973; Simmel, 1955). More recently, Hocker and Wilmot (1995) have argued that the escalation of conflict is often necessary for the effective management of conflict issues. Engaging in avoidance and accommodation for the purposes of maintaining relational harmony may turn out in the end to be more harmful than helpful. For example, Lloyd and Cate (1985) showed that conflict about role performance often leads to the construction of a "better" relationship than is created by avoiding discussions of roles.

Possible Contributions of a Dialectical View of Contradiction

In what ways can an understanding of contradiction and opposition in relational interaction benefit scholarship concerning relationship satisfaction? First, there is a strong need to investigate oppositional tendencies of satisfaction and dissatisfaction, and to comprehend how current assumptions in the literature tend to limit the investigation of these oppositions. In their discussion of the nature of opposition, Baxter and Montgomery (1996) have asserted that an understanding of opposition resides not only in the recognition of logical opposites, or mutually exclusive and exhaustive oppositions, such as the popular "A" and "not-A" opposition; it also resides in the acknowledgment of functional opposites, or what are described as nonexhaustive, mutually exclusive oppositions (Baxter & Montgomery, 1996; Werner & Baxter, 1994). Functional, nonexhaustive, mutually exclusive oppositions refer to all forms of contradiction that are found in everyday interaction. For example, functional opposites of satisfaction might include disagreement, conflict, emotional distance, autonomy needs, social constraint, or any other *lived* experience that functions as an opposition to satisfaction.

Research on relational interactions has tended to focus on one of two general areas of inquiry: (1) individual and/or psychological variables such as affective, behavioral, and physiological responses (Broderick & O'Leary, 1986; Karney, Bradbury, Fincham, & Sullivan, 1994; Gottman, 1994; Krokoff, 1990; Levenson & Gottman, 1983, 1985; Smith, Vivian, & O'Leary, 1990); and (2) relational and social exchange models, including but not limited to research on attachment and love styles (see Hendrick, Hendrick, & Adler, 1988; Martin, Blair, Nevels, & Fitzpatrick, 1990; Pistole, 1989), relational comparisons and exchange orientations (see Buunk & VanYperen, 1991), fairness and reward level (see Cate, Lloyd, Henton, & Larson, 1982), communication behaviors (see Markman et al., 1993; Siavelis & Lamke, 1992; Ting-Toomey, 1983), and conflict management issues (see Heavey, Layne, & Christensen, 1993; Gottman, 1993; Kurdek, 1994, 1995; Yelsma, 1984). To date, very little research has been conducted on the nature of oppositions and satisfying relational interactions.

Second, recognizing the potential for ongoing contradiction in relationships would suggest that people's everyday interaction does not necessarily conform to the ideal relational type or to consistent positive interactions over time. Contradictions may be found in the desire for the ideal versus the real (i.e., tensions that result from either seeking the relational ideal or reconstructing new rules and strategies for relational change). At the very least, a dialectical philosophy embraces the assumption that competing tendencies—the basic interplay between centripetal and centrifugal forces—are fundamental for understanding and coping with change. For relational partners, then, seeking creative alternatives for coping with ongoing tensions, or embracing rather than denying "negative episodes," may be an important step in relational growth. In addition, our notions of what it means to have satisfying relationships are constructed and reconstructed through the ongoing dialogue with others—a process, by the way, that requires both unity and division, agreement and opposition.

Change and Relationship Satisfaction

Dialectical scholars embrace a perspective of change as critical to and inherent in all social interaction. Questions about how and why changes occur must take into account sociohistorical conditions (Ochs, 1993) as well as temporal elements of interaction (Bakhtin, 1981; Werner & Baxter, 1994). Although relationship satisfaction researchers acknowledge the need for longitudinal research (e.g., Fincham & Bradbury, 1993; Gottman, 1991; Smith et al., 1990), the primary assumption is that change over time can ultimately be predicted, traced, and generally understood. Predicting change in relationships requires that the conditions (the subject of investigation) at Time 1 are knowable and measurable, and that those stable dimensions can be compared with conditions at Time 2. One notable corollary of this orientation includes the individual as knowable, as having a relatively stable identity. From a dialectical perspective, stability and change constitute an important dimension of social interaction, and consistently privileging one over the other disregards the dynamic relationship between the two. Before identifying how change is construed within a dialectical perspective, we examine two emphases with regard to "change" within the satisfaction literature.

The Emphasis on Stability

There is no question about the benefits of understanding what relational partners view as predictable and stable within the relationship, though it is likely that such perceptions of stability are *active* psychological processes that help humans to deal with uncertainty (Duck, 1994). Previous research has disregarded behaviors and interactions that are novel, unusual, or unpredictable as it develops an effort—parallel to the one observable in other areas of human life—to create predictability and stability in representations of relational interaction. Relationship satisfaction researchers generally seek to determine the level of satisfaction at Time 1 in relation to some other variable without measuring changes or, more importantly, variance over time (Duck, 1994). Gottman (1993), for example, indicated that of the approximately 2,000 studies examining divorce or marital separation, only 3 were longitudinal. (Gottman also noted that deterioration of satisfaction did not predict divorce or separation.) Of the studies reviewed for this chapter, only a handful were of longitudinal design. Using satisfaction as a focal point for understanding issues of quality, longevity, and stability in relationships must not be based on representations of interaction that project a completely static characterization onto the relationship on the basis of one "snapshot" measurement (Duck, 1994).

The concern for "reliability," and the prevalence of one-time measurement, do not mean that scholars have not attempted to account for change in relational satisfaction (see Fincham & Bradbury, 1993; Gottman & Krokoff, 1989; Huston & Vangelisti, 1991; Markman et al., 1993). Generally, though, the reasons for change in satisfaction levels can be accounted for either by some type of individual cognitive transformation (a psychological perspective), or by some social or cultural circumstance. An example of this research can be found in the work on attribution theory, where satisfaction researchers generally attempt to establish a connection between individual characteristics and assessments of relational satisfaction. The importance of individual cognitions and affective states, and of subsequent attributions made by relational partners about marital events, is a central concern (e.g., Fincham, Bradbury, & Scott, 1990). Bradbury and Fincham (1988), however, examined the role of context as a potential mediating variable in the relationship between attributions and relational satisfaction. Unfortunately, the notion of "context" was reduced to a definition of the psychological variables or conditions that affect behavior in interaction. A fundamental premise of the psychological perspective in this research is "that beliefs and attributions influence behavior" (Fincham et al., 1990, p. 142). Even within this framework, the individual is construed as knowable and stable, thus raising a more fundamental question of identity (Duck, West, & Acitelli, 1996).

The Emphasis on a "Fixed" Identity

The theoretical lens through which much of the research on satisfaction in personal relationships has been conducted is psychological or social-psychological in nature. A psychological perspective implicitly (if not explicitly) regards the individual psyche as the source of behavior and action in relational interaction; the person becomes the birthplace of motives and reasons for action.

A strictly psychological perspective has been criticized for its construction of the self as inflexible and constant. In fact, Shotter (1989) has argued that psychological research has been dominated and limited by the duality of self–other, in which individual experience, or ego, is separate and distinct from social influence. "In this Cartesian sense, it is 'the self' as a 'thing' which becomes the ultimate, unconditioned source of thought, meaning and, strangely, of language and speech also" (p. 137). The construction of the self is also described, not as a unitary entity, but as a "fluid process of becoming" (Baxter, 1994, p. 26). In addition, Slugoski and Ginsberg (1989) have argued that identity is paradoxical, in that "at any moment we are the same as, yet different from, the persons we once were or ever will be" (p. 36). Change represents an ongoing process in which dimensions of "self" are constructed and reconstructed through time (Erbert, 1995). Identity is constructed through processes in which both stability and change are present, and in which one "blends" and "bleeds" within and between the other.

Possible Contributions of a Dialectical View of Change

How does a dialectical view of change differ from what has been described by satisfaction researchers? By contrast to psychological or social-psychological perspectives, a dialectical perspective, as we conceive of it here, generally regards social interaction (and dialogic process) as fundamental to processes of relating. Social interaction is sustained via a series of utterances by which self and other are in an ever-changing, dynamic dialogue. It is the communicative interaction between self and other that creates conditions of satisfaction and dissatisfaction, harmony and conflict, avoidance and engagement, and so forth. What happens in a relationship is not owned by one person or the other, but is a product of the relational system, which is constituted in and through dialogic processes—in particular, the everyday talk that occurs there (Duck, 1994). Relational partners might benefit from a dialectical perspective by attempting to understanding how their interaction and dialogue serve to sustain both positive and negative dimensions of interaction. For example, if a husband views his wife as essentially negative and "at fault" in an interaction, he may seek to distance himself from responsibility for any portion of the negative episode.

When investigators are considering issues of satisfaction and dissatisfaction, a dialectical perspective is valuable as a tool for examining cycles of stability and change or satisfaction and dissatisfaction. Compared to only two measurements across time, measurements of cyclical activity at multiple time periods within a relationship may result in better understanding of the regularity, duration, frequency, and amplitude of relational issues (see Altman et al., 1981; VanLear, 1991), especially those activities regarded as positive, negative, or both. For example, research on the "demand–withdraw" patterns in marital conflict and satisfaction (Christensen & Heavey, 1990; Heavey et al., 1993) could be extended by an analysis of the duration, frequency, regularity, and amplitude of the demand–withdraw cycles. In addition, we might ask, "In what ways are dissatisfied (or satisfied) couples different yet similar with regard to these four cyclical issues?"

These and other types of questions can provide a greater understanding of not only cycles of interaction, but the extent and nature of relational change, as well as one-time change. They also indicate a need to understand ongoing communicative practices and interactive behaviors—that is, praxis issues of interaction.

Praxis and Relationship Satisfaction

As noted earlier, the term "praxis" refers to conditions of interaction in which persons are both free to act, yet potentially constrained by those same actions. As Baxter and Montgomery (1996) have argued, relationship parties make communicative choices based on their unique history together, but these choices serve to alter future interaction. For example, when intimate couples engage in patterns of destructive conflictual interaction, which results in negative outcomes, they are constrained by that particular history of conflict (or past destructive episodes); however, the communicative choices in each subsequent conflictual interaction can also be the springboard for both positive and negative conflictual interactions in the future. The focal point here consists of the temporal qualities of past, present, and future as they affect couples' interaction. An important question satisfaction researchers must address more fully is how to classify, organize, and explain human experience with regard to specific contradictions faced by partners through any relationship's history. To date, research has privileged central tendencies rather than individual instances of interaction.

The Emphasis on Generalizability

The search for generalizable conclusions about satisfaction in personal relationships is based on a premise that central tendencies provide a social and cultural framework from which to understand intimate interaction. It is a "top-down" as opposed to a "bottom-up" approach to understanding satisfaction in personal relationships, and the focus on central tendencies and generalizable conclusions has effectively silenced any discussion of the idiosyncratic, novel, or highly variable dimensions of relational interaction. What scholars tend to do in the study of close personal relationships is to privilege central tendencies over the variability that may characterize individual instances (Duck, 1994). Within couple types, for example (Gottman, 1993; Fitzpatrick, 1988), how often do couples display behaviors that could be classified as belonging to all three of Fitzpatrick's or all five of Gottman's couple types? Researchers' own constructions of the critical questions to ask may, paradoxically, serve to constrain the nature of their inquiries. The focus on generalizability may lead to a type of unity or consensus about the best ways to gather data, view relational satisfaction, or behave during conflict—all of which exemplify a centripetal bias that Bakhtin worked to dispel.

Generalizations about intimate interaction may prove more limiting than beneficial. Consider for example, how generalizations provide a picture of interaction that is then construed as "normalized" behavior. Conclusions can be reached about how an individual should or may behave in interactive circumstances. If satisfaction in personal relationships is desired, laypersons may look toward generalized standards as a guide to achieving satisfaction (McCall, 1988; Prusank, Duran, & DeLillo, 1993; Simmel, 1950); in this case, the goal of happiness is achieved by engaging in behaviors that are reported to be "productive" or "satisfying" for others. Interestingly, John Gray's (1992) self-help book on intimate relationships, *Men Are from Mars, Women Are from Venus*, promotes an ideal relational type in which partners are advised to be agreeable and not argue. In this way, generalizations may serve as a constraining mechanism for individuals, rather than allowing for the construction of alternative routes for accomplishing relational satisfaction. "Perhaps we are in too much of a hurry to come to conclusions about human behavior anyway, and thereafter to stop wondering what un-disclosed potentialities it has" (Kelly, 1966/1970, p. 12). According to Kelly, behavior is the way in which people ask questions; problems arise when the *meaning* that we assign to behavior is rigidly placed in categories or judged as simply appropriate or inappropriate. If contradictory process-es are indeed part of the deep structure of all social experience, then exploring contradictory forces necessitates examining the concrete prac-tices of people at specific moments in couples' relational histories. This does not preclude seeking central tendencies, but would suggest a more balanced research picture.

Possible Contributions of a Dialectical View of Praxis

How can issues of praxis benefit the investigation of satisfaction in close relationships? First, researchers need to examine the types of symbolic or communicative codes that are produced and reproduced in intimate interaction and that lead to satisfy and dissatisfying outcomes (Duck, 1994). Second, it is important to determine what types of contradic-tions are manifested in the assessment, judgment, and evaluation of satisfying *and* dissatisfying relational interactions (Duck & Wood, 1995).

Third, questioning how people respond to the various contradic-tions they face should also concern satisfaction theorists. When con-fronted with contradictions, people may respond with a number of strategies designed to help them "cope" with the ensuing tension. Bax-ter (1988, 1990) has argued that at least six fundamental responses ex-ist with regard to three contradictions, autonomy–connection, open-ness–closedness, and predictability–novelty. The six responses have been grouped into four basic types: (1) selection—attempting to make one pole or condition dominant; (2) separation—coexistence of both poles, but denial that the two are interdependent; (3) neutralization—diluting the intensity of the contradiction by moderation or disqualification; and (4) reframing—transforming the elements of the contradiction. There is some evidence to suggest that satisfaction is related to the type of response used (Baxter, 1990); however, the specific nature of the rela-tionship is preliminary. That is, Baxter (1990) argued that satisfaction is correlated with reframing, but also suggested that the short relation-al histories of study participants may have played a part in that out-come. Relational participants themselves might attempt to expand their understanding of relational contradictions and seek creative and/or al-ternative approaches to problem solving within the relationship. Recog-nition of the valuable role of "negative episodes" might help alleviate the conception that the relational pair function in an "ideal" state of happiness and bliss. What the work of Baxter and colleagues (e.g., Baxter,

1990; Baxter & Dindia, 1990; Baxter & Montgomery, 1996) indicates is a need for a fuller understanding of responses to ongoing relational contradictions such as autonomy and connection. Satisfaction researchers can begin to explore how types of responses to contradictions are linked to both positive and negative assessments of interaction. In addition, assessing the potential constraining affects of patterns or responses to contradictions on the relational system may provide insight about the interdependent nature of individuals within the system. Other questions might include these: In what ways do responses change or vary over time? How do intervening variables such as third-party involvement or other contingent conditions (work, child care, etc.) affect the assessment of satisfaction? These questions certainly indicate the need to examine satisfaction issues within the confines of the relational system—that is, a more holistic picture of contradictory forces in intimate interaction.

Totality and Relationship Satisfaction

Baxter and Montgomery's (1996) interpretation of dialectical theory regards totality not as a holistic picture of interactive practices among people, but as one form of wholeness that helps us understand the "knot" of contradictions existing in ongoing relational interaction. Generally speaking, researchers have attempted to understand relational systems by examining a number of social and or cultural "artifacts" as a way to account for outside influences on the intimate relationship; however, what has emerged is a fragmented picture of relational systems.

The Emphasis on Accumulated Fragmentalism

Attempts to construct a holistic picture of relational interactions and the system in which those interactions take place are daunting if not unrealistic endeavors, especially if "the whole" is assumed to be well represented by an accumulation of fragments rather than by some consideration of their connections and contexts (Kelly, 1969). Thus, satisfaction researchers are forced to incrementally include or exclude "variables" that may potentially influence satisfaction in close relationships, without fully understanding their dynamic interplay. Most of these variables or issues are conceived of as part of the larger social and cultural conditions that affect satisfaction. Such investigations include, but are not limited to, the following: leisure activity patterns (Holman & Jacquart, 1988; Smith, Snyder, Trull, & Monsma, 1988), household division of labor (Benin & Agostinelli, 1988; Suitor, 1991; Yogev & Brett, 1985), family life and/or child care issues (Blair, 1993; Lye &

Biblarz, 1991; Steinberg & Silverberg, 1987), employment and work-related issues (Blair, 1993; Rotheram & Weiner, 1983; Vannoy & Phil-liber, 1992), and gender roles and expectations (Fowers, 1991; Langis, Sabourin, Lussier, & Mathieu, 1994; Lye & Biblarz, 1991; Rotheram & Weiner, 1983). Hence, a very fragmented picture of what influences satisfaction and dissatisfaction is presented.

Possible Contributions of a Dialectical Approach to Totality

How might embracing a dialectical approach to totality help improve scholarship in the satisfaction literature? First, a focus on totality reem-phasizes the importance of context, and all that context implies, for intimate relationships. "Context is not an independent phenomenon, apart from the relationship. Instead, communication between relation-ship parties, and with third-party outsiders and social institutions, shapes the dynamic boundary that distinguishes the 'inside' from the 'outside' of a relationship" (Baxter & Montgomery, 1996, p. 45). Espousing a "totalizing" philosophy implies that scholars consider context, explore the dialogue between self and other(s), discover contradictory process-es over time, and entertain multiple points of view (from the multi-vocality implied in dialogic processes).

Second, relational partners are not simply faced with one contradic-tion per se, but with a number of potential contradictions in intimate relationships. For example, a couple may experience tensions or con-tradictions that entail issues of autonomy and connection, certainty and uncertainty, and stability and change, all within a single interaction episode. A preliminary study using interview and questionnaire data on contradictions and conflict (Erbert, 1996) reveals that married cou-ples report the presence of multiple internal as well as external con-tradictions during conflictual interaction episodes. Conflict participants appear to engage in conflicts directly related to the relational pair, or internal relational concerns (Baxter, 1990, described internal contradic-tions as autonomy–connection, predictability–novelty, and openness–nonopenness), as well as external concerns (e.g., third-party open-ness–nonopenness, integration–separation, and conventionality–unique-ness) that involve in-laws, work issues, and child care. The "knot" of contradictions emerging in this research suggests that a multiplicity of contradictory forces is at work during episodes of conflict.

Third, the issues linking satisfaction to an assortment of social and cultural factors, as noted above, could be extended to include assess-ments of contradictions in intimate relationships. For example, what are the contradictory processes involved in child care? Work-related conflict? Problems with in-laws? What contradictions might arise for couples when socially constructed expectations for behavior (e.g., how to rear children or how to fulfill gender role expectations) clash with the need for unique solutions to dilemmas in the relational system? These questions highlight the need for better comprehension of contradictory processes in relational interaction.

Fourth, perhaps we should question the utility of assessing the state of intimate relations by asking for global evaluations of levels of happiness. After all, a global assessment of the relationship requires participants to construct a simplified, relatively abstract construction of a unique relational history. It may be theoretically useful to ascertain what other types of evaluative referents may be made about intimate interaction. For example, why not ask participants about relationship change, transformations, challenge, crises, or growth as indicators of relational "health"? Perhaps satisfaction has outlived its usefulness for determining why and how relationships "work" or are supposed to work.

Fifth, a dialectical perspective does not imply that any one methodological approach is superior to any other, yet it is obvious that self-report methods have dominated the satisfaction literature. Perhaps qualitatively based approaches, or combining quantitative and qualitative methods, might provide an alternative voice to research that is exclusively quantitative. However, when researchers attempt to "immerse" themselves in the relational systems of others via interviews, diaries, and/or direct observational techniques, a number of practical if not ethical dilemmas emerge. Tension may arise between violating others' privacy and needing to violate this privacy to comprehend unique dyadic systems. By examining conflictual and negative events, researchers also run the risk of promoting or at least instigating the recurrence of unresolved issues. On the other hand, the boundaries between the private and the public are already blurred for couples seeking help, therapy, and intervention about intimate relations.

Totality does not imply that a complete picture or understanding of relational systems can be achieved. What totality does represent is an attempt to comprehend the unpredictability (and predictability) of everyday interaction, while paying close attention to the interdependencies of a variety of individual, relational, social, and communicative factors.

CONCLUDING REMARKS

The purpose of this chapter has been to explore how dialectical theory might realistically intersect with, and improve upon, research on satisfaction in close relationships. We recognize that our rendering of dialectical theory does not represent the voice of all (or even most) dialectical theorists. Perhaps if people were to embrace the ubiquity of ongoing contradictions, the pressure to conform to an unattainable relational ideal, or to definitively resolve all relational tensions, would be reduced. Our purpose has been to generate questions about the nature of relational interaction and researchers' construction of what satisfaction is and what it should come to mean to others. As Kelly (1964) once remarked, "a pat answer is the enemy of a fresh question" (p. 115).

REFERENCES

Acitelli, L. K. (1992). Gender differences in relationship awareness and marital satisfaction among young married couples. *Personality and Social Psychology Bulletin, 18*, 102–110.

Altman, I. (1993). Dialectics, physical environments, and personal relationships. *Communication Monographs, 60*(1), 26–41.

Altman, I., Vinsel, A., & Brown, B. B. (1981). Dialectic conceptions in social psychology: An application to social penetration and privacy regulation. In L. Berkowitz (Ed.), *Advances in experimental social psychology* (Vol. 14, pp. 107–160). New York: Academic Press.

Bakhtin, M. M. (1981). *The dialogic imagination: Four essays by M. M. Bakhtin* (M. Holquist, Ed.; C. Emerson & M. Holquist, Trans.). Austin: University of Texas Press.

Bakhtin, M. M. (1986). *Speech genres and other late essays* (V. W. McGee, Trans.). Austin: University of Texas Press.

Baxter, L. A. (1988). A dialectic perspective on communication strategies in relationship development. In S. W. Duck (Ed.), *Handbook of personal relationships* (pp. 257–273). New York: Wiley.

Baxter, L. A. (1990). Dialectic contradictions in relationship development. *Journal of Social and Personal Relationships, 7*, 69–88.

Baxter, L. A. (1994). Thinking dialogically about communication in personal relationships. In R. L. Conville (Ed.), *Uses of "structure" in communication studies* (pp. 23–37). New York: Praeger.

Baxter, L. A., & Dindia, K. (1990). Marital partners' perceptions of marital maintenance strategies. *Journal of Social and Personal Relationships, 7*, 187–208.

Baxter, L. A., & Montgomery, B. M. (1996). *Relating: Dialogues and dialectics.* New York: Guilford Press.

Baxter, L. A., & Wilmot, W. W. (1983). "Secret tests": Social strategies for acquiring information about the state of the relationship. *Communication Monographs, 50*, 264–272.

Benin, M. H., & Agostinelli, J. (1988). Husbands' and wives' satisfaction with the division of labor. *Journal of Marriage and the Family, 50*, 349–361.

Billig, M. (1987). *Arguing and thinking: A rhetorical approach to social psychology.* Cambridge: Cambridge University Press.

Blair, S. L. (1993). Employment, family, and perceptions of marital quality among husbands and wives. *Journal of Family Issues, 14*(2), 189–212.

Bradbury, T. N., & Fincham, F. D. (1988). Individual difference variables in close relationships: A contextual model of marriage as an integrative framework. *Journal of Personality and Social Psychology, 54*(4), 713–721.

Broderick, J. E., & O'Leary, L. D. (1986). Contributions of affect, attitudes, and behavior to marital satisfaction. *Journal of Counseling and Clinical Psychology, 54*(4), 514–517.

Buunk, B. P., & VanYperen, N. W. (1991). Referential comparisons, relational comparisons, and exchange orientation: Their relation to marital satisfaction. *Personality and Social Psychology Bulletin, 17*(6), 709–717.

Cate, R. M., Lloyd, S. A., Henton, J. M., & Larson, J. H. (1982). Fairness and reward level as predictors of relationship satisfaction. *Social Psychological Quarterly, 45*(3), 177–181.

Christensen, A., & Heavey, C. L. (1990). Gender and social structure in the demand/withdraw pattern of marital conflict. *Journal of Personality and Social Psychology, 59*(1), 73–81.

Conville, R. L. (1983). Second-order development in interpersonal communication. *Human Communication Research, 9*(3), 195–207.

Conville, R. L. (1988). Relational transitions: An inquiry into their structure and function. *Journal of Social and Personal Relationships, 5,* 423–437.

Cornforth, M. (1968). *Materialism and the dialectic method.* New York: International.

Deutsch, M. (1973). *The resolution of conflict: Constructive and destructive processes.* New Haven, CT: Yale University Press.

Duck, S. W. (1994). *Meaningful relationships: Talking, sense, and relating.* Thousand Oaks, CA: Sage.

Duck, S. W., West, L., & Acitelli, L. K. (1996). Sewing the field: The tapestry of relationships in life and research. In S. W. Duck, K. Dindia, B. Ickes, B. Milardo, R. Mills, & B. Sarason (Eds.), *Handbook of personal relationships* (2nd ed., pp. 1–23). Chichester, England: Wiley.

Duck, S. W., & Wood, J. T. (1995). For better for worse, for richer for poorer: The rough and smooth of relationships. In S. W. Duck & J. T. Wood (Eds.), *Understanding relationship processes 5: Confronting relationship challenges* (pp. 1–12). Thousand Oaks, CA: Sage.

Erbert, L. A. (1995). *Personal construct theory and relational dialogue: The construction and reconstruction of identity.* Paper presented at the annual meeting of the Speech Communication Association, San Antonio, TX.

Erbert, L. A. (1996). Conflict and dialectics: Retrospective accounts of primary contradictions in marital conflict (Doctoral dissertation, University of Iowa, 1996). *UMI Dissertation Services,* 9639970.

Fincham, F. D., & Bradbury, T. N. (1987). The assessment of marital quality: A reevaluation. *Journal of Marriage and the Family, 49,* 797–809.

Fincham, F. D., & Bradbury, T. N. (1993). Marital satisfaction, depression, and attributions: A longitudinal analysis. *Journal of Personality and Social Psychology, 64*(3), 442–452.

Fincham, F. D., Bradbury, T. N., & Scott, C. K. (1990). Cognition in marriage. In F. D. Fincham & T. N. Bradbury (Eds.), *The psychology of marriage: Basic issues and applications* (pp. 118–149). New York: Guilford Press.

Fitzpatrick, M. A. (1988). *Between husband and wife: Communication in marriage.* Beverly Hills, CA: Sage.

Fowers, B. J. (1991). His and her marriage: A multivariate study of gender and marital satisfaction. *Sex Roles, 24*(3–4), 209–221.

Glenn, N. D. (1990). Quantitative research on marital quality in the 1980's: A critical review. *Journal of Marriage and the Family, 52,* 818–831.

Goldsmith, D. (1990). A dialectic perspective on the expression of autonomy and connection in romantic relationships. *Western Journal of Speech Communication, 54,* 537–556.

Gottman, J. M. (1991). Predicting the longitudinal course of marriages. *Journal of Marital and Family Therapy, 17*(1), 3–7.

Gottman, J. M. (1993). The roles of conflict engagement, escalation, and avoidance in marital interaction: A longitudinal view of five couple types. *Journal of Consulting and Clinical Psychology, 61*(1), 6–15.

Gottman, J. M. (1994). *What predicts divorce?* Hillsdale, NJ: Erlbaum.

Gottman, J. M., & Krokoff, L. J. (1989). Marital interaction and satisfaction: A longitudinal view. *Journal of Consulting and Clinical Psychology, 57*(1), 47–52.

Gottman, J. M., & Levenson, R. W. (1992). Marital processes predictive of later dissolution: Behavior, physiology, and health. *Journal of Personality and Social Psychology, 63*(2), 221–233.

Gray, J. (1992). *Men are from Mars, women are from Venus.* New York: HarperCollins.

Heaton, T. B., & Albrecht, S. L. (1991). Stable unhappy marriages. *Journal of Marriage and the Family, 53,* 747–758.

Heavey, C. L., Layne, C., & Christensen, A. (1993). Gender and conflict structure in marital interaction: A replication and extension. *Journal of Consulting and Clinical Psychology, 61*(1), 16–27.

Hendrick, S. S., Hendrick, C., & Adler, N. L. (1988). Romantic relationships: Love, satisfaction, and staying together. *Journal of Consulting and Clinical Psychology, 54*(6), 980–988.

Hocker, J. L., & Wilmot, W. W. (1995). *Interpersonal conflict* (4th ed.). Dubuque, IA: Brown & Benchmark.

Holman, T. B., & Jacquart, M. (1988). Leisure-activity patterns and marital satisfaction: A further test. *Journal of Marriage and the Family, 50,* 69–77.

Holquist, M. (1983). Answering as authoring: Mikhail Bakhtin's translinguistics. *Critical Inquiry, 10,* 307–319.

Honeycutt, J. M. (1986). A model of marital functioning based on an attraction paradigm and social-penetration dimensions. *Journal of Marriage and the Family, 48,* 651–667.

Huston, T. L., & Vangelisti, A. L. (1991). Socioemotional behavior and satisfaction in marital relationship: A longitudinal study. *Journal of Personality and Social Psychology, 61*(5), 721–733.

Johnson, D. R., Amoloza, T. O., & Booth, A. (1992). Stability and developmental change in marital quality: A three-wave panel analysis. *Journal of Marriage and the Family, 54,* 582–594.

Karney, B. R., Bradbury, T. N., Fincham, F. D., & Sullivan, K. T. (1994). The role of negative affectivity in the association between attributions and marital satisfaction. *Journal of Personality and Social Psychology*, 66(2), 413–424.

Kelly, G. A. (1979). The language of hypothesis: Man's psychological instrument. In B. Maher (Ed.), *Clinical psychology and personality: The collected papers of George Kelly* (pp. 147–162). New York: Wiley. (Original work published 1964)

Kelly, G. A. (1979). Ontological acceleration. In B. Maher (Ed.), *Clinical psychology and personality: The collected papers of George Kelly* (pp. 7–45). New York: Wiley. (Original work published 1969)

Kelly, G. A. (1970). A brief introduction to personal construct theory. In D. Bannister (Ed.), *Perspectives in personal construct psychology* (pp. 1–29). New York: Academic Press. (Original work published 1966)

Krokoff, L. J. (1990). Hidden agendas in marriage. *Communication Research*, 17(4), 483–499.

Kurdek, L. A. (1994). Areas of conflict for gay, lesbian, and heterosexual couples: What couples argue about influences relationship satisfaction. *Journal of Marriage and the Family*, 56, 923–934.

Kurdek, L. A. (1995). Predicting change in marital satisfaction from husbands' and wives' conflict resolution styles. *Journal of Marriage and the Family*, 57, 153–164.

Langis, J., Sabourin, S., Lussier, Y., & Mathieu, M. (1994). Masculinity, femininity, and marital satisfaction: An examination of theoretical models. *Journal of Personality*, 62(3), 393–414.

Levenson, R. W., & Gottman, J. M. (1983). Marital interaction: Physiological linkage and affective exchange. *Journal of Personality and Social Psychology*, 45(3), 587–597.

Levenson, R. W., & Gottman, J. M. (1985). Physiological and affective predictors of change in relational satisfaction. *Journal of Personality and Social Psychology*, 49(1), 85–94.

Lloyd, S. A., & Cate, R. M. (1985). The developmental course of conflict in dissolution of premarital relationships. *Journal of Social and Personal Relationships*, 2, 179–194.

Locke, H. J., Wallace, K. M. (1959). Short marital adjustment and prediction tests: Their reliability and validity. *Journal of Marriage and the Family*, 21, 251–255.

Long, E. C. (1993). Perspective-taking differences between high- and low-adjustment marriages: Implication for those in intervention. *American Journal of Family Therapy*, 21(3), 248–259.

Long, E. C. J., & Andrews, D. W. (1990). Perspective taking as a predicator of marital adjustment. *Journal of Personality and Social Psychology*, 59(1), 126–131.

Lye, D. N., & Biblarz, T. J. (1993). The effects of attitudes toward family life and gender roles on marital satisfaction. *Journal of Family Issues*, 14(2), 157–188.

Markman, H. J., Renick, M. J., Floyd, F. J., Stanley, S. M., & Clements, M.

(1993). Preventing marital distress through communication and conflict management training: A 4- and 5-year follow-up. *Journal of Consulting and Clinical Psychology, 61*(1), 70–77.

Marks, S. R. (1989). Toward a systems theory of marital quality. *Journal of Marriage and the Family, 51,* 15–26.

Martin, J. D., Blair, G. E., Nevels, R., & Fitzpatrick, J. H. (1990). A study of the relationship of styles of loving and marital happiness. *Psychological Reports, 66,* 123–128.

McCall, G. J. (1988). The organizational life cycle of relationships. In S. W. Duck, D. F. Hay, S. E. Hobfoll, W. J. Ickes, & B. M. Montgomery (Eds.), *Handbook of personal relationships* (pp. 467–486). Chichester, England: Wiley.

Montgomery, B. M. (1993). Relationship maintenance versus relationship change: A dialectical dilemma. *Journal of Social and Personal Relationships, 10,* 205–224.

Morson, G. S., & Emerson, C. (1990). *Mikhail Bakhtin: Creation of a prosaics.* Stanford, CA: Stanford University Press.

Noller, P., & Fitzpatrick, M. A. (1990). Marital communication in the eighties. *Journal of Marriage and the Family, 52,* 832–843.

Norton, R. (1983). Measuring marital quality: A critical look at the dependent variable. *Journal of Marriage and the Family, 45,* 141–151.

Ochs, E. (1993). Constructing social identity: A language socialization perspective. *Research on Language and Social Interaction, 26*(3), 287–306.

Pistole, M. C. (1989). Attachment in adult romantic relationships: Style of conflict resolution and relationship satisfaction. *Journal of Social and Personal Relationships, 6,* 505–510.

Prusank, D. T., Duran, R. L., & DeLillo, D. A. (1993). Interpersonal relationships in women's magazines: Dating and relating in the 1970's and 1980's. *Journal of Social and Personal Relationships, 10,* 307–320.

Rawlins, W. K. (1983). Negotiating close friendship: The dialectic of conjunctive freedoms. *Human Communication Research, 9*(3), 255–266.

Rawlins, W. K. (1992). *Friendship matters: Communication, dialectics, and the life course.* New York: Aldine/de Gruyter.

Rotheram, M. J., & Weiner, N. (1983). Androgyny, stress, and satisfaction: Dual-career and traditional relationships. *Sex Roles, 9*(2), 151–158.

Rychlak, J. F. (1976). *Dialectic: Humanistic rationale for behavior and development.* New York: Karger.

Sabatelli, R. M. (1988). Measurement issues in marital research: A review and critique of contemporary survey instruments. *Journal of Marriage and the Family, 50,* 891–915.

Shotter, J. (1989). Social accountability and the social construction of 'you'. In J. Shotter & K. J. Gergen (Eds.), *Texts of identity* (pp. 133–151). Newbury Park: Sage.

Siavelis, R. L., & Lamke, L. K. (1992). Instrumentalness and expressiveness: Predictors of heterosexual relationship satisfaction. *Sex Roles, 26*(3–4), 149–159.

Simmel, G. (1950). *The sociology of Georg Simmel* (K. Wolff, Trans.). New York: Free Press.

Simmel, G. (1955). Conflict. New York: Free Press.

Slugoski, B. R., & Ginsberg, G. P. (1989). Ego identity and explanatory speech. In J. Shotter & K. J. Gergen (Eds.), Texts of identity (pp. 36–55). Newbury Park: Sage.

Smith, G. T., Snyder, D. K., Trull, T. J., & Monsma, B. R. (1988). Predicting relationship satisfaction from couples' use of leisure time. American Journal of Family Therapy, 16(1), 3–13.

Smith, D. A., Vivian, D., & O'Leary, K. D. (1990). Longitudinal prediction of marital discord from premarital expressions of affect. Journal of Counseling and Clinical Psychology, 58(6), 790–798.

Steinberg, L., & Silverberg, S. B. (1987). Influences on marital satisfaction during the middle stages of the family life cycle. Journal of Marriage and the Family, 49, 751–760.

Suitor, J. J. (1991). Marital quality and satisfaction with the division of household labor across the family life cycle. Journal of Marriage and the Family, 53, 221–230.

Ting-Toomey, S. (1983). An analysis of verbal communication patterns in high and low marital adjustment groups. Human Communication Research, 9(4), 306–319.

VanLear, C. A. (1991). Testing a cyclical model of communicative openness in relationship development: Two longitudinal studies. Communication Monographs, 58, 337–361.

Vannoy, D., & Philliber, W. W. (1992). Wife's employment and quality of marriage. Journal of Marriage and the Family, 54, 387–398.

Volosinov, V. N./Bakhtin, M. M. (1973). Marxism and the philosophy of language (L. Matejks & I. R. Titurnik, Trans.). Cambridge, MA: Harvard University Press.

Werner, C. M., Altman, I., & Brown, B. B. (1992). A transactional approach to interpersonal relations: Physical environment, social context and temporal qualities. Journal of Social and Personal Relationships, 9, 297–323.

Werner, C. M., Altman, I., Brown, B. B., & Ginat, J. (1993). Celebrations in personal relationships: A transactional/dialectic perspective. In S. Duck (Ed.), Social context and relationships (pp. 109–138). Newbury Park, CA: Sage.

Werner, C. M., & Baxter, L. A. (1994). Temporal qualities of relationships: Organismic, transactional, and dialectical views. In M. L. Knapp & G. R. Miller (Eds.) Handbook of interpersonal communication (2nd ed., pp. 323–379). Thousand Oaks, CA: Sage.

Yelsma, P. (1984). Functional conflict management in effective marital adjustment. Communication Quarterly, 32(1), 56–61.

Yogev, S., & Brett, J. (1985). Perceptions of the division of household and child care and marital satisfaction. Journal of Marriage and the Family, 609–618.

Zuo, J. (1992). The reciprocal relationship between marital interaction and marital happiness: A three-wave study. Journal of Marriage and the Family, 54, 870–878.

PART 3

CONFLICT AND
SATISFACTION IN
CLOSE RELATIONSHIPS

CHAPTER 9

Angry at Your Partner?: Think Again

CLIFFORD I. NOTARIUS
SAMUEL L. LASHLEY
DEBRA J. SULLIVAN

Intimate relationships provide fertile ground for interpersonal conflict. These conflicts can ultimately lead partners to break their promise to love, honor, and cherish each other forever. Research over the last decade has convincingly demonstrated that the way couples handle their disagreements is the best predictor of the long-term success of their relationships (Gottman, 1994b; Notarius & Markman, 1993). Surprisingly, it is not how loving the partners are to each other in good times that makes or breaks a marriage; it is how the partners deal with conflict.

Since the management of conflict is such an important area for couples, it is essential to understand the nature of anger in intimate relationships. Anger is the fuel that fires relationship conflict, and its heat can either forge adaptive relationship change or melt down the foundation of the relationship. Our goal in this chapter is to give you, our readers, a framework for understanding the experience of anger in your relationships.

People who turn to the shelves of their local bookstore in search of advice for dealing with anger will find ample titles ready to take on all comers. Although there are many offerings, there is little agreement on the best way to deal with anger toward a loved one. Religious faith, psychotherapy, sociology, anthropology, and the self-help movement all provide inspiration to the authors. Readers of these books are encouraged to (1) release their anger or suffer physical and mental consequences of suppression (Rubin, 1969); (2) regulate their anger by first recognizing and then altering the kinds of thoughts and unrealistic expectations of others that cause one to become angry (McKay, Rogers, & McKay, 1989); (3) use their anger as a signal to inform them of needs or goals that are not being met, and then plan a course of action that will maximize the likelihood of achieving their goals (Lerner, 1985); (4) focus on changing themselves rather than on changing their partners (Wetzler, 1992); (5) take personal responsibility for their behavior and anger, and abide by virtues consistent with Christian teachings (Carter & Minirth, 1993); and (6) follow a Twelve-Step program to remedy a "rageaholic's" behavioral addiction to anger (Potter-Efron, 1994).

Part of the reason for such contradictory advice lies in the complexity that underlies human anger. To avoid adding to this confusion, we begin our discussion of anger in intimate relationships with a definition of anger and consideration of prominent theoretical perspectives that have been proposed in attempts at better understanding this basic emotion.

ANGER DEFINED

In day-to-day discourse, people tend to use the word "anger" to describe a variety of related emotional states. A formal definition will help clarify the experiences we are focusing on, as well as illustrate the complex nature of an emotion such as anger. *Webster's New Collegiate Dictionary* (1960) defines anger as "a strong passion or emotion of displeasure, and usually antagonism, excited by a sense of injury or insult" (p. 34). Although it is a simplification to divide the world of emotion into "positive" and "negative" reactions (a step often taken in empirical studies of emotion), this definition makes it clear that anger is a "negative" emotional state. As with other negative emotional states (e.g., disgust), a person so aroused will be motivated to take action to minimize the subjective displeasure. The ways people respond to alleviate this displeasure will have consequences for their well-being, and, in the context of interpersonal relationships, for the well-being of the relationships.

Emotions are not always felt one at a time. Often they are experienced simultaneously—for example, feelings of joy and jealousy at someone else's success. Perhaps for this reason, many related emotions are at times incorrectly assumed to be synonymous with anger. Although they may occur simultaneously, differentiating these related emotions from anger will allow us to explore the role of discrete emotions in relationship satisfaction more clearly.

"Contempt," for example, is defined in *Webster's* (1960) as "the feeling with which one regards that which is esteemed mean, vile, or worthless" (p. 180). In contempt, there is thus a direct message that the target of the communication is worthless. In anger, however, the person experiencing the anger is the one who feels a measure of worthlessness, stemming from his or her perception of injury or insult. Thus, when angry, a person may blame a partner for hurting him or her, but will not deem that partner worthless. Conversely, contempt has as its intent the communication that the receiver is in fact, at that moment, deemed worthless by the speaker. Such a message may indeed leave the receiver feeling angry.

There are obviously other emotions (e.g., disdain) that carry a similar negative or hostile tone. Nevertheless, this example illustrates the importance of specificity when one is investigating the role of anger in intimate relationships. The distinction between anger and contempt can help partners clarify their goals in an encounter and facilitate constructive expression of their emotional experiences. For example, an angry message expressed without contempt (or disdain) has the possibility of moving a couple toward mutual understanding of personal wants, desires, disappointments, and vulnerabilities. On the other hand, when one lover is contemptuous or disdainful toward the other, it is very costly to the relationship because it is a communication that the other is deemed worthless—at least momentarily. This is a far more destructive message between intimate partners than is an angry message that signifies hurt and disappointment.

COMPONENTS OF ANGER

Another way to define anger is to consider the components that combine to form the multidimensional emotional response we experience as anger. The experience of anger involves a specific set of thoughts, bodily reactions, facial expressions, and behavioral actions. Unfortunately, there is no definitive theory that links all these aspects into a coherent portrait of anger. Instead, disparate findings speak to the independent operation of the components more than they do to how the pieces fit together to give rise to a discrete emotional reaction we might call "anger."

Physiology

In terms of bodily reactions, there is both diffuse and specific physiological activation with anger. The diffuse arousal results from sympathetic nervous system activity that is part of the body's preparation for flight or fight—labeled by Cannon (1929) as the "emergency reaction." It includes an increase in heart rate, an increase in blood flow to the muscles, an increase in sweat gland activity, a decrease in the flow of saliva, dilation of the pupils, and deeper and faster respiration. This nonspecific arousal reaction can also occur with fear, pain, and hunger.

More specific reaction patterns have been found to be associated with fear and anger. For example, relatively large increases in diastolic blood pressure and heart rate have been found to accompany anger, but not fear (Ax, 1953; Schwartz, Weinberger, & Singer, 1981). Researchers have also found increased skin temperature—the result of peripheral vasodilation—when subjects were expressing anger (Ekman, Levenson, & Friesen, 1983); by contrast, with fear there is a decrease in skin temperature (Levenson, Ekman, & Friesen, 1990). These findings support the everyday saying "I was so angry I could feel my blood beginning to boil." They also help us to understand the physical discomfort that often accompanies anger and propels a person into actions aimed at reducing the distress. Unfortunately, these immediate responses tend to inhibit reflective discussion, which can foster intimacy and change in the long run.

Facial Expression

The classic facial expression of anger includes a frown with the muscles of the brow moved inward and downward (Izard, 1977). The eyes are fixed in a stare at the object of the anger. "The nostrils dilate and the wings of the nose flare out. The lips are opened and drawn back in a rectangle-like shape, revealing clinched teeth. Often the face flushes red" (Izard, 1977, p. 330). It is worth trying to pose this facial expression, for if the pose is accurate you are likely to feel a measure of anger. With a mirror in front of you, you can easily sense how potent this expression can be during relationship conflict.

Thoughts

The thoughts that precede, accompany, and maintain anger are essential components of this emotional response. Lazarus (1991) has perhaps given the greatest attention to defining these thoughts as part of his cognitive model of emotion. He contends that individuals get angry when the goal of "protection or enhancement of self-esteem" (Lazarus, 1994, p. 212) is threatened. The ego identity, or self, is made up of the set of beliefs, values, and commitments that a person deems important. It encompasses what people think about themselves and how they

think they should be treated by others. Anger is the reaction that ensues when another's actions are perceived as a "demeaning offense against
me and mine" (Lazarus, 1991, p. 222). In other words, angry people feel
that someone has directly insulted or disrespected their values and beliefs, who they are, and what is important to them.

In an intimate relationship, this slight is especially painful because
of the importance intimate partners place on being positively valued
by their mates. Partners want and expect each other's love, respect, and
acceptance. When one partner's behavior forces the other even momentarily to question that love and acceptance, the questioner is thrust into
the uncomfortable position of wondering whether he or she is worthy
of the partner's love. At this moment, the questioner may use anger
in order to focus his or her attention on the external world (e.g., "You
know I wanted to go to the movies instead of having dinner with the
Wolffs, and yet *you* went ahead and made dinner plans anyway"), rather
than on disquieting inner turmoil (e.g., "Most of the time when we have
dinner with the Wolffs I feel unloved and unworthy, because you wind
up criticizing me in front of them. I feel put down and miserable, and
it really hurts").

Behavior

The behavioral expressions of anger are varied and can range along a
continuum from explosive rage (both verbal and physical) to simmer-
ing, fuming, and silent discontent that are unmistakable as anger, and
yet the person so predisposed may overtly deny being angry about anything. The nature of the behavioral response will be influenced by the
strength of the physiological reaction, by an individual's beliefs about
the consequences of his or her actions, and by the individual's social
and personal standards of conduct (Lazarus, 1991). The behavioral
response is also shaped by the person's goals in an encounter. In close
interpersonal relationships, there are likely to be at least two competing goals: the preservation of self-esteem or personal well-being, and
the preservation of the relationship.

It is precisely the balance of these two goals that can lead either
to the gateway to greater intimacy and understanding, or the trap door
to increased defensiveness and resentment. When people risk being vulnerable in their relationships, they create opportunities to give and
receive the support and acceptance they desire. Alternatively, if they
allow hidden concerns over self-esteem to prevail, they may temporarily succeed in deflecting a psychologically wounding attack, but they
increase the likelihood that interactions with their partners that lead
to such attacks will be repeated. This is the consequence of tit-for-tat

negative exchanges in a relationship. Thus the behavior that seems easiest to carry out, and most effective in protecting one person's self-esteem at that moment, is paradoxically the least effective in making an intimate connection with the other person and strengthening self-esteem in the long run.

ANGER: A VIGNETTE

We'd like to introduce you to Beverly and Andy, who are about to find themselves in conflict. Their argument puts the various components of anger that we have discussed into motion. On a rainy Saturday, Beverly and Andy have decided to spend the day cleaning. This is a chore that Beverly has been wanting to do for a long time and Andy has been actively avoiding. Before they start cleaning, Andy makes a point of asking Beverly to go through their accumulated magazines and throw out the ones she doesn't want. After several hours of hard work for both of them, Andy sits down in the living room and notices that the big pile of magazines is still on the coffee table. He calls out to Beverly, "Hey, what about the magazines in here?" She responds, "I'll do it later." With a furrow in his brow, Andy thinks to himself, "I have to do everything on her schedule, but the one thing that I ask, she doesn't have time for it."

Although Andy may or may not be fully aware of precisely what is bothering him, at the base of his concerns is doubt about Beverly's respect for his wishes and priorities. As he sits brooding, he becomes angrier and more agitated as his bodily arousal increases, but he tries to contain the arousal and doesn't say anything to Beverly. He may not even be aware of just how physiologically aroused he is (Cacioppo & Petty, 1986). When Beverly is finishing up, she passes Andy and asks with a smile, "Want to go to the movies tonight?" Ignoring or perhaps not seeing her smile, he simply says, "No."

Beverly can easily sense his negative tone of voice, and she feels a knot forming in her stomach. She has no way of knowing what he is upset about, but she begins to anticipate an argument, based on her experience in hearing Andy's tone of voice. She thinks to herself, "He is sitting in front of the magazine pile. That is what he must be mad about. It's just like him to get upset about something so minor. I'm not giving in this time; I'll just see what happens." She asks, "Is something wrong?" Andy scowls and says, "Nothing!" rather pointedly. Andy's (destructive) silent pouting can be seen to reflect two competing goals. The active anger reflects his disappointment and hurt that his wishes have not been attended to by his mate. His anger will distract him from feeling ignored and hurt. Although anger is not a particularly pleasant emotion, it is better than feeling ignored, vulnerable, and unloved. Andy's silent stewing reflects his goal to preserve the relationship and not threaten his primary source of support and caring. What he most needs from Beverly is for her to acknowledge her respect for and valuing of him, and also to acknowledge that her oversight has hurt him. However, his angry and indirect response toward her leaves her confused and defensive.

At this point Beverly feels attacked, but she is not sure why. Andy also feels that he has been purposefully devalued by Beverly. Both may be too highly aroused to discuss their feelings in a way that enhances mutual understanding. If Beverly and Andy do discuss the magazines, Beverly may not understand that his anger does not stem simply from the fact that she hasn't done anything about the magazine pile. Rather, the intensity of Andy's reaction stems from his interpretation that his wishes are unimportant to his wife, and that, ultimately, he is unimportant.

Andy, maintaining his angry, defensive posture, may not be able to say he's hurt. Instead, he may prefer to feel the power of his anger rather than the pain of his hurt. Given this stance, the conflict will not be resolved; instead, both partners will feel hurt, angry, and frustrated, and each will blame the other for being unreasonable.

This vignette illustrates well how all the components of anger—thoughts, behavior, feeling, expression, and physiology—interact to produce the phenomenological experience of anger. As we have noted above, it may seem like an overstatement to describe Andy as so hurt by this encounter. Yet it is our belief that couples invest so much energy in these types of simple everyday events because they evoke the themes of love, respect, caring, status, and influence, and therefore take on inordinate personal significance. As subjective interpretations of events tap into these themes, a personal wound is opened, and the hurt from this wound is too difficult to acknowledge. Anger is then used to cover the hurt with the full force of righteous indignation: "I can't believe she ignored the magazines. This time I'm right and she's wrong, I'm being mistreated and it is not fair." Hence, attempts to cope with anger are often not successful because people are focused on the surface issue and not on the underlying interpretations. When this happens, the angry behavior can become contemptuous, or it can be submerged as defensive stewing. Either way, it pushes people further away from what they want, rather than drawing them closer to their desires for care, respect, equality, and understanding.

WHAT TRIGGERS ANGER?

It is useful to keep in mind a catalog of relationship events that can trigger anger between partners. Several efforts at developing such a catalog have been made (Buss, 1989; Snell, McDonald, & Koch, 1991). Buss (1989) identified 15 categories of behavior that can evoke anger:

Condescending
Abusive
Moody
Unfaithful
Inconsiderate
Sexualizes others
Disheveled
Emotionally constricted or
   sexually withholding/rejecting

Possessive/jealous/dependent
Physically self-absorbed
Neglecting/rejecting/unreliable
Insulting of partner's appearance
Sexually aggressive
Self-centered
Related to alcohol abuse

The categories are broad and include many of the behaviors both men and women complain are anger-provoking—especially when exhibited by a relationship partner. Although not a complete list, it does illustrate the wide range of upsetting behaviors people engage in, and by implication what some of the vulnerabilities of angered persons may be. In some cases, the behavior and the threat it represents appear fairly straightforward. If your partner acts inconsiderately, you are likely to feel unimportant or unloved, and may defend against this devaluation through anger. A partner's self-centered behavior, on the other hand, may constitute a less obvious or more indirect threat to your self-esteem. For example, when your partner tells a series of tasteless jokes during dinner with your family, you may begin to get concerned that your entire family will lose respect for you ("What's wrong with Emily that she married such a loser?").

Any list of specific behaviors that trigger anger will be incomplete. However, we believe that underlying these discrete behaviors is a much smaller list of threats to the self. Appreciating these vulnerabilities in yourself *and* your partner will begin the process of moving beyond destructive arguments over petty behavior and into a more fruitful discussion of particular sensitivities that so often lie below the surface of anger.

HOW TO UNDERSTAND YOUR ANGER

The model of anger that we are developing places primary importance on the interpretations that you make of each situation you confront. A naive view of anger holds that an event is the immediate cause of emotion. Imagine that you are waiting in line to pay for a purchase in a large department store, and the clerk takes someone who has just walked to the front of the line. In this situation (which we have adapted from Lazarus, 1994), you may experience yourself as getting "steamed"; if asked why, you might say, "Because that person cut in front of the line and I was here first." The implicit model of anger underlying this view looks like this:

Event (person cut in line) → Anger

Along with your focus on the triggering event, there will be various thoughts that help fuel your sense of injustice. These thoughts might include any or all of the following: "What's so special about this person? Why does she get to cut in line? What makes her time more precious than mine? I have a busy life too!"

Now imagine standing in line and stewing for a few minutes until you get to the cash register. When you hand your things to the cashier, she says, "Thanks for being so patient with the person who cut in line. Her daughter was just taken to the hospital, and she was buying her a robe that she needed. I know it was an inconvenience for you." Your anger is likely to ebb, although you may still feel frustrated and annoyed. At this point, you realize that there is a good explanation for why the woman was able to cut to the front of the line, and it has nothing inherently to do with the store clerk's perception that she is a more worthy person than you, or that her time is more valuable than yours. Thus, silent interpretations of events, and not the events themselves, are the immediate antecedents of an emotional response. Thus a more accurate model would look like this:

Event → Interpretation → Anger

In the scenario we have been describing, the model would look like this:

Woman cuts in line → "I was here first. This is unfair.
What makes her better than me?" → Anger

As we have noted above, there are specific themes behind the interpretations that give rise to anger. The primary theme is stated well by Lazarus (1994): "What makes us angry is that we have been taken for less than we want to be by someone who is being inconsiderate or malevolent" (p. 212). Furthermore, anger will be fueled by blaming the other person for his or her actions. With blame, an angry person holds the other accountable for his or her actions and assumes that the other had control to act otherwise (Fincham & Jaspers, 1980; Lazarus, 1991).

The concept of self-esteem is much overused in psychology, and yet it plays an undeniable role in the onset of anger. When you are "taken for less than [you] want," you are in essence identifying a momentary experience that leaves you feeling worse about yourself, or at least doubting your competence in a relevant area under perceived attack. However, as is evident in the example above, it is entirely possible that the person who cut in line had no intent to threaten your well-being; you were able to construct an esteem-lowering interpretation all by yourself. The woman who cut in line did not perceive you as less worthy than she. She was simply preoccupied with her daughter. Nevertheless, her actions caused you to question your self-worth, and as a result you became angry.

This model is useful because it provides a basis for understanding how the unique characteristics of a person can either increase or decrease the likelihood of anger in response to the *same* external event. Since challenges to self-esteem are the wellspring of anger, people need some way of systematically understanding what it is about certain events that cause them to experience a momentary threat to their personal sense of well-being, competence, or security and then become angry. Not surprisingly, childhood experiences with parents provide both the source of personal strength to protect people from these powerful feelings, and the vulnerability that opens people up to hurt. The application of childhood attachment theory (Bowlby, 1973, 1980, 1982, 1988) to adult romantic relationships provides a basis for understanding how a particular encounter with a partner can lead to anger.

ORIGINS OF VULNERABILITY AND ANGER: ATTACHMENT THEORY

Childhood Attachment

Attachment theory focuses on early interactions between parent and child, although interactions throughout life with intimate others retain the potential to alter the outcome of these early experiences. Human infants are born into a state of complete dependency on adults to meet basic needs (food, touch, comfort); without these provisions, survival is threatened. In order to facilitate the bond between infant and caregiver, attachment theorists have proposed that an infant is born with a set of behaviors designed to maintain proximity with the primary caretaker. Aspects of this behavioral system include smiling, crying, and visual tracking. Any parent can readily attest to the power these infant behaviors have for influencing nearby adults. According to the theory, adult responsiveness is also a biological given. When infant and caretaker are sufficiently close to each other, and the caretaker is responsive to the infant's needs, the infant will experience a sense of security and love.

With satisfaction of this "attachment system," the infant or child is free to engage other behavioral systems that are part of social competence and personal well-being. These other behavioral systems include exploration of the unknown (a willingness to tolerate some anxiety when confronting the unfamiliar), affiliation, giving care to others, and eventually sexual mating. If, on the other hand, the infant or child perceives the caretaker as unavailable, inattentive, or disapproving, a state of anxiety is created. This will lead the infant or child to attempt to reengage the attachment system in order to kindle proximity and caretaking from the primary caregiver. At such times, other behavioral systems (e.g., exploration) are compromised as the child devotes his or her energy to establishing an adequate attachment relationship. If this effort is successful, a feeling of security will return. If it is not successful, the child will begin a process of adaptation to the disturbed attachment relationship in an effort to get his or her caretaking needs met.

Over time the child and caretaker will have thousands of "attachment encounters"; as a result of these, the child will begin to form a set of expectancies about how significant others will react to his or her needs. These expectancies have been labeled an "internal working model," and they provide the child with a set of predictions about how the caregiver will meet or fail to meet his or her attachment needs. As long as the caretaker meets the child's attachment needs most of the time, the child will develop an internal working model that he or she is worthy of getting these needs met. If the caretaker does not reliably meet the child's needs, the child will develop an internal working model that he or she is not worthy of getting these needs met, or that he or she is asking for too much from the caretaker and must adjust himself or herself to suit the needs of the caretaker.

When the attachment encounter is unsuccessful, a child attempts to establish or reestablish the connection in the following manner. Initially, the child protests with a display of behaviors designed to show the child's unhappiness with the unfulfilled attachment yearning: crying, searching for proximity to the attachment figure, and protest against others' efforts to provide comfort. After protest, the child shows sadness and decreased effort to regain closeness. With continued absence of closeness with the provider of care, the child will become emotionally detached. The child moves back and forth through these stages as a function of the relation with the attachment figure. Thus repeated failures may lead the child to become emotionally detached much of the time. An emotionally detached person has a hard time showing anyone his or her needs for being taken care of, and an equally hard time providing such care to an intimate partner in need.

From both attachment and psychodynamic perspectives, the relationship that develops with the caregiver not only serves as a model for how significant others will respond in times of need; it also serves as the basis for self-esteem. If a child's needs are reliably and consistently met, the child will develop a sense of the self as worthy and deserving of care, the world will be seen as fair and safe, and trust in others will be fostered. If, on the other hand, a child's needs go unmet or there is a lack of responsiveness to the child's needs, then the dependent child will come to see the world as unpredictable or nonresponsive, and he or she will develop a view of the self as unworthy and undeserving (of closeness, support, and caring). The development of self-esteem thus parallels the development of internal working models for how significant others in the child's world will react to his or her most basic needs: "Experiencing the parent as available, sensitively responsive, and affectively accepting leads the child to develop simultaneously both a secure attachment and the sense that, as one who merits such treatment, he or she must be inherently worthy" (Cassidy, 1988, p. 122).

The reason for taking you through this developmental model should now be apparent. People's early attachment relationships with primary caretakers shape the internal working models they bring with them to other significant relationships. Thus early "attachment encounters" give rise to scripts that guide people's reactions to unmet needs. These early working models have been shown to have considerable stability over time (Main, Kaplan, & Cassidy, 1985) and to be resistant to change (Hazan & Shaver, 1994). However, awareness of established scripts in the context of a supportive intimate relationship can provide an opportunity for revising the script and evolving an updated working model.

For example, Mark often became sullen and withdrawn when Lauren turned down his invitation for sex. In the day or two that followed, Mark frequently became annoyed and angry at Lauren for something trivial, and a lengthy argument would ensue. During therapy, Mark realized that when he approached Lauren with a need for closeness and connection and was rejected, he equated this with the rejection he often felt from his parents as a child. He also responded to Lauren the way he typically responded as a child—by withdrawing and letting his anger seep out indirectly. In Mark's early childhood, he was frequently punished for expressing his anger directly; therefore, not only were his needs not met, but his attempts to express himself directly were discouraged. After making this connection to his childhood experiences, Mark came to see his withdrawal and then anger as protests against unmet needs. He also realized that this destructive reaction was learned in childhood.

When Mark and Lauren were able to identify this pattern, Mark was able to revise his internal script to be more in line with his relationship with Lauren in the here and now, rather than his relationship with his parents in the past. He learned that the best way to fulfill his needs was to remain available and open to Lauren and not to withdraw into himself. Sometimes he would approach her again, and at other times he would talk about his feelings without blame and anger. Lauren came to realize that when she turned down Mark's invitation for sex, he often felt deeply hurt as a result. Being sensitive to this, Lauren was able to listen to Mark's feelings nondefensively and sometimes make herself more available, and at other times explain to Mark why she wasn't available. Mark learned that his wife's reasons for being unavailable often had nothing to do with him. Through risking these interactions, Mark also realized that Lauren did not respond to his anger and hurt in the same way his parents had. Lauren was open to communication, and at times would meet his needs even if initially she had declined. As these corrective experiences led to intimacy and closeness, Mark's relationship with Lauren slowly moved beyond the stage where he would withdraw and become angry when his immediate desires went unfulfilled and he was hurting.

Adult Attachment

At this point you may be wondering about your own attachment history and what internal working models are predominant in your relationship with an intimate partner. The precise assessment of attachment history and working models is a difficult task. However, it is possible to gain an overview of your general characteristics. Read the following three descriptions and pick the one that best describes your feelings:

> I find it relatively easy to get close to others and am comfortable depending on them and having them depend on me. I don't often worry about being abandoned or about someone getting too close to me.

> I am somewhat uncomfortable being close to others; I find it difficult to trust them completely, difficult to allow myself to depend on them. I am nervous when anyone gets too close, and often, love partners want me to be more intimate than I feel comfortable being.

> I find that others are reluctant to get as close as I would like. I often worry that my partner doesn't really love me or won't want to stay with me. I want to merge completely with another person, and this desire sometimes scares people away. (Hazan & Shaver, 1987, p. 515)

If you endorsed the first statement, then you are likely to be among the 60% of the population whose attachment history has imparted a stable base. You are likely to view yourself as competent in personal relationships, to see your needs and desires as legitimate, and to have trust in others' meeting these needs. You are likely to be proactive with your partner, letting your partner know what you want and need in an assertive manner without being overly critical. If your partner fails to meet your needs, you may be disappointed, but you are unlikely to be deeply hurt. Instead, you will continue to accept the legitimacy of your needs and continue to restate your desires as you give your partner the opportunity to meet your requests.

If you subscribed to either of the second two descriptions, you are likely to be part of the remaining 40% of the population whose attachment histories were filled with some level of disappointment as significant others did not provide consistent and reliable caregiving. You coped with this disappointment in one of two ways. If you endorsed the second description, you probably tended as a child toward the use of detachment to deal with an unresponsive caregiver. Now as an adult, when your needs go unmet, you may prefer to avoid contact with a partner rather than to state (and restate if necessary) what you want. Over time, if things do not change, you may become more and more withdrawn from your partner and feel more and more resentful and angry that your needs are not being met. However, you are still unlikely to ask assertively for what you wish. When your needs go unfulfilled, and you feel unloved or uncared for, you are likely to become a "silent steamer"— holding in your anger (Notarius & Markman, 1993).

If you endorsed the third description, you are likely to have had a history with caretakers who alternated between being unavailable and unresponsive at times and intrusive and invasive at other times. In your current relationship, when your needs are being met, the relationship may seem quite satisfying and stable. When your needs go unmet, however, very strong emotional reactions and expressions can be triggered. Despite the obvious signs of distress you show, you may not be easily comforted. The relationship may take on a rather chaotic character, going from supreme satisfaction when things are going well to extreme distress when there is conflict and frustrated needs.

With just these three types of attachment histories, there are many possible mating patterns between two partners. And given that these types may not be discrete, but may vary along a continuum, it is unlikely that any given relationship will ever be precisely described in terms of these patterns. Nevertheless, we believe that these broad types are useful, in that they suggest a beginning point for looking at prototypical responses to unmet needs—a fact of life in even the best of relationships.

Self-esteem is likely to be the most robust among individuals who find the first description most like them, and lower among persons endorsing either of the next two descriptions. Thus we might expect strong negative emotions to be a more prominent feature in relationships where one or both partners have had less than ideal childhood experiences with primary caregivers. Furthermore, as suggested above, the manner in which these emotions are experienced and expressed may vary across the three attachment types.

As a given, we expect that partners' needs, wants, and desires will be in conflict from time to time in all relationships. When this happens within the context of a relationship where both partners feel a secure, stable base, we expect that the disappointment that results from unfulfilled needs will be channeled into assertive negotiations as the partners work toward a mutually satisfying accommodation of each other's perspectives. Partners who endorse the second statement above are likely to avoid this negotiation process. They are more likely to feel that their partners *should* know what they want and need, and when these provisions are not forthcoming, they will feel resentful, unfulfilled, and unwilling to do anything about their unmet desires. Should one partner make a demand, it is likely to elicit thoughts of inequity in the other: "I'm not getting what I want, and yet I'm expected to do X, Y, and Z, for you . . . forget it." Not surprisingly, with this process in full gear, conflict is likely to escalate and become entrenched.

Partners who endorse the third description as characteristic of themselves are likely to be emotionally reactive and to have relationships with marked emotional extremes (Hazan & Shaver, 1987). When needs are being met and the partners are in agreement, there will be no threat to self-esteem, and consequently there can be a feeling of joyous union without threat and with slight anticipation of future problems. However, when disagreements and disappointments surface, these can be experienced as profound threats to self-worth and corresponding anger will ensue: "If you loved and understood me, you would know what I want and need. I wouldn't have to ask for it. Since you are not giving me what I need, you must not love me, and I must be unlovable." It is easy to see how such a train of thought can lead to both conflict and misery.

If a significant number of people endorse the second or third descriptions, it may seem surprising that so many people get past their own defenses, low self-esteem, and lack of trust in others in order to come together as couples. And yet we know that many of the 40% of the population who are insecurely attached do find their way into relationships. Why would they want to risk so much, if their past experiences have left them feeling insecure? Some believe that "mutual attraction and sexual interest can get couples together, but if partners fail to satisfy each other's needs for comfort and security, dissatisfaction will likely result" (Hazan & Shaver, 1994, p. 11.).

Satir (1967), an experienced family therapist, offers a similar explanation:

> Once puberty brought adult sexuality to the fore, they risked relationship in spite of all their fears. Also, they were in love which, for the time, enhanced their self-esteem and made each feel complete. Each said: "You seem to value me . . . I am lucky to have you . . . I need you in order to survive . . . I am complete if you are around." Both ended up living for each other and, in doing so, entered into a "survival pact." Each said privately to himself: "If I run out of supplies I will take from you. You will have enough, in an emergency to serve us both." The trouble is, when choosing each other as mates, that Mary and Joe did not communicate their fears (of worthlessness) to each other. (p. 9)

And Satir argues that consequently, over time, neither partner will be able to meet the unrealistic needs of the other, and resentment and hurt will ensue. Certainly sexuality is a strong reinforcer for relationship development. However, sexuality is only one reason why people seek intimate relationships. Other reasons—such as a continued desire for attachment to a primary caregiver, as well as the reciprocal role of providing care to someone else (a role that can enhance self-esteem)—have been suggested as equally important. What remains essential to remember is that these fears and insecurities have power in people's lives solely because of their desire to connect with others and to be valued. These desires can be so strong that individuals may, as Satir suggests, temporarily suppress their disappointments and anger in the service of attracting a partner. Thus we might expect to see insecurely attached persons exert increased control over negative emotions, including anger, during courtship so as not to jeopardize the relationship. This in fact was found to be the case in a recent study (Feeney, 1995). It still remains to be studied whether, over time, the emotional control demonstrated in courtship yields to less control as disappointments and discord come to dominate the relationship. Whatever the reasons people join in intimate relationships, continued satisfaction in these relationships will be directly affected by their ability to negotiate the daily give-and-take process of meeting each other's needs.

ANGER AND RELATIONSHIP SATISFACTION

No relationship will be or should be free of anger. Its occurrence simply heralds a transaction that has left at least one partner feeling a little bit worse about himself or herself, and thinking that the other person acted intentionally and therefore deserves to be blamed for the transgression. Exactly how the anger is expressed, responded to, and worked through holds the key to whether or not an angry exchange is constructive or destructive for a relationship. In addition, the frequency of these types of encounters is likely to be a factor in relationship satisfaction. Few relationships will benefit from frequent encounters that leave one or both partners feeling threatened or attacked. On the other hand, subtle put-downs that diminish self-esteem, and that are stored away without comment, will also eventually erode relationship satisfaction.

The triggers that evoke a threat to self-esteem and the resultant anger lie in the day-to-day interactions that partners have with each other. These interactions include everyday conversations, problem-solving discussions, and daily deeds (see Buss's [1989] list on p. 226). Interactions that lead to anger will often be accompanied by a negative voice tone, an angry facial expression, and perhaps a hostile gesture. These types of behaviors are much more common in distressed, unhappy relationships than they are in happy unions (Gottman, 1994b; Gottman, Markman, & Notarius, 1977; Margolin & Wampold, 1981), suggesting that the signs of anger in a relationship deserve careful attention.

Despite the evidence associating marital distress with anger, there is also recent evidence showing that appropriately expressed anger can be a harbinger of marital satisfaction over time (Gottman & Krokoff, 1989). If your partner is doing something that leaves you feeling hurt and angry, it is obviously not constructive simply to ignore the offensive behavior and hope that it goes away. It is better to disclose your anger to your partner in a manner that maximizes the opportunity for your partner to learn what impact his or her behavior has had upon you. This is most likely to be accomplished if you state clearly and assertively: "When you did X, I was angry and hurt because I felt unappreciated and put down; I felt that what I had done was worthless in your eyes, and I need you to value me." If your anger leads you to respond in a contemptuous way toward your partner, or if your anger is explosively charged, you are much more likely to provoke a defensive response from your partner than to maximize the opportunity for understanding. Any encounter that leaves you feeling hurt and angry, and your partner feeling attacked and engaged in defensive maneuvers, is likely to be destructive. This is equally true for both males and females in close personal relationships, despite some recent focus on sex differences in marriage. Thus, although anger can be a positive force for relationship change, it needs to be expressed in such a way that it fosters mutual understanding and responsive change (Notarius & Markman, 1993).

HOW TO DEAL WITH ANGER

We believe that there are several good resources available for helping couples deal constructively with their anger (e.g., Gottman, 1994a; Notarius & Markman, 1993). The expression of anger that promotes relationship satisfaction requires careful attention to and monitoring of words, thoughts, and physiological or bodily arousal. A detailed plan is mapped out in a recent book (Notarius & Markman, 1994). Here we concentrate on a metaphor that we have used with some success to move couples into a better position to understand and deal with their anger. (Warning: This metaphor is not for the squeamish.)

We ask partners to imagine a scenario in which one person is in the kitchen cutting up some vegetables for dinner right after the partners have had a huge fight and are not talking to each other. The anger in the relationship is palpable. Just as one partner happens into the kitchen, the person cutting the vegetables slips and badly cuts a finger. There is blood spurting everywhere. At this point we ask both partners to state what would happen. With no exception to date, all couples report that there would be caretaking—every effort would be made to do whatever was necessary to take care of the wounded partner. In this scenario, there is a physical wound, and the wounded partner's body is taking care of alerting the other that attention is required. When one partner bleeds, the other takes care of him or her. If the other stood by and watched him or her bleed without providing care, this would be a powerful message indeed.

Now we ask couples to consider a similar scenario in which a partner suffers a psychological wound that causes "internal bleeding." The hurt is not visible to the world, and therefore support will not be immediately forthcoming. Instead, the injured party must "emotionally bleed" in order to get support. The likelihood of getting support in this scenario will be directly related to the clarity of the "emotional bleeding." If the wounded person decides to bare his or her teeth as some wounded animals do, then this is likely to keep away a potential caretaker. If, on the other hand, the wounded person decides to show the wound plainly to another, to "bleed," then caretaking will most likely follow. Thus, the advice we offer to couples is for partners to "bleed" when they are psychologically hurt. We say, "Show your wounds to your partner, and just as if you were physically bleeding, more often than not you will receive the caretaking you desire."

There are two other aspects of this metaphor to consider. The primary difference between cutting oneself while slicing vegetables and suffering an emotional wound is that in the latter case, the other partner is usually held responsible for the injury. And in this case, the "emotional bleeding" that we encourage will be directed at the person blamed for the injury, who is *also* the potential caregiver. We find it useful to have the "bleeding" partner focus primarily on his or her own wound rather than on blaming the other for the injury. We remind couples that the goal is caretaking, and that at that moment anything that interferes with it will be self-destructive.

Second, we encourage couples to think through the scenario in which the injured partner plays the role of a hurt animal and snarls at anyone who attempts to provide care. Such behavior certainly minimizes the opportunity for another to provide care, but it need not preclude caregiving. Accordingly, if a partner finds that his or her wounded mate is pushing others away, successful approach and caregiving under these adverse circumstances can be an opportunity to show an extra amount of caring. In essence, it conveys this message: "I love you in spite of all of your efforts to suffer alone and to push me away. I will not be pushed away." Of course, if this becomes a predictable pattern in the relationship rather than an infrequent opportunity for showing extra caring, it may be difficult for the caregiver to keep overcoming the initial barriers to providing care. It is hard enough to be a caregiver without having to overcome the obstacles of a partner in need who rejects succor.

Beyond the empathetic approach to handling anger illustrated in this metaphor, anger can be used to enhance relationship satisfaction once a couple learns to approach conflict wisely. To return to Beverly and Andy's conflict, it should now be apparent that both partners have opportunities throughout their interaction to change a destructive, angry episode into a relationship-enhancing one. As Andy sits staring at the magazines, his hostile thoughts toward someone he loves, his angry facial expressions, or his growing discomfort from physiological arousal can cue him into his feeling of being devalued by Beverly. At this point he may either reappraise the importance of a stack of magazines to his self-esteem, or begin a conversation with Beverly about his vulnerability to her apparent disregard for him in this instance. Following an exposure of personal vulnerability such as this, Beverly will be much more likely to be open to constructive problem solving than if she is feeling defensive because of the tension and passive withdrawal on Andy's part.

Beverly also has opportunities to change the destructive outcome of their Saturday morning activity. When she takes notice of Andy's negative tone of voice, instead of becoming defensive herself and preparing to fend off any insinuation from Andy that there is anything wrong with her or the way she is cleaning the house, she can acknowledge that Andy's anger is probably the result of something more meaningful than the magazines. Beverly can then approach him and ask him what he is angry about. When he responds, "The damn magazines," she can then ask him sincerely whether he feels she is disregarding the things he feels are important, and explain that it was simply an unintentional oversight. Andy will then discover that his wife does honor his requests and is happy to move the magazines.

Often, moving to this stage of interaction is difficult because both partners are feeling attacked. Even if they know how to resolve the issue, they may still think, "I am the one who was wronged here. He [or she] should have to make the first attempt to reconcile." The first problem with this thinking is that if both partners feel this way, they will not be able to reach a satisfactory resolution. The second problem is the conflict between wanting to resolve the issue and being unwilling to do what is necessary to achieve it. In the end, it does not matter who initiates the resolution; the benefits will still be as sweet for both partners. Over time, we encourage both partners to play the role of caregiver.

If the behaviors suggested above for the resolution of anger seem highly unlikely to happen in your relationship, you are not alone. Even though there are ample suggestions for how to deal with anger in life and in relationships, we are struck by an unshakeable clinical reality in our work with couples: It is difficult to change a lifelong pattern for dealing with the hurt that underlies so much of the anger that emerges in the context of close personal relationships. We have seen many couples learn the appropriate strategies for dealing with their anger, and even experience considerable success trying these out in their relationships. Yet there comes a time when doing this is not enough. One or both members of such a couple, in the security of the therapy room, can chart out with calm insight what steps they needed to take to resolve a painful conflict encounter that left both feeling hurt, angry, and resentful, and what barriers were erected to prevent this action. Despite having these novel insights and new behavioral strategies, the partners turn to one of us and say, "But I just couldn't do it. I know what I was supposed to do. I know in the past when I did it, it worked. But I was just too angry to try this time." Thus we think it essential to turn our attention to helping couples at this stage of their work to master unremitting relationship anger.

WHY IT IS SO HARD TO CHANGE

You now have some understanding of why you get angry at your partner and why your partner gets angry at you. You've used suggestions on how to deal with anger, and you've found them helpful to a point. So why is it so difficult to change these patterns when you need to the most—when you are so angry you can't do anything about it, other than attack your partner in a defensive rage or withdraw into a funk? What stops you from saying, "When you say or do X, it makes me angry because it feels like an attack on who I am. I feel put down, belittled, and treated unfairly and without respect. Do you understand?" What stops you from responding to this type of statement from your partner by saying, "Okay, when I did X, you felt like I was treating you unfairly, with no respect, and you felt under siege. Do I have it? Let's talk about how we can understand and work through this." This would set the stage for closeness and problem solving. Instead, the same old troubling patterns play out. Both you and your partner have a good idea about what you are supposed to do, but neither of you can carry out these new behaviors when you need it most—in the midst of an argument when both of you are feeling hurt. Why?

We think there are three interrelated forces that conspire to make changes in dealing with anger in an intimate relationship so difficult. All three can be traced back to the interactions you had as a child with parents, siblings, and perhaps other significant adults. The three forces, which we discuss in turn, are as follows: the permanence of self-esteem; the manner in which caregivers responded to you when you needed caretaking and support; and the way your parents modeled angry interactions.

The Permanence of Self-Esteem

As attachment theory suggests, the origins of self-esteem can be traced back to the adequacy with which significant adults reliably met or failed to meet the needs of a child. If attachment needs are consistently met, self-esteem is promoted. If needs are not consistently met, then the development of self-esteem will be compromised as the child's view of the world becomes dominated by concerns that he or she must not be worthy of caring and support. Since these emotional tracks are laid down early in life, they are tough to move.

According to the model of anger that we have developed, the interpretations that people construct for events in their lives will help determine the consequent emotion that is generated following the event. Individuals with low self-esteem will be primed to interpret events as threats to personal well-being because they are so unsure of themselves and expect that people think the worst of them. The strength of anger, whether expressed outwardly or held silently, protects the fragile self from feeling horrible about oneself. As you probably know, it is always easier to look externally and blame another for what has not gone to your liking than to examine honestly how you feel about yourself and your possible contribution.

We believe that these core beliefs about the self, formed in childhood in interaction with parents, will not yield easily to experiences later in life that affirm competence. Many clients we see can speak at length about how competent they feel, and freely describe themselves as having high self-esteem. Nevertheless, below the bravado of accomplishment lie nagging doubts that their parents did not value them or held a sibling in higher regard, or that their achievements were never quite good enough to please Mom or Dad. Thus, as children, they did not internalize a positive image of themselves as seen through the eyes of their parents. Later in life, they may understand intellectually that not being valued by their parents does not mean they are unworthy, but their emotional core remains frightened about failure and overly sensitive to criticism. If this is an accurate description of your experience, you can see why it is very difficult to alter the automatic and well-rehearsed response patterns involved in anger among intimate partners. Above all else, you may crave the unshakeable love of an intimate partner, and if this person disappoints you, criticizes you, ignores you, or behaves in any manner that pokes at your self-esteem, before you know it you will become angry and blame him or her for your bad feelings.

The Manner in Which Caregivers Responded to You When You Needed Caretaking and Support

One of the developmental challenges facing children is the task of putting powerful thoughts and feelings into words. Parents can facilitate this task by taking time to talk with their children about concerns and to listen to their feelings in an open way that encourages further talk. When children go to a parent with powerful feelings and do not receive a receptive ear, they are being taught that strong emotions cannot be discussed and must be dealt with privately. Even well-meaning parents who pat a child on the back and happily chide, "Cheer up," are invalidating an inner experience that is troubling. Over time, such training leads the child to withdraw into himself or herself rather than to risk rejection and further hurt. If this was your childhood experience, is it any wonder that when you are hurt as an adult, you don't know how to elicit or receive the support and caretaking needed from a partner? You may have had little opportunity to break what is likely to be a well-learned, well-rehearsed pattern of coping with hurt.

Let's follow an example that traces these childhood experiences into adulthood. We meet Tim as a 15-year-old in the midst of adolescence, pushing for more independence from his parents while at the same time wanting the security of their guidance and support. Tim is friends with two buddies who are slightly older, and the three friends decide to plan an overnight bicycle trip. They write away for maps, choose possible destinations, and have great fun together planning the big adventure. To this point, none of the boys have talked about the trip with their parents. Once they have settled on a 100-mile trip, the day comes when each will present the trip to his parents.

Tim chooses to begin the discussion over dinner. If some magic "truth meter" could be placed on his inner thoughts, it would reveal that Tim is actually petrified about the thought of this bicycle trip. He is scared about his physical ability to pedal 100 miles; he is scared about being away from home for several nights; he is scared about camping out; and he is scared that his friends will think less of him if he doesn't go on the trip. But an observer would never know that these are his thoughts. Instead, he boldly launches into a description of the trip and all the work he and his friends have done to plan it. He doesn't get too far before his mother glances at his father, and his father says, "You're not going. Tell Mark and Ralph that you are not going with them. Case closed." Tim takes solace in the anger he directs at his parents. Feeling unfairly treated, his fears about the trip give way to righteous indignation about how miserable his parents are. He argues his case for a few minutes and then storms away from the dinner table and loudly slams the door to his room. The whole house shakes. Here, at this moment, is an opportunity for Tim to learn about anger, to seek and receive care, and to talk through his feelings. Tim has made his move, and his parents must make theirs.

If his parents let Tim stew in his room alone and do not break the silence, Tim will learn that his anger has no safe outlet and that it has no use. He may attempt to bring up the issue again, and each time his parents may say, "No, and that is final." If this has been a consistent pattern of behaving and responding to needs and feelings in Tim's family, he will have learned that his emotions (in this case, fear and anger) and his needs (for guidance and support) are not legitimate. Tim will never have to confront his fears about doing something he is scared of, and will never get the opportunity to puzzle out his often contradictory feelings and options with his parents. He will miss the opportunity to talk about his anger, to understand it better, and to resolve it with his parents. He will not learn how to "bleed" when he is hurt, and instead will learn how to put up a stone wall against others when he is angry.

Years later, Tim's wife is likely to learn this pattern pretty quickly. For example, suppose Tim has an issue that he wants to discuss with her, but he is unsure of his feelings and is feeling somewhat vulnerable about the matter. As he starts to test the waters, wondering whether his wife will be supportive, he may take a slight hesitation or well-meaning questioning from her as a sign that he will not be supported. He may rapidly explode into a rage, leave the room, and slam the door. In essence, Tim is equating his wife's hesitation with parental rejection. His hurt and anger will come automatically, because the behavior pattern and associated feelings have been ingrained over the years when dealing with his parents. Not understanding Tim's "overreaction," his wife may become defensive herself and have a difficult time knowing what to do or how to comfort him. Because Tim perceives his wife's behavior as similar to his parents' behavior, he is going to have a hard time letting down the defensive wall that protects his vulnerable self-esteem. He is going to have a hard time letting his wife provide the comfort and support he wants but cannot admit wanting.

There is an alternative and more constructive outcome for Tim's adolescent scenario. Shortly after Tim slams the door, his father comes up, knocks on the door, and says, "I'd like to talk. Can I come in?" Tim thinks it over and mumbles, "Okay." His father starts off in this way: "I don't like it that you left the dinner table, ran upstairs to your room, and then slammed the door. Getting up like you did and slamming the door like you did is disrespectful to your mother and me. However, I realize that for you to behave like that, something must be bothering you. Why are you so angry with us?" Tim may then feel freer to respond, "I'm sorry that I slammed the door, but I really want to go on this trip. You never let me do anything I want to do. You don't trust me. We have this trip all planned out."

Tim's father might then say, "I know you really want to go on this trip. And, yes, I do trust you in many things. Perhaps I should have listened to your plans before just saying 'No.' I guess the reason I jumped in so fast is that I was scared that the trip would not be safe for you and that it was a little unrealistic. But I do know how much you want to go. What would it be like for you to tell Mark and Ralph we won't let you go?"

With that said, Tim begins to feel that his father—though disapproving of his behavior at the dinner table—understands him, and his anger slowly gives way to unexpressed fear. Tim confides, "Well, you know, part of me really wants to go, and part of me is really terrified. I'm not sure it is a good idea, but after we started planning I didn't want to be the one who was backing out."

The conversation still has a way to go, and it is unlikely to play out as smoothly as we have described it here, but it is firmly on track to allow Tim to seek support from his father and for his father to provide a nurturing ear. In the process, Tim's anger is transformed into an opportunity for intimacy with his father and an opportunity for learning how anger can lead to constructive outcomes. People who grew up in environments like this will have learned constructive ways to communicate when angry and will be more able to get their needs met when they are scared, hurt, or challenged.

The Way Parents Modeled Angry Interactions

Children's parents (or primary caregivers) are their first role models for how adults react to and deal with powerful emotions. Children are especially sensitive to adults' display of angry behavior, and so will be particularly alert to how adults deal with this emotion (Cummings & Davies, 1994). The ways in which parents communicate with each other when angry serves as the model for how adults deal with anger and conflict. Over time and many angry conflicts, children learn their parents' way of communicating around anger. If angry conflicts are resolved — that is, if the parents each state their positions in the encounter, and a child witnesses them arriving at a mutually acceptable solution — then the child's model for dealing with angry conflict will be a constructive one. If, on the other hand, the parents model ineffective conflict resolution tactics when angry, then the child may not learn how to deal effectively with anger in relationships.

Consider the following scenario. Nancy's parents have a history of arguing over being on time to appointments with each other. One night, Nancy's father, Ted, plans to come home early to prepare a nice dinner for the family. He leaves a message for Mary, Nancy's mother, to let her know his plans. When he gets home, he finds a message that she has to run a business errand, that she will be home at 6:00, and that she is looking forward to dinner. Mary's appointment goes a little longer than she expected, and she starts to get nervous about another fight with Ted over being on time. She thinks about calling home to let him know she is going to be late, but doesn't want to get off the road to make the call. When Mary finally walks in the door, 35 minutes late, Nancy is witness to the following scene:

Her father is standing in front of the oven staring at an overcooked roast. Her mother says, "Smells good. What are we having?"

"Charred leather. Where the hell have you been? Why can't you ever be on time?"

Mary responds, "How was I supposed to know *today* was the day you were going to come home early and cook? You leave me a message at 4 and expect the whole world to revolve around you. I've got work to do too. I thought I could get home, but everything took longer than I expected. And why must you get so angry? I am sick and tired of it."

"Fine. Forget me coming home early and cooking. I try to help out, and this is what I get. I'm going back to work."

Mary shouts out after him, "Who are you helping out? This is your family too!"

Nancy and her mother eat dinner together in silence. Afterwards, Nancy goes up to do her homework, but she and her mother say little. Eventually, her father returns home and sleeps on the couch in the den. Over the next couple of days, there is tension in the house, but eventually things return to "normal" with no conversation about the ruined dinner.

In this scenario, both parents explode and then retreat into an angry silence. Each thinks the other is being irrational and unjustified in his or her anger, and each holds firmly to his or her respective position. If you grew up in a similar environment, when faced with angry conflicts with significant others you may only know how to explode or withdraw, and believe you have to hold tightly to your "correct position." You may have witnessed no alternatives. Even if you didn't agree or like the way your parents responded to each other when angry, you were exposed again and again to this destructive method of conflict resolution. Learning a new method of resolving angry conflict will take hard work, as the old patterns involving thoughts, arousal, and behaviors have become ingrained over time.

Suppose that Nancy is fortunate enough to witness a different pattern of conflict between her parents. Suppose one of her parents stops the argument early and says, "I know you are really upset here, so let's stop this fight. You go first and tell me why you are so upset, and I'll listen. Then I'll let you know what upset me. Okay?" The parents then share their different sides of the conflict, while Nancy has a chance to observe how conflict between partners can be discussed and can lead to closeness instead of being avoided and ending in distance.

If you grew up with these types of role models, you will have learned more constructive ways of communicating angry feelings with significant others and will be able to bring those skills to your present family. Inevitably, parents will not always model ideal communication around conflict and anger. But when they do, they provide their children with the opportunity to see anger dealt with adaptively, and they enhance their children's resources for dealing with anger in their adult lives.

SOME FINAL THOUGHTS ON CHANGE

What, then, can you do if your parents or other caretakers left you with vulnerabilities in the mantle of self-esteem, more often than not were unavailable for caregiving, and did not provide you with good models for coping with anger or communicating effectively when angry? The key to change is threefold. First, you have to acknowledge those aspects of yourself that you consider weaknesses, and to understand the source of these vulnerabilities. If you frequently felt criticized by a parent and felt that the only way you could defend yourself was through an angry attack or withdrawal, then you may respond to an innocent statement from your partner as if it were a pointed criticism from a parent. In essence, you are responding to voices from the past rather than to the person beside you. At this moment, understanding the source of your anger, searching for the underlying wound, and sharing the hurt with your partner can go a long way toward changing the pattern. In addition, your efforts to strengthen competence and build self-esteem will increasingly make anger a less likely response to hurt.

Second, while working on increasing your self-esteem and differentiating between your parent's and your partner's behaviors, you need to start taking risks to behave and communicate more effectively with your partner. Suggestions for how to do this are provided in the earlier section "How to Deal with Anger," and in recent books for couples (Gottman, 1994a; Notarius & Markman, 1994). If you find you are having trouble putting these suggestions into practice in your relationship, we suggest you seek the professional help of a couple therapist to help get you on the right track.

Third, it is necessary to practice, practice, and practice alternative responses to anger. Your characteristic way of responding to anger did not develop overnight, and a new pattern will also not develop overnight—no matter how much you may wish it could. Instead, repeated rehearsal of the old pattern has formed a linked network of thoughts or interpretations, physiological reactions, words spoken, and actions taken when angered. This well-orchestrated response can happen so quickly as to seem automatic. The best way to change it is to begin practicing alternative ways of thinking (e.g., replacing "hot thoughts" that generate anger with "cool thoughts" that promote conversation and problem solving—Notarius & Markman, 1994); quieting physiological arousal with relaxation techniques (e.g., Benson, 1976); and avoiding critical remarks that make others defensive in favor of listening and understanding, which promote closeness and intimacy (Notarius & Markman, 1994).

Everyone has had the experience of learning a new behavior. It is easiest to master the new behavior when arousal is low. For example, it is easier to master a new golf or tennis swing in the privacy of a lesson than it is on the tee or court, when people are watching, the pressure is high, and you want to do well and avoid embarrassment. The principles are the same when you are trying to master new interpersonal behaviors. You will have an easier time practicing new behaviors when pressure is low than in the midst of intense conflict. Therefore, we suggest that you and your partner begin to practice new ways of dealing with anger when arousal is not too high. Repeated practice in low-conflict situations will make it easier to use new resources when they are needed in more challenging times. It is also helpful to realize that dealing with anger is a "team sport." You will make it harder on yourself if your behavior is so provocative to your partner that it stretches the partner's resources beyond his or her current capabilities to respond adaptively. Instead, if you each try to help the other person master a new way of dealing with anger, and do this repeatedly, you will find the old patterns giving way to change. Risking new behaviors can lead not only to protecting your self-esteem, but also to getting the love, acceptance, and support from your relationship for which you yearn.

REFERENCES

Ax, A. F. (1953). The psychological differentiation between fear and anger in humans. *Psychosomatic Medicine*, *15*, 433–442.

Benson, H. (1976). *The relaxation response*. New York: Avon.

Bowlby, J. (1973). *Attachment and loss: Vol. 2. Separation: Anxiety and anger*. New York: Basic Books.

Bowlby, J. (1980). *Attachment and loss: Vol. 3. Loss: Sadness and depression*. New York: Basic Books.

Bowlby, J. (1982). *Attachment and loss: Vol. 1. Attachment* (2nd ed.). New York: Basic Books.

Bowlby, J. (1988). *A secure base: Parent–child attachment and healthy human development*. New York: Basic Books.

Buss, D. M. (1989). Conflict between the sexes: Strategic interference and the evocation of anger and upset. *Journal of Personality and Social Psychology*, *56*, 735–747.

Cacioppo, J. T., & Petty, R. E. (1986). Social processes. In M. G. H. Coles, E. Donchin, & S. W. Porges (Eds.), *Psychophysiology: Systems, processes, and applications* (pp. 646–679). New York: Guilford Press.

Cannon, W. B. (1929). *Bodily changes in pain, hunger, fear, and rage*. New York: Appleton.

Carter, L., & Minirth, F. (1993). *The anger workbook*. Nashville, TN: Thomas Nelson.

Cassidy, J. (1988). Child–mother attachment and the self in six-year olds. *Child Development*, *59*, 121–134.

Cummings, E. M., & Davies, P. T. (1994). *Children and marital conflict: The impact of family dispute and resolution*. New York: Guilford Press.

Ekman, P., Levenson, R. W., & Friesen, W. V. (1983). Autonomic nervous system activity distinguishing among emotions. *Science*, *221*, 1208–1210.

Feeney, J. A. (1995). Adult attachment and emotional control. *Personal Relationships, 2,* 143–159.

Fincham, F. D., & Jaspers, J. M. (1980). Attribution of responsibility: From man the scientist to man the lawyer. In L. Berkowitz (Ed.), *Advances in experimental social psychology* (Vol. 13, pp. 81–138). New York: Academic Press.

Gottman, J. M. (1994a). *Why marriages succeed or fail.* New York: Simon & Schuster.

Gottman, J. M. (1994b). *What predicts divorce?: The relationship between marital processes and marital outcomes.* Hillsdale, NJ: Erlbaum.

Gottman, J. M., & Krokoff, L. J. (1989). Marital interaction and satisfaction: A longitudinal view. *Journal of Consulting and Clinical Psychology, 57,* 47–52.

Gottman, J. M., Markman, H., & Notarius, C. (1977). The topography of marital conflict: A sequential analysis of verbal and nonverbal behavior. *Journal of Marriage and the Family, 39,* 461–477.

Hazan, C., & Shaver, P. R. (1987). Romantic love conceptualized as an attachment process. *Journal of Personality and Social Psychology, 52,* 511–524.

Hazan, C., & Shaver, P. R. (1994). Attachment as an organizational framework for research on close relationships. *Psychological Inquiry, 5,* 1–22.

Izard, C. E. (1977). *Human emotion.* New York: Plenum Press.

Lazarus, R. S. (1991). *Emotion and adaptation.* New York: Oxford University Press.

Lazarus, R. S. (1994). Appraisal: The long and short of it. In P. Ekman & R. J. Davidson (Eds.), *The nature of emotion: Fundamental questions* (pp. 208–215). New York: Oxford University Press.

Lerner, H. (1985). *The dance of anger.* New York: Harper & Row.

Levenson, R.W., Ekman, P., & Friesen, W.V. (1990). Voluntary facial action generates emotion-specific autonomic nervous system activity. *Psychophysiology, 27,* 363–384.

Main, M., Kaplan, N., & Cassidy, J. (1985). Security in infancy, childhood, and adulthood: A move to the level of representation. In I. Bretherton & E. Waters (Eds.), Growing points of attachment theory and research. *Monographs of the Society for Research in Child Development, 50*(1–2, Serial No. 209), 66–104.

Margolin, G., & Wampold, B. E. (1981). Sequential analysis of conflict and accord in distressed and nondistressed marital partners. *Journal of Consulting and Clinical Psychology, 49,* 554–567.

McKay, M., Rogers, P. D., & McKay, J. (1989). *When anger hurts: Quieting the storm within.* Oakland, CA: New Harbinger.

Notarius, C. I., & Markman, H. J. (1993). *We can work it out: Making sense of marital conflict.* New York: Putnam.

Notarius, C. I., & Markman, H. J. (1994). *We can work it out: How to solve conflicts, save your marriage, and strengthen your love for each other.* New York: Perigee.

Potter-Efron, R. (1994). *Angry all the time.* Oakland: New Harbinger.

Rubin, T.J. (1969). *The angry book.* New York: Collier.

Satir, V. (1967). *Conjoint family therapy.* Palo Alto, CA: Science & Behavior Books.

Schwartz, G. E., Weinberger, D. A., & Singer, J. A. (1981). Cardiovascular differentiation of happiness, sadness, anger and fear following imagery and exercise. *Psychosomatic Medicine, 43,* 343–364.

Snell, W. E., McDonald, K., & Koch, W. R. (1991). Anger provoking experiences: A multidimensional scaling analysis. *Personality and Individual Differences, 12,* 1095–1104.

Webster's new collegiate dictionary. (1960). Springfield, MA: G. & C. Merriam Co.

Wetzler, S. (1992). *Living with the passive–aggressive man.* New York: Fireside.

CHAPTER 10

Conflict and Satisfaction in Couples

ANDREW CHRISTENSEN
PAMELA T. WALCZYNSKI

Perhaps the most significant transformation that ordinary adults go through during their lives is the transition from a loving, romantic relationship to a breakup. Most adults experience at least one romantic relationship that ends—whether it involves the breakup of boyfriend and girlfriend, the termination of wedding plans, or separation and divorce. This transition typically moves people from a stage of intense love and satisfaction, in which partners fantasize a life together and may pledge commitment "till death do us part," to a stage of anger and dissatisfaction, in which the partners may wish they had never met or hope they will never interact again. Understanding this transformation will tell us much about relationship satisfaction and treatments to improve it.

Psychological research has examined the possible reasons for this transformation by investigating the concurrent and longitudinal correlates of relationship satisfaction and stability (see Karney & Bradbury, 1995, for a review of longitudinal predictors of marital quality and stability). Various personality factors, such as neuroticism and impulsivity, have been implicated in this transformation (Kelly & Conley, 1987). Attributional tendencies in a partner that place the cause and responsibility for negative events upon the other partner can predict the decline of marital quality (Bradbury & Fincham, 1990). Communication skills deficits are also correlated with current and future satisfaction (Weiss & Heyman, 1990; Karney & Bradbury, 1995).

Although the evidence for all of these variables, as well as others, is convincing, they are dissatisfying in a couple of respects. First, because these variables refer to stable characteristics (personality traits, skills, cognitive tendencies), they do not yield a dynamic explanation for why, when, and how the transformation from love to breakup takes place. Consider, for example, the personality trait of neuroticism. If one or both partners in a couple are high on neuroticism, they were presumably neurotic throughout their relationship, from the days of intense love to breakup. How and when did this stable characteristic turn the love of courtship and early marriage into the anger of breakup? Similarly, their communication skills were presumably present (or lacking) from the first days of their relationship (Lindahl, Clements, & Markman, in press). How and when did these skills transform their relationship? Second, these variables are often distal from the immediate factors that lead to breakup. Typically, partners break up because they get into seemingly unresolvable conflict about particular issues, such as their sexual relations, their attention to each other's needs, their child-rearing strategies, and so forth. Often the partners point to these particular conflicts ("She couldn't keep her parents out of our relationship," "He couldn't tolerate an intimate relationship") as the cause of their breakup.

In this chapter we argue that once a relationship has been well established, conflict is the most important proximal factor affecting satisfaction in the relationship and ultimately its course. We say "once a relationship has been well established," because we do not believe that conflicts are usually influential in the early stages of a relationship. The factors that attract two people to each other and the pleasure they take in each other are much more likely than conflict to determine whether or not a relationship develops. However, once a relationship has been established, the nature and level of conflict become important determinants.

Empirical evidence supports our view about the importance of conflict to satisfaction. Several diary and self-report studies have focused on the amount of conflict in relationships, and have found that distressed spouses experience more frequent conflicts than nondistressed spouses (e.g., Christensen & Margolin, 1988; Schaap, Buunk, & Kerkstra, 1988). Schaap and his colleagues suggest that the higher frequency of conflict about certain topics in distressed relationships may indicate that such problems remain unresolved in these relationships.

Observational studies of conflict in couples also support a linkage between the nature and intensity of conflict and relationship satisfaction. In these studies, researchers typically have each couple discuss an area of disagreement, and the couple's interaction is coded by observers along various dimensions. Results from such studies indicate that the communications of distressed couples differ in quality and in intensity from those of nondistressed couples. Among the most consistent findings in this area are that distressed partners criticize and disagree with each other more often than nondistressed partners, and that they reciprocate negative behaviors to a greater extent than nondistressed couples (e.g., Gottman, 1979; Schaap et al., 1988). Margolin (1988) summarizes the differences between distressed and nondistressed couples with respect to conflict as follows: "The conflict style of distressed couples includes a higher frequency and longer chains of punitive behaviors, as well as less productive outcomes" (p. 197).

In addition to these cross-sectional data, there are substantial longitudinal data supporting the notion that conflictual interactions predict marital dissatisfaction and breakup (see Karney & Bradbury, 1995, for a review). For example, a recent study (Heavey, Christensen, & Malamuth, 1995) that examined the predictability of the "demand–withdraw" pattern of interaction (Christensen & Heavey, 1993) showed that over a 2½-year period, the extent of "wife demand–husband withdraw" interaction at Time 1 predicted a decline in marital satisfaction even after initial levels of marital satisfaction were statistically controlled. Perhaps the most extensive longitudinal investigation of the effects of conflict patterns on marital satisfaction and divorce has been conducted by Markman and his associates (e.g., Lindahl et al., in press). They have shown that behaviors coded during conflict discussions, such as emotional invalidation, predict marital outcomes up to 8 years later.

Thus, there is a substantial body of evidence supporting our proposition that argument, conflict, and negativity are strongly associated with marital dissatisfaction, both concurrently and longitudinally. We now need to look more closely at such conflict to understand it better. First, we propose the broad outlines of a behavioral theory of conflict development that can explain how partners can enter a relationship with such hope and love but leave with such pain and disappointment. Then we discuss behavioral therapies that attempt to repair these destructive processes in couples.

ANALYSIS OF CONFLICT

To understand conflict, an important distinction must be made between the "structure of conflict" and the "process of conflict." By structure of conflict, we mean the conflict of interest between the partners—the incompatibility of needs or desires that characterize a particular struggle. For example, Joan wants to spend more time with her family of origin, whereas Derrick prefers to visit Joan's family infrequently. A particular conflict of interest such as this one may be exacerbated by various circumstantial factors. Perhaps Joan's family lives nearby while Derrick's lives far away; therefore, her family presents the possibility of more frequent contact. Furthermore, let us assume that Joan's family has special needs that require more frequent contact (e.g., her parents' age and disability make it impossible for them to leave the house on their own). These situational factors, as well as the difference in their desire for contact, constitute a dilemma for this couple and define what we mean by the structure of the conflict.

By the process of conflict, we mean the actual interaction that takes place between the pair around the conflict of interest. For example, Joan may try to convince Derrick that it is his obligation to visit her family frequently; Derrick may disavow obligations to her family. It is important to note that any particular conflict of interest can lead to a variety of conflictual processes. For example, Derrick may berate Joan's family as a means of explaining and justifying his infrequent visits there, while Joan defends her family. Conflictual processes may involve little or no verbal interaction at all. At some point Joan may just visit her family by herself without even inviting Derrick, but she may be especially distant and cold to him upon her return.

Development of Incompatibility

People do not seek out partners with whom they are incompatible or with whom they have conflicts of interest. From a behavioral/social learning perspective, partners seek out mates with whom they experience and anticipate reinforcement. Evidence indicates that people tend to marry partners of similar background (Broderick, 1992), which may make mutual reinforcement more likely. For example, if Denise and Rick are both fiscally conservative, they will reinforce these views in each other in a variety of ways. They will compliment each other for saving money; they will endorse each other's opinions about avoiding risky investments; and they will mutually ridicule others who lose money on risky propositions.

Certain differences between partners may also increase the likelihood of reinforcement. For example, if Laura is ambitious and energetic and Walter is relaxed and "laid back," they may find gratification in each other's personal qualities. Laura's energy and enthusiasm may motivate and support Walter in getting a career direction in his life.

Walter's ability to set aside responsibilities and enjoy life may make it possible for Laura to enjoy her leisure time more.

This common notion that differences are appealing or that "opposites attract" was represented scientifically in Winch's (1958) theory of complementary needs in mate selection. According to Winch, an individual selects a partner from his or her "field of eligibles" who provides the maximum need gratification for the individual and whose own needs are complementary to the partner's needs. "Complementarity of needs" refers to a condition in which the needs being gratified by one partner are different in kind or intensity from the needs being gratified in the other partner. In the example just above, Laura and Walter's relationship would be complementary if Laura's need for dominance is gratified by giving directions to Walter, who in turn receives gratification from being given guidance.

Although Winch (1958) offered empirical support for his theory of complementary needs in mate selection, the vast majority of studies examining need complementarity have either found no relationship between the needs of spouses or have found evidence in favor of "homogamy," or similarity of needs in mate selection (see review by Barry, 1970). It is our contention, however, that the need complementarity hypothesis has not yet been adequately tested and may actually be an important factor in mate selection. In previous studies, data analysis has generally been accomplished by correlating a specific need of the husband (e.g., dominance) with the complementary need of the wife (e.g., submission) in a sample of couples. The problem with this approach is that an overall nonsignificant correlation for a complementary need pair (e.g., dominance–submission) might have included many couples for whom the dominance–submission complementarity was irrelevant, as well as some couples for whom the dominance–submission complementarity was significant, leading to an overall finding of no relationship. We would therefore argue that because the basis for complementarity is likely to be different for different couples, we must assess couples individually to determine what characteristics are important and relevant for each couple.

Behaviorally oriented theorists have suggested that satisfaction in relationships decreases over time because of "reinforcement erosion" (Jacobson & Margolin, 1979). Through repetition, reinforcers may lose their rewarding power. Whether reinforcement is based on similarity or complementarity, it may fade over time. For instance, the 100th time that Denise and Rick find they agree in their fiscal conservatism may be less reinforcing than the first time they discover their agreement.

We suggest additional and more complex processes through which initial reinforcement and satisfaction may be undermined. Some of the similarities and differences between partners, which were sources of initial attraction, may eventually lead to incompatibilities between them. The basis for initial attraction may also be the source of later conflict. Let us consider first the similarities between partners. The mutual reinforcement that partners provide each other on the basis of their similarities may lead them to an extreme and unbalanced position that may be costly for them and lead to conflict. In their fiscal conservatism, Denise and Rick may mutually reinforce and accentuate each other's aversion to financial risk. Therefore, they may decide to delay buying a house until they have saved a substantial portion of its cost and have sufficient income to pay the mortgage. But home prices appreciate so fast that they find a few years later that even with their higher savings, they cannot afford the house today that they could have afforded a few years ago if they had been willing to risk taking on the mortgage. One partner may then blame the other for their financial conservatism and insist that the other should have provided a counterpoint and balance to their own financial hesitations.

The attraction of differences may serve more commonly than the attraction of similarities as a breeding ground for later incompatibility and conflict. What originally seemed attractive to the partner may take on a darker aspect later. Consider, for example, ambitious Laura and laid-back Walter. Laura's energy and ambition, which earlier seemed attractive to Walter, may translate into pressure and demands upon him that he comes to find aversive. Likewise, Walter's laid-back style, which initially seemed appealing to Laura, may seem more like laziness to her later on. They may have conflicts of interest about whether Walter should change jobs or seek a promotion as opposed to staying where he is, or whether they should go away for the weekend or work on fixing up the house.

Many of the incompatibilities that present dilemmas for partners were not part of their original attraction to each other. They simply result from the fact that two different people are trying to live life together. No matter how careful people are in their mate selection, mates will be different from each other and will not always want the same thing, at the same time, and in the same intensity. Moreover, there will be times when these differences are important and cannot be easily dismissed. The partners will have stumbled upon an important conflict of interest; the stage is then set for conflictual interaction.

During courtship, potential incompatibilities are probably minimized. The partners are likely to be on their best behavior. Areas of potential incompatibility are often avoided. However, as the partners increase their exposure to each other—as they spend more time together in more diverse circumstances, as they meet each other's families and friends—the exposure of incompatibilities becomes more and more likely.

Up until now, we have discussed incompatibilities that were there from the very beginning, but that did not raise their ugly heads until later in the relationship. However, incompatibilities may develop over time as the partners change, based on their life experiences. First, partners may generate incompatibilities through their shared experiences. For example, the members of a couple may seem perfectly compatible in their views on children. They plan on how many they will have, when they will have them, and how they will rear them. However, the experience of having children may generate unpredictable and incompatible reactions in the couple. Monica and Rodney may have both planned that Monica would return to work 6 weeks after the birth; once the baby arrives, however, Monica may find the thought of turning over her baby's care to another abhorrent, while Rodney can't imagine curtailing their lifestyle in the drastic way that a loss of Monica's income would require.

Second, partners may generate incompatibilities through their individual experiences as well as through their shared experiences. Personal experiences in each partner's work world or social world apart from the other may create new needs and desires that conflict with the partner's. For example, Ann and Daren may have been compatible on issues of closeness and time together throughout their courtship and early marriage. However, later in the relationship, Ann makes an important career change that moves her into a demanding but exciting position. She spends long hours at the office and no longer has the time for Daren that she used to have.

Whatever their source and however they come about, incompatibilities between partners create conflicts of interest. She wants it one way; he wants it the other way. They create genuine dilemmas for partners because they may lead to deprivation and punishment for one or both. If Monica stays with the baby rather than returning to work, Rodney will have to curtail his and their lifestyle; if Monica returns to work, she must face the pain and anxiety of not being with her baby. Similarly, Daren must either suffer the loss of some time together and closeness with Ann, or Ann must suffer the fear and anxiety of not meeting her career demands. Both couples are likely to experience a series of unpleasant discussions or arguments about their issues.

The Process of Conflict: Coping with Incompatibility

Early in courtship, it is likely that partners try to accommodate each other when they face incompatibilities, particularly if those incompatibilities are not too important. They may not want to rock the boat of their relationship; the rewards from the early relationship are more important than the temporary loss of other gratifications. However, as partners become more used to each other, as they experience some "rein-forcement erosion" in the relationship, and as they face important in-compatibilities, they may be less willing to accommodate each other. They may resort to coercion to solve conflicts of interest.

Coercion

As developed by Patterson (e.g., Patterson & Hops, 1972), coercion theory describes several behavioral processes that operate in conflicts of interest between partners. In its essence, coercion involves the simul-taneous operation of positive and negative reinforcement. One part-ner applies aversive stimulation to the other until the other complies. For example, Mark criticizes and belittles Dena for being "socially iso-lated" and "unsupportive" of him until she agrees to go to a party at his company. Mark gets positively reinforced for his criticism and be-littling (Dena goes to the party with him, which he wanted), while Dena gets negatively reinforced (the criticism and belittling terminate once she has complied). Thus, on future occasions both may be expected to repeat their actions. However, the process can become much more com-plicated than this simple illustration implies. If Dena finds certain so-cial events uncomfortable and thus avoids them, giving in to Mark terminates his aversive behavior but exposes her to the uncomfortable experience of the party. She may refuse to attend certain parties that she feels particularly averse to, but in so doing she provides Mark with a more powerful intermittent reinforcement for his criticism. Further-more, she may unintentionally "shape" his criticism into higher inten-sities. Early in the relationship, she may respond with compliance to slight indications of his disapproval at her hesitation to accept social invitations. However, as she becomes habituated to his subtle signs of disapproval and experiences the discomfort of compliance with his in-vitations, she may not comply until he engages in more and more criti-cism and belittling. Also, coercion is not one-sided. Dena may engage in coercive efforts with Mark to get some of the things that she wants from him. She may use different types of aversive stimulation in response to different issues. She may, for example, withdraw from Mark when he does not spend what she feels is appropriate time with their son. Even though different behaviors are involved, it is still a coercive process. Over time, as both engage in coercive efforts, their relationship becomes more and more marked by negative interactions.

Vilification of Differences

As partners get into more and more coercive interchanges, they are likely to think about these conflictual interactions. They will make judgments about the causes of these interactions and who is responsible for them. Based on attribution theory and research (Bradbury & Fincham, 1990), we can predict that each partner in a coercive conflict is likely to find the cause for the conflict in the other and to find the other responsible for the problem. Dena may conclude that Mark is very selfish and inconsiderate, and that this is why he insists on going to these superficial parties and ignores her feelings about them. This selfishness and inconsiderateness also explain to her why he doesn't interact with their son more. Mark, on the other hand, may conclude that Dena is insecure and neurotic, which is why she is so intimidated by social events. Also, he worries that she is going to make their son the same way by overprotecting him, insisting on so much parental contact, and not allowing the boy to develop independence. Thus, the differences between them become vilified. They are no longer differences; now they are deficiencies.

Partners are also likely to share these attributions with each other. Mark and Dena's conflicts about going to social events and about Mark's amount of contact with their son will be filled with accusations of insecurity, selfishness, and inconsiderateness, defenses against these attacks, and counterattacks. Increasingly, the conflicts will involve disagreements about their attributions for the problem (Kelley, 1979). Mark and Dena will fight not just about social events and time with their son, but about the unsavory motives behind each other's positions.

Polarization

Partners may become more polarized in their positions over the course of their conflicts. The conflicts lead to deprivations by each, which may intensify their desires. As Mark is deprived of going to social events with his wife, he may give more attention to those events and develop more elaborate justifications for those events. On the other hand, as Dena experiences more pressure from Mark and engages in more effort to defend her position, any desire for such social events on her part may be lost. It begins to look as if Dena has no desire at all for social contact, while such contact is the most important thing in Mark's life. As a result of their coercive process of coping with their differences, they may begin to seem even more different than they were to begin with.

Another process of polarization may occur through the division of labor and specialization that accompany incompatibilities between partners. Partners may become more and more skilled at activities for which they are fighting, and less and less skilled at activities for which their partners are fighting. Dena spends more time with their son than does Mark. She knows her son better than Mark does, is more comfortable with him, and can engage him in mutually enjoyable activities better than Mark can. Dena's and Mark's conflicts about time with their son are likely to increase this skill disparity. For example, to make up for the lack of contact between Mark and their son, Dena may spend more time than she might otherwise with their son. Mark's efforts with their son may be no match for Dena's and may be easy for Dena to criticize—all of which may lessen Mark's activities with him, and ultimately Mark's comfort and skill with those activities.

Through these processes of coercion, vilification, and polarization, inevitable differences between partners may set the stage for escalating conflict and apparent "irreconcilable differences" that destroy relationship satisfaction and, in the extreme, set the stage for separation and divorce. We now consider a detailed example of these processes.

An Example: Incompatibility in Closeness

"Closeness" has been proposed as an essential dimension of relationships (Kelley et al., 1983); in the present context, this dimension refers to the extent to which the lives of partners are interdependent. Incompatibilities in the degree of closeness desired by partners can take different forms. For example, one partner may want to spend more time together, while the other partner may want to spend more time alone or with friends. Also, one partner may want more sharing of thoughts and feelings in the relationship, while the other may want to keep thoughts and feelings more private. One partner may want greater contact with friends and family than the other wants.

A number of clinical theorists have focused on the difference in closeness desired by partners as a central problem for many couples seeking therapy (e.g., Christensen, 1987; Jacobson & Margolin, 1979). Empirical evidence is consistent with the idea that incompatibilities in closeness are tied to relationship dissatisfaction and distress. For example, Christensen (1987, 1988) has shown in a community sample of married and cohabiting couples that a discrepancy between partners in desired closeness is highly correlated with a measure of relationship satisfaction. Christensen and Shenk (1991) also found an association between a difference in desired closeness and the clinical status of couples, such that nondistressed couples reported less of a discrepancy in desired closeness than did distressed (clinic-referred and divorcing) couples.

To illustrate how an incompatibility in closeness may result in relationship distress, consider the following case. Early in their 10-year relationship, Mike and Jenny enjoyed spending all of their free time together, sharing their most intimate thoughts and feelings, and engaging in shared activities. Over the years, however, Mike became more involved in his career and in his long-time interest in chess, while Jenny maintained her interest in a close intimate relationship. Although he continued to enjoy contact with Jenny, Mike had less time for this contact. Then two major events happened that exacerbated this growing incompatibility between them. First, Mike got a major promotion in his job, which meant a considerable salary increase but long hours and much travel. Then Jenny got pregnant with twins. Even though Jenny had a career of her own, they decided that she should stay home with the twins. Mike made enough money now to support the family alone. However, these events initiated a major change in their roles: Mike was now the hard-working sole breadwinner, whereas Jenny was the busy stay-at-home mother with twins. These shifts in roles were accompanied by shifts in what each wanted from the other. Jenny wanted Mike to be at home more and to be more involved with her and the children. Mike felt caught between the pressures at work and at home. Although he wanted to help Jenny with the children, his work demands were more intense than they had ever been. Also, he felt more confident and assured at work than he did at home. He could run a business meeting far better than he could quiet a crying baby. Jenny got more and more distressed at what she felt was her absent husband and father. She would try to talk to Mike about the problem, but in her anger at his absence and at his apparent reluctance even to discuss the problem, she often became upset, critical, and demanding. Mike would be defensive and try to avoid or end these conversations. He saw no way to please her other than by damaging or destroying his career. As their negative interaction cycle of her demanding and his withdrawing (Christensen & Heavey, 1993) became more polarized, their positions on closeness also became more polarized and rigid. It seemed as if Jenny only wanted family contact and had no needs for independence; it seemed as if Mike only wanted the independence and achievement his job provided and had no needs for closeness and intimacy. At this point, their incompatibilities seemed overwhelming.

Factors That Influence the Conflict Process

We have described some general processes that may affect conflict in couples. One might ask: Why don't all couples travel this route? If all couples are faced with incompatible differences, why is it that only some escalate into severe conflict that leads to unhappiness, separation, and divorce? Why is it that some couples manage to deal effectively with their incompatibilities? What distinguishes those partners who are successful in marriage from those who are not? We believe there are several variables that combine to affect the course of marital conflict: the match between partners, the personalities of each, the conflict resolution skills of each, and the stressful circumstances they encounter.

Match between Partners

Through luck or search, some matches are better than others. Some partners have fewer incompatibilities than others. Their interests and habits mesh. Their initial match or their life courses generate fewer conflicts of interest. Alternatively, the initial match provides such powerful mutual reinforcement that the couple is able to manage conflicts in other areas. We can imagine a couple with such a powerful physical/sexual attraction to each other that they are greatly motivated either to work out their conflicts or to tolerate them. General support for these ideas is provided by research showing that personality and attitudinal similarity predict positive marital outcomes (Karney & Bradbury, 1995) and that compatibility between partners in leisure interests and role preferences predicts positive marital outcomes (Huston & Houts, in press).

Personality

A second variable that affects the likelihood of incompatibilities' escalating into greater and greater conflict is the personality of each partner. Considerable research has shown that neuroticism in either spouse is associated with decreased marital satisfaction and stability (see Karney & Bradbury, 1995, for a review). In fact, by far the lengthiest longitudinal study of marriage showed that neuroticism predicted decline in satisfaction and separation across 40 years of marriage (Kelly & Conley, 1987). We suggest that neuroticism affects marital satisfaction and stability by complicating the resolution of incompatibilities. Neurotic partners are likely to overreact emotionally to conflicts of interest, to engage in coercion, or to avoid or withdraw from discussion of conflictual topics. These reactions are likely to escalate the conflict and make it more difficult to resolve.

In addition to neuroticism, research has implicated attributional tendencies as important for the outcome of marriage. A number of investigations have demonstrated both cross-sectional and longitudinal associations between maladaptive attributions and marital satisfaction (see Bradbury & Fincham, 1990, for a review). We suggest that cognitive tendencies to attribute responsibility for problems to one's partner complicate the resolution of conflicts of interest. Partners are likely to blame and accuse each other during conflictual discussions, which will escalate those discussions and make them more difficult to resolve.

Conflict Resolution Skills

Research has demonstrated powerful cross-sectional and longitudinal associations between interactional behaviors of partners on the one hand and marital stability and satisfaction on the other. As expected, positive behavior predicts stability and satisfaction, whereas negative behavior predicts dissatisfaction and breakup (Weiss & Heyman, 1990; Karney & Bradbury, 1995). Because most of this research assesses positive and negative behaviors in conflict situations, we believe that these data represent, in part, differing levels of conflict resolution skills in the couples being investigated. If partners have little skill at conflict resolution, then their attempt to resolve the inevitable differences that arise during marriage will frequently fail, leading to mounting conflicts. If, on the other hand, their conflict resolution skills are sophisticated, they may be able to handle especially difficult incompatibilities.

Stressful Circumstances

Major life stressors and daily stressors take their toll on relationship satisfaction. For example, research on the transition to parenthood has shown that this major life event is associated with a decline in marital satisfaction (e.g., Belsky & Pensky, 1988). In addition, several studies have shown that daily stressors are associated with more negative marital interactions. For example, in a study of air traffic controllers, Repetti (1989) showed that high-workload days were associated with greater negative interaction between spouses.

Christensen and his colleagues (Christensen & Pasch, 1993; Christensen & Shenk, 1991) have suggested two mechanisms to explain why stress may increase conflict and dissatisfaction in relationships. First, stress is liable to increase partners' need for support while it simultaneously decreases their ability to provide support. Stressful events can create negative affective arousal and then fatigue (Repetti, 1989), which increase partners' need for emotional support and concrete assistance. If one spouse has stayed up most of the night with a crying baby, that spouse may need comfort from the other, as well as release from his or her usual daily tasks. Also, stressful events may create cognitive processing distortions (e.g., Jarvis, 1982) and a greater self-focus (e.g., Wood, Saltzberg, & Goldsamt, 1990), which make stressed partners less available to understand and appreciate each other's point of view.

A second way in which stressful events can increase conflict and dissatisfaction in relationships is by exacerbating old conflicts of interest or creating new ones. Consider the example of the transition to parenthood. Common conflicts of interest about household tasks can be easily exacerbated by the increased demands that a new baby makes on a couple. If a wife wanted a husband to do more housework before their first child, she may well increase her demands, since she may have less time available for housework. Also, new conflicts will inevitably arise, such as differences over who will do child care when.

At this point, we have (we hope) established that conflicts are inevitable in couples; that these conflicts have a major impact on satisfaction in relationships; and that a number of variables, such as stressful circumstances and personality factors, influence the course of these conflicts. We now turn to therapeutic treatments for couple conflict. Consistent with our analysis of conflict, our focus is on behavioral approaches to treatment.

BEHAVIORAL TREATMENTS FOR COUPLES

Behavioral treatments have been developed to assist couples in resolving their conflicts and improving their satisfaction. Here we discuss both the traditional behavioral treatment of couples and a new therapy designed to improve the outcome of the traditional approach.

Traditional Behavioral Couple Therapy

In traditional behavioral couple therapy (TBCT; Jacobson & Margolin, 1979; Stuart, 1980), change is the means for dealing with incompatibilities. Partners are taught positive strategies for accommodating and compromising, so that each makes changes in the actions that cause the other distress. During an assessment period, the therapist carefully pinpoints those behaviors by each partner that contribute to the other's unhappiness, as well as the behaviors that are a source of strength and attraction between them. During this period the therapist also promotes a "collaborative set"—a shared responsibility for the problems and an attitude of cooperation so that they can work together to solve the problems (Jacobson & Margolin, 1979). The assessment period ends with a feedback session in which the therapist shares the behavioral conceptualization of the problem and the treatment plan for ameliorating the problem. The couple is encouraged to comment on the therapist's conceptualization and treatment plan and to provide corrective feedback.

TBCT consists of three primary strategies: "behavior exchange," "communication training," and "problem-solving skills training." Typically, treatment starts with behavior exchange. In this strategy, partners first specify a list of noncontroversial behaviors that would be pleasing for each and that could be provided with relatively little effort. A back rub, a special meal, and a greeting card are examples. Partners might be asked either to generate lists of behaviors that would be pleasing for each other or to generate lists that would be pleasing for themselves. Once such lists are generated, the therapist directs the couple to increase the frequency of these positive behaviors. The therapist might prescribe particular days, such as "caring days" (Stuart, 1980), during which a particular partner is to provide an especially high level of these behaviors to the other. Or the therapist might encourage the couple to increase the frequency of these behaviors over the course of the week. During subsequent sessions, the therapist debriefs the assignment by finding out what the partners did for each other, how they each felt about it, and whether and how each expressed appreciation for the other's efforts. Based on these behavior exchange experiences, changes are made in the lists of positive behaviors, and additional assignments to increase the frequency of these behaviors are given. The goal of behavior exchange is to increase the exchange of positively reinforcing activities. In so doing, the partners may be in a more positive position to approach their conflicts.

The goal of the second strategy, communication training, is to teach partners a positive way of talking about their problems without allowing the discussion to degenerate into blame, defensiveness, and distortion. Partners are taught expressive speaking skills and receptive listening skills. Under expressive skills, partners are taught to focus on their own feelings in reaction to each other's specific behavior. Instead of focusing on what the other partner does or does not do and expressing that with a blaming "you message" (e.g., "You never do . . . "), partners are taught to focus on what they are feeling and express that with a nonblaming "I message" (e.g., "I feel excluded when . . . "). Partners are taught to take responsibility for their own feelings (e.g., they are taught to say "I feel guilty . . . " rather than "You make me feel guilty . . . "). Partners are also taught to relate their feelings to the specific behavior of the other rather than to some general trait of the other. For example, one partner may be taught to say, "I feel disappointed when you don't sit down and talk to me when you get home from work," rather than "I feel disappointed that you are such a closed, selfish person."

In addition to expressive speaking skills, partners are taught receptive listening skills. First, the therapist makes sure that the listener is attentive to the speaker. The listener needs to be oriented to the speaker and maintain eye contact with the speaker. Then the therapist asks the partners in turn to demonstrate that they have listened by paraphrasing or summarizing the speaker's comments before making their own comments. This requirement ensures that partners listen to each other rather than formulate their next comments. It also slows communication, which is often helpful during the discussion of controversial issues. Paraphrases and summaries are to focus on what the speaker said and are not to include editorial commentary by the listener. The therapist may also train each partner to reflect the emotions the speaker is feeling. All summaries, paraphrases, and reflections of feeling must meet with the speaker's approval before the listener is allowed to proceed. Thus, a listener who does not have the speaker's ideas right can be corrected immediately. Once the speaker has communicated a piece of what he or she has to say, the roles are changed and the former speaker now becomes the listener, following the same guidelines to summarize and paraphrase.

The goal of the third strategy, problem-solving skills training, is to teach couples a positive method for negotiating changes in their relationship. In problem solving, couples first agree upon a definition of the problem, which delineates the specific situations and behaviors that are problematic. Then the couple brainstorms possible solutions to the problem, withholding judgments about the relative worth of each solution. After all possible solutions have been generated, the couple discusses the pros and cons of each solution. Based on this discussion of pros and cons, the couple negotiates a written agreement that specifies what each will do to try to solve the problem. Once a written agreement is reached, the couple attempts to implement it in the following week. At the next session, these efforts are reviewed, and modifications to the agreement are made as needed.

As a result of this training in communication and problem-solving skills, couples ideally will resolve some of the specific problems that brought them into therapy. However, TBCT therapists have a more optimistic goal than simply the resolution of presenting problems: They hope to instill in their couples sufficient interpersonal skills to enable these couples to handle future difficulties on their own, using these same communication and problem-solving skills. To promote this goal, therapists gradually decrease their active intervention, shifting more and more responsibility to couples as the couples gain these communication and problem-solving skills. Toward the end of treatment, therapists may gradually fade their influence, seeing the couples less frequently until final termination of therapy.

Considerable research has been conducted on TBCT—indeed, more than on any other approach to couple therapy. About two dozen clinical trials have been conducted in several countries, such as the United States, Great Britain, Germany, and Australia. Studies have consistently shown the superiority of TBCT to various control conditions (Jacobson & Addis, 1993; Hahlweg & Markman, 1988). In fact, because of its history of empirical research, TBCT has been designated by a task force of the Clinical Psychology Division of the American Psychological Association (Division 12) as an empirically validated treatment. Despite this positive record, research has shown that about a third of couples show no changes as a result of treatment (Jacobson & Follette, 1985). Furthermore, some of the successfully treated couples relapse, so that only about one-half of couples improve during treatment and maintain their improvement for a 1- to 2-year period following treatment termination (Jacobson, Schmaling, & Holtzworth-Munroe, 1987). Not surprisingly, those couples that fail to respond to TBCT and those that relapse tend to be the most distressed couples (Jacobson, Follette, & Pagel, 1986). Thus, although TBCT has demonstrated success in treating couples, there is plenty of room for improvement.

Clinicians treating couples with traditional behavioral approaches face several difficulties that probably lead to the lack of success with many couples. First, some couples are unwilling or unable to make the changes required in TBCT. Second, even if couples do make changes during treatment, they may fail to maintain those changes during follow-up. And finally, some changes that a couple makes in treatment are not satisfying to one or both partners. For example, let's assume that Susan is unhappy because Ed is not more physically affectionate with her. Anxious to improve his relationship, Ed agrees to increase the frequency of affection to Susan. He follows through with his agreement and methodically kisses her each morning before leaving for work, each evening on his return, and before going to sleep at night. However, he gets little from Susan for all his efforts. She complains that "he is just going through the motions," and that "he doesn't really mean it."

From a behavioral perspective, the problem is that TBCT creates change through "rule-governed" behavior as opposed to "contingency-shaped" behavior (Skinner, 1966). In rule-governed behavior, a rule or plan for behavior is verbally specified, and people obtain reinforcement for matching their behavior to the rule. The rule in the example above is for Ed to be more physically affectionate to Susan; he matches his behavior to that rule, and then looks expectantly for Susan and the therapist to reinforce him appropriately. In contingency-shaped behavior, the contingencies in the environment shape particular behavior in people, instead of people's matching their behavior to verbal rules. For instance, Ed will kiss Susan because the circumstances elicit that from him, not because he is trying to remember to follow a rule. Even though the rule-governed kiss and the contingency-shaped kiss may look very similar to an outside observer, they may feel very different to the participants. In the former, Ed does what he is supposed to do; in the latter, he does what he feels like. There is likely to be a spontaneity in the latter that is missing in the former, and this spontaneity makes the contingency-shaped behavior far more reinforcing.

Integrative Behavioral Couple Therapy

Because of the clinical inadequacies of TBCT and its limited ability to promote relationship satisfaction, Christensen and Jacobson developed integrative behavioral couple therapy (IBCT; Christensen, Jacobson, & Babcock, 1995; Christensen & Jacobson, in press; Jacobson & Christensen, 1996). The purpose of IBCT is to supplement the change strategies of TBCT with strategies for promoting acceptance between partners. Unlike TBCT, IBCT assumes the existence of incompatibilities in many (perhaps most) couples that cannot be resolved by accommodation and compromise. Instead, these differences are best accepted by each partner. Furthermore, the often difficult process of understanding and ultimately accepting differences between partners may actually create greater closeness and intimacy. IBCT also assumes that a combination of change and acceptance will be more powerful than either alone. If partners experience acceptance from each other, they may be more willing to change. Likewise, if they experience change from each other, they may be more willing to accept each other. Finally, IBCT suggests that the strategies for promoting acceptance may expose partners to previously unnoticed aspects of their relationship that may bring about spontaneous changes—contingency-shaped behavior—that may ameliorate some of the problems between them.

Like TBCT, IBCT consists of an initial set of several assessment sessions followed by a feedback session and then treatment sessions. IBCT can employ any of the assessment or treatment strategies of IBCT; however, an emphasis on emotional acceptance marks it as unique. "Emotional acceptance" means, at the very least, tolerance for each other's problematic behavior. At its best, emotional acceptance involves an appreciation of the partners' differences, even though those differences at times create pain and difficulty. Emotional acceptance does not refer to submission to each other's negative behavior or even resignation to that behavior. Rather, the accepting partner tolerates—and, in the best of circumstances, even embraces—the other's unpleasant behavior, because the accepting partner sees and experiences it in the larger context of the other and of their relationship together.

Here we briefly describe the three main strategies used to promote acceptance. For additional information on IBCT, the reader should consult Christensen et al. (1995), Christensen and Jacobson (in press), and Jacobson and Christensen (1996). In the first strategy, called "emotional acceptance through empathic joining," an IBCT therapist tries to generate discussions about problems that will elicit compassion in each partner for the other. This is no easy feat, since members of a couple in therapy often enter into discussions about problems with considerable anger, attributions that blame each other for the problem, and little sympathy for each other's plight. As a first step in moving the couple to a more compassionate stance, the therapist gathers information about the problem and reformulates it in a way that shows each partner in a sympathetic position—as acting in an understandable way when faced with difficult conditions. Typically, the IBCT therapist reformulates the problem in terms of differences between partners and their ways of handling the differences that, although understandable, have polarized them and made the differences even more problematic. For example, Joan may see the problem she and Martin have about his mother as stemming from Martin's unhealthy dependency on his mother and her inability to "cut the apron strings." Martin may see the problem as generated by Joan's insecurity about being left out and by Joan's tendency to be overcritical of others, especially his mother. In a formulation of this problem, an IBCT therapist would focus first on the difference in attachment that the two have toward Martin's mother and the difference in the closeness each has with his or her family of origin. Joan is not close to her parents and wants a very strong connection with Martin. Although Martin wants a strong bond with Joan, he is very close to his parents, particularly his mother. Then the IBCT therapist would focus on how their understandable attempts to cope with this difference have created even bigger problems for them. Because of this difference, Joan feels she is not the central figure in Martin's life. Unable to get Martin to understand her experience and the pain it brought, she has begun to criticize his mother and him. Threatened by the idea that Joan might be demanding that he end his close relationship with his mother and stung by Joan's criticism of his mother, Martin has taken on a defensive role—defending his mother and himself, occasionally attacking Joan for being so critical, but mostly withdrawing from her. This withdrawal, of course, has only exacerbated Joan's sense of exclusion from Martin's world. Stuck in these roles of criticizer and defender/withdrawer, they have each escalated their behavior, and neither is able to hear the pain the other is experiencing.

The therapist's presentation of this formulation and the couple's acceptance of it is just the first step toward promoting empathic joining in relation to the problem. During treatment sessions, the couple is encouraged to discuss salient incidents from the past week that may illustrate the problem. The therapist encourages the reporting of positive incidents, in which the partners handled the problem better, as well as negative incidents, in which they repeated their unpleasant patterns; however, negative incidents are likely to predominate during the early stages of therapy. Upcoming incidents are especially important to discuss, because they allow the possibility of anticipating and perhaps circumventing problems. For example, if Martin and Joan have been invited to his parents' house for dinner this coming Sunday, a discussion about potential dangers in this upcoming event may well be helpful. IBCT prefers a focus on concrete incidents in the immediate past or future, because these incidents represent the current manifestation of their problem and because the emotions surrounding these incidents are often easily accessible. However, IBCT also encourages a general discussion of the pattern between the couple, especially if there is no immediate, relevant incident.

In order to promote emphatic joining in regard to the problem during these discussions, IBCT therapists focus on "soft experiences" rather than "hard experiences." Hard experiences are emotions and thoughts that reveal the self as strong, closed, and resistant. Examples are emotions such as anger, resentment, and disgust, and thoughts such as "I won't be walked on any more" and "I am not going to let myself be manipulated." Soft experiences reveal the self as vulnerable and open. Examples are emotions such as disappointment, hurt, and sadness, and thoughts such as "I wasn't sure if you would like it" or "I didn't know how you would respond." IBCT assumes that hard and soft emotions and thoughts are equally legitimate and are both part of most emotional experiences. IBCT therapists do not deny the hard experiences or punish the expression of those experiences. Instead, they elicit and highlight the softer experiences, because these experiences are often not expressed and because they have the potential to spontaneously elicit empathic responding. If Martin sees how excluded and alone Joan feels in their relationship, and how her anger and criticism may spring from this sense of exclusion, Martin may be more empathic toward Joan and more accepting of her anger and criticism. Likewise, if Joan sees how beaten down Martin is by her attacks, she may feel empathy for him. The increased empathy may promote not only acceptance, but also spontaneous change. Martin may be more motivated to include Joan in his confidences; Joan may find herself less critical of Martin.

The second strategy for promoting acceptance is though "unified detachment" from the problem. Whereas the first strategy emphasizes a close-up, emotionally tender discussion of the problem, the second strategy emphasizes a more distant, intellectual, descriptive discussion of the problem. The first focuses on emotional expression; the second centers on intellectual analysis. Although the two strategies are conceptually distant, they are often interwoven together in interventions with couples. They both focus on the same material—recent, salient incidents relevant to the current problem.

To promote acceptance via detachment, an IBCT therapist asks the partners to focus on the sequence of problematic behavior between them, emphasizing the triggers that activate each partner. For example, Joan and Martin's sequence typically begins with some mention of Martin's mother. Through her voice tone or her words, Joan will provide some negative assessment of the situation or of Martin's mother. In response, Martin will defend his mother or offer some positive assessment of her. Even if Joan says nothing, Martin will often rise in defense against what he senses Joan is thinking. After some argumentative discussion, both Joan and Martin withdraw in hurt and anger. "Hot buttons" or "triggers" for Martin are any direct attacks on his mother or implications that his relationship with her is pathological; for Joan, they are any indications that Martin is seeking support or advice from his mother. If partners have a clear and correct analysis of their problem, they are less likely to engage in a blaming discussion of it. They are more likely to see it as a problem that they both have, rather than as a problem that one partner has foisted on the other. They are more likely to be more accepting of each other as they see that each is caught in a dilemma. They may thus be more open to problem solving spontaneously.

IBCT therapists try to use humor and metaphor to provide couples with some distance from their problems. If part of the sequence between Martin and Joan is for Martin to disguise contact with his mother and for Joan to seek evidence for it, the therapist might comment on Joan's becoming more like a detective in this relationship and Martin's becoming more like a spy, covering his contact with the secret agent, his mother. These metaphors of "detective," "spy," and "secret agent" may allow the two of them some humorous perspective on their dilemma. Of course, therapists must be careful not to be disrespectful of clients or to diminish clients by promoting a humorous angle on their problems.

As partners obtain both intellectual understanding of their pattern and emotional distance from it, they may find it easier to accept the problematic behavior that each partner brings to the pattern. This acceptance may not be obvious in the immediate presence of the problematic behavior; the partners may still get upset and angry. However, they may be able to recover from an incident more quickly because they understand the dynamics involved. For example, Martin may still get angry when Joan criticizes his mother, but he may be able to get over that upset in much less time than before therapy.

A third strategy for promoting acceptance is "tolerance building." When partners find certain behaviors in each other unacceptable, it is usually because those behaviors are so painful for them. Often such a behavior itself is not reprehensible; it is not violent or cruel or of malicious intent. Instead, it causes pain in part because of the sensitivity of the other partner to that behavior (or lack of behavior). For example, a husband's lack of physical affection to his wife or a wife's inattention to her husband is not in itself a despicable, deplorable act. However, in the context of the relationship and given the partner's sensitivities, it can be acutely painful. If the partner could become less sensitive to this response (or lack of response), he or she could tolerate it better and perhaps be more accepting of it. The third strategy has that goal in mind.

One way to promote tolerance is to engage the couple in a discussion of the possible positive features of each partner's negative behavior. This discussion does not deny that there are serious negative features of the behavior for its recipient, nor does the discussion try to create positive features where none exist. However, it is often the case that problematic behavior has important positive features. In fact, as we have discussed earlier, sometimes one partner is attracted to features of the other partner that later show a negative, unpleasant side. Consider Martin and Joan. Joan finds Martin's close communication with his mother a problem. Yet Martin's ease in expressing his feelings, his lack of pretense, and his openness in describing his weaknesses and vulnerability are all features that Joan originally found endearing in him. These are the very features that were fostered in his relationship with his mother. For his part, Martin at first found Joan's assertion and strength of character very appealing. She was not one to let anyone take advantage of her or dismiss her. Of course, it is just that assertiveness that now makes her so vocal in her complaints to Martin about his mother. A discussion of these possible positive features of each partner's problematic behavior will not suddenly make each embrace those negative aspects of the other. However, it provides some perspective on their struggle and may make them more tolerant of each other.

Another strategy for promoting tolerance is to role-play aversive behavior. An IBCT therapist will request that partners exhibit the very qualities that are upsetting to each other in the session. If the partners comply, they will express these behaviors in a very different context than that in which they are usually expressed. A third person, the therapist, is present. The behaviors are stimulated by a request from the therapist, rather than by a provocative incident. Also, the therapist may interrupt the expression of these behaviors by finding out the emotional reactions of each. Because of this different context, the aversive behaviors are less likely to have their usual sting. Sometimes couples find the whole situation amusing. Tolerance for these aversive behaviors may be fostered in this new context. Even if the behaviors create the distress that they normally do, the therapist is there to interrupt the usual sequence and explore each partner's reactions, using strategies described above for fostering acceptance.

Comparison of the Traditional
and Integrative Approaches

IBCT is designed to assist couples in coping with their differences by fostering change and accommodation to these differences and by fostering acceptance of these differences. Whether IBCT can improve relationships through these dual processes of change and acceptance can only be evaluated through outcome research. Currently, Jacobson and Christensen are conducting a clinical trial comparing IBCT with TBCT. At this point 16 couples meeting the criterion of moderate to severe marital distress have been randomly assigned to either IBCT or TBCT and have completed their respective treatments. Treatment consisted of 20–25 sessions of therapy conducted by five professional therapists chosen and supervised by Jacobson and Christensen. Each therapist saw an equal number of cases in each condition. On our primary outcome measure, the Global Distress scale of the Marital Satisfaction Inventory (MSI; Snyder, 1979), repeated-measures analyses of variance revealed an interaction between time and treatment condition that was significant for husbands and approached significance for wives, despite the small sample size. Both husbands and wives showed greater increases in marital satisfaction in IBCT than they did in TBCT. In addition, other analyses indicated that wives in IBCT rated their husbands' behavior as being significantly more acceptable to them at the end of treatment than did wives in TBCT. Ratings by IBCT husbands were in the same direction but not statistically significant.

We also evaluated our results according to the more demanding criteria of clinical significance and long-term follow-up. By "clinical significance," we mean that a couple not only improved but improved so much as to score more like normal couples than like distressed couples on standard satisfaction questionnaires such as the MSI (Jacobson & Truax, 1991). On the MSI, 50% of husbands and wives in IBCT met our criteria of clinical significance, whereas only 13% of husbands and 38% of wives met those criteria in TBCT. Furthermore, at a 6-month follow-up, husbands and wives in IBCT showed significantly more improvement than their counterparts in TBCT. At a 1-year follow-up, three TBCT couples but no IBCT couples had separated or divorced.

Obviously, these data must be interpreted cautiously, since they are based on such small samples. We continue to gather data on the effectiveness of IBCT as well as of TBCT. However, the current data certainly have supported our belief that IBCT, with its combined strategy of promoting acceptance and change in couples, is a powerful treatment for helping couples resolve the problems posed by their differences.

SUMMARY

In this chapter we have argued that conflict is the most important proximal determinant of satisfaction in established relationships. Although the empirical literature does not offer good comparative information about which factors are most important in determining satisfaction, research has consistently shown that conflict and negative behavior are cross-sectionally and longitudinally associated with satisfaction at a substantial level. We have also offered a behavioral theory of how conflict develops in relationships, which emphasizes inevitable incompatibilities between partners. We have analyzed how these incompatibilities develop over time, how partners cope with them, and how personality and circumstances affect them. Finally, we have presented two behavioral approaches to couple therapy, both of which attempt to ameliorate conflict in couples. TBCT focuses on making positive change in couples through behavior exchange procedures, communication training, and problem-solving training. IBCT assumes that there are some incompatibilities in most or all couples that will not be resolved by active change. It therefore promotes acceptance of differences as well as active change. Early data from an ongoing study comparing the two treatments suggest that the integrative approach may be more powerful than the traditional approach in helping couples cope with conflict and thus improve relationship satisfaction.

REFERENCES

Barry, W. A. (1970). Marriage research and conflict: An integrative review. *Psychological Bulletin, 73,* 41–54.

Belsky, J., & Pensky, E. (1988). Marital change across the transition to parenthood. *Marital and Family Review, 12,* 133–156.

Bradbury, T. N., & Fincham, F. D. (1990). Attributions in marriage: Review and critique. *Psychological Bulletin, 107,* 3–33.

Broderick, C. B. (1992). *Marriage and the family.* Englewood Cliffs, NJ: Prentice-Hall.

Christensen, A. (1987). Detection of conflict patterns in couples. In K. Hahlweg & M. J. Goldstein (Eds.), *Understanding major mental disorders: The contribution of family interaction research* (pp. 250–265). New York: Family Process Press.

Christensen, A. (1988). Dysfunctional interaction patterns in couples. In P. Noller & M. A. Fitzpatrick (Eds.), *Monographs in social psychology of language: No. 1. Perspectives on marital interaction* (pp. 31–52). Clevedon, England: Multilingual Matters.

Christensen, A., & Heavey, C. L. (1993). Gender differences in marital conflict: The demand–withdraw interaction pattern. In S. Oskamp & M.

Costanzo (Eds.), *Gender issues in contemporary society* (pp. 113–141). Newbury Park, CA: Sage.

Christensen, A., & Jacobson, N. S. (in press). *When lovers make war: Building intimacy from conflict through acceptance and change.* New York: Guilford Press.

Christensen, A., Jacobson, N. S., & Babcock, J. C. (1995). Integrative behavioral couple therapy. In N. S. Jacobson & A. S. Gurman (Eds.), *Clinical handbook of couple therapy* (pp. 31–64). New York: Guilford Press.

Christensen, A., & Margolin, G. (1988). Conflict and alliance in distressed and nondistressed families. In R. A. Hinde & J. Stevenson-Hinde (Eds.), *Relationships within families: Mutual influences* (pp. 263–282). Oxford: Oxford University Press.

Christensen, A., & Pasch, L. (1993). The sequence of marital conflict: An analysis of seven phases of marital conflict in distressed and nondistressed couples. *Clinical Psychology Review, 13,* 3–14.

Christensen, A., & Shenk, J. L. (1991). Communication, conflict, and psychological distance in nondistressed, clinic, and divorcing couples. *Journal of Consulting and Clinical Psychology, 59,* 458–463.

Gottman, J. M. (1979). *Marital interaction: Experimental investigations.* New York: Academic Press.

Hahlweg, K., & Markman, H. J. (1988). The effectiveness of behavioral marital therapy: Empirical status of behavioral techniques in preventing and alleviating marital distress. *Journal of Consulting and Clinical Psychology, 56,* 440–447.

Heavey, C. L., Christensen, A., & Malamuth, M. M. (1995). The longitudinal impact of demand and withdrawal during marital conflict. *Journal of Consulting and Clinical Psychology, 63,* 797–801.

Huston, T. L., & Houts, R. M. (in press). The psychological infrastructure of courtship and marriage: The role of personality and compatibility in romantic relationships. In T. Bradbury (Ed.), *The developmental course of marital dysfunction.* New York: Cambridge University Press.

Jacobson, N. S., & Addis, M. E. (1993). Research on couples and couple therapy: What do we know? Where are we going? *Journal of Consulting and Clinical Psychology, 61,* 85–93.

Jacobson, N. S., & Christensen, A. (1996). *Integrative couple therapy: Promoting acceptance and change.* New York: Norton.

Jacobson, N. S., & Follette, W. C. (1985). Clinical significance of improvement resulting from two behavioral marital therapy components. *Behavior Therapy, 16,* 249–262.

Jacobson, N. S., Follette, W. C., & Pagel, M. (1986). Predicting who will benefit from behavioral marital therapy. *Journal of Consulting and Clinical Psychology, 54,* 518–522.

Jacobson, N. S., & Margolin, G. (1979). *Marital therapy: Strategies based on social learning and behavior exchange principles.* New York: Brunner/Mazel.

Jacobson, N. S., Schmaling, K. B., & Holtzworth-Munroe, A. (1987). A component analysis of behavioral marital therapy: Two-year follow-up and prediction of relapse. *Journal of Marital and Family Therapy, 13,* 187–195.

Jacobson, N. S., & Truax, P. (1991). Clinical significance: A statistical approach to defining meaningful change in psychotherapy research. *Journal of Consulting and Clinical Psychology, 59,* 12–19.

Jarvis, I. L. (1982). Decision-making under stress. In L.Goldberger & S. Brezmitz (Eds.), *Handbook of stress: Theoretical and clinical aspects* (pp. 69–87). New York: Free Press.

Karney, B. R., & Bardbury, T. N. (1995). The longitudinal course of marital quality and stability: A review of theory, method, and research. *Psychological Bulletin, 118,* 3–34.

Kelley, H. H. (1979). *Personal relationships: Their structures and processes.* Hillsdale, NJ: Erlbaum.

Kelley, H. H., Berscheid, E., Christensen, A., Harvey, J. H., Huston, T. L., Levinger, G., McClintock, E., Peplau, L. A., & Peterson, D. R. (1983). *Close relationships.* New York: Freeman.

Kelly, E. L., & Conley, J. J. (1987). Personality and compatibility: A prospective analysis of marital stability and marital satisfaction. *Journal of Personality and Social Psychology, 52,* 27–40.

Lindahl, K., Clements, M., & Markman, H. (in press). The development of marriage: A nine-year perspective. In T. Bradbury (Ed.), *The developmental course of marital dysfunction.* New York: Cambridge University Press.

Margolin, G. (1988). Marital conflict is not marital conflict is not marital conflict. In R. deV. Peters & R. McMahon (Eds.), *Marriage and families: Behavioral treatment and processes* (pp. 193–216). New York: Brunner/Mazel.

Patterson, G. R., & Hops, H. (1972). Coercion, a game for two: Intervention techniques for marital conflict. In R. Ulrich & P. Mountjoy (Eds.), *The experimental analysis of social behavior* (pp. 424–440). New York: Appleton-Century-Crofts.

Repetti, R. L. (1989). Effects of daily work load on subsequent behavior during marital interaction: The roles of social withdrawal and spouse support. *Journal of Personality and Social Psychology, 57*(4), 651–659.

Schaap, C., Buunk, B., & Kerkstra, A. (1988). Marital conflict resolution. In P. Noller & M. A. Fitzpatrick (Eds.), *Monographs in social psychology of language. No. 1. Perspectives on marital interaction* (pp. 203–244). Clevedon, England: Multilingual Matters.

Skinner, B. F. (1966). An operant analysis of problem solving. In B.Kleinmuntz (Ed.), *Problem solving: Research method teaching* (pp. 225–257). New York: Wiley.

Snyder, D. K. (1979). Multidimensional assessment of marital satisfaction. *Journal of Marriage and the Family, 41,* 813–823.

Stuart, R. B. (1980). *Helping couples change: A social learning approach to marital therapy.* New York: Guilford Press.

Weiss, R. L., & Heyman, R. E. (1990). Observation of marital interaction. In F. D. Fincham & T. N. Bradbury (Eds.), *The psychology of marriage: Basic issues and applications* (pp. 87–117). New York: Guilford Press.

Winch, R. F. (1958). *Mate-selection: A study of complementary needs.* New York: Harper.

Wood, J. V., Saltzberg, J. A., & Goldsamt, L. A. (1990). Does affect induce self-focused attention? *Journal of Personality and Social Psychology, 58,* 899–908.

CHAPTER 11

———••———

Marital Quality:
A New Theoretical Perspective

FRANK D. FINCHAM
STEVEN R. H. BEACH
SUSAN I. KEMP-FINCHAM

Changing economic and social circumstances at the beginning of the
20th century called public attention to problems in family relationships.
Although initial research on the marital relationship focused on sexual problems, the most frequently studied aspect of this relationship concerns what has been variously labeled "satisfaction," "adjustment,"
"success," "happiness," "companionship," or some other term reflective
of the quality of the marriage. This is perhaps not surprising, because
approximately 40% of the problems for which people seek professional
help in the United States concern dissatisfaction with their spouses or
marriages (Veroff, Kulka, & Douvan, 1981), and the deleterious effects
of such problems on mental and physical health are well documented
(Burman & Margolin, 1992; Fincham, in press; Gotlib & McCabe,
1990). Notwithstanding the attention paid to it, the concept of marital quality remains poorly understood. The present chapter therefore
offers a new conception of marital quality that is designed to address
problems in prior work and ground the construct more firmly in the
broader psychological literature, particularly research on attitudes. Before turning to our analysis, we first provide a brief overview of current
knowledge regarding marital quality, which highlights the need for a
new approach to the concept.

MARITAL QUALITY: CURRENT STATUS

Marital quality has gained the attention of researchers from a number of disciplines, and the literature on this topic is vast. Rather than attempt to provide a review of pertinent theory and research (for such a review, see Glenn, 1990), we highlight features of the literature that lead us to offer a new conception of marital quality.

The first important feature of writings on marital quality is that they focus almost exclusively on Western, and more particularly North American, marriages. This is both a strength and a weakness. It is a strength in that there is widespread agreement (though not consensus) in North American society that marriage is primarily for the benefit of the spouses, rather than the extended family, society, the ancestors, the deity or deities, and so on. Widespread agreement on the hedonic purpose of marriage has the potential to simplify the task of researchers engaged in assessing and understanding marital quality, and thereby to promote advances in understanding. On the other hand, there is the strong temptation to insert in measures of marital quality items that may not be applicable in other cultures. For example, an assessment of marital quality that asks whom respondents would marry if they had their lives to live over again (as in one of the most widely used measures of marital quality, the Marital Adjustment Test [MAT; Locke & Wallace, 1959]), is clearly not applicable in cultures where arranged marriages are accepted practice. Likewise, questions assessing degree of interspousal agreement may be poor indicators of marital quality in cultures where open disagreement with a spouse is discouraged. Although no single set of items assessing marital quality is likely to have universal applicability, how marital quality is defined will determine the potential applicability of the concept across cultures.

Second, the literature on marital quality is characterized by a lack of adequate theory. As will become increasingly evident in the paragraphs below, conceptual confusion is widespread. In addressing this issue, some scholars have even called for elimination of such terms as "marital satisfaction" and "marital adjustment" (Lively, 1969; Trost, 1985). This feature of the literature most likely reflects the fact that research on marital quality has never been heavily theoretical. As Glenn (1990) points out in his review, most research is justified on practical grounds "with elements of theory being brought in on an incidental, ad hoc basis" (p. 818). Lack of attention to theory has had unfortunate consequences. For example, Spanier (1976) eliminated items from his influential Dyadic Adjustment Scale (DAS) when they were positively skewed, thereby assuming that items reflective of marital quality approximate a normal distribution. But as Norton (1983) points out, such items may be less critical indicators or even irrelevant to marital quality if marital quality, inherently involves skewed data because spouses tend to report "happy" marriages. Moreover, if the outcome predicted by marital quality is itself skewed (e.g., aggression), then a skewed predictor may be best (Heyman, Sayers, & Bellack, 1994).

Third, the relative absence of adequate theory is reflected in the disjuncture that exists between theoretical statements and measures of marital quality. There are many measures of marital quality available, but few appear to be derived from theory. Moreover, where there is a theoretical foundation, the link between the theory and the measure is often tenuous. For example, the widely used DAS defines adjustment as both a process and an outcome of the same process, thus creating substantial conceptual difficulties. The relative lack of adequate theory is less of a problem when measures are derived empirically and, on the basis of actuarial data, promote the development of a theoretical framework. However, as Snyder (1982) notes, the absence of naturally occurring criterion groups limits the use of a purely empirical approach to establishing the validity of measures of marital quality. In any event, even empirically constructed measures of marital quality are inadequate, as actuarial data relating to them are the exception rather than the rule.

Fourth, it is not clear what most instruments of marital quality actually measure. Most frequently, measures consist of a polyglot of items, and responses to them are not conceptually equivalent. For example, widely used measures (e.g., the MAT, the DAS) include a variety of items ranging from reports of specific behaviors that occur between spouses to evaluative inferences regarding the marriage as a whole. Typically, an overall score is computed by summing over the items, but it is not clear how such a score should be interpreted. Although this problem was identified in the marital literature over 25 years ago (see Nye & MacDougall, 1959), it remains an issue. Dahlstrom (1969) describes three levels at which responses to self-report inventories can be interpreted: they can be seen (1) as veridical descriptions of behavior (e.g., responses regarding frequency of disagreement reflect the actual rate of disagreement between spouses); (2) as potential reflections of attitudes (e.g., frequently reported disagreement may reflect high rates of disagreement, but may also reflect the view that the partner is unreasonable, that the spouse feels undervalued, or some other attitude); and (3) as behavioral signs whose meaning can only be determined by actuarial data (e.g., rated disagreement may reflect time spent together, respondent's self-esteem, frequency of sexual intercourse, or a host of other variables). Few measures of marital quality address the level at which responses are to be interpreted.

Fifth, our knowledge base of the determinants and correlates of marital quality includes (an unknown number of) spurious findings. This is because of overlapping item content in measures of marital quality and measures of constructs examined in relation to marital quality. For example, Banmen and Vogel (1985) found a significant association between communication (as assessed by Bienvenu's [1970] Marital Communication Inventory; e.g., "Do the two of you argue a lot over money?"; "Do you and your and your spouse engage in outside activities together?") and marital quality (as assessed by the DAS; e.g., "Indicate the extent of agreement or disagreement between you and your partner on: handling family finances," "Do you and your mate engage in outside interests together?"). The resulting tautological association hinders theory construction and affects the credibility of research findings. Fincham and Bradbury (1987) discuss the dilemma caused by overlapping item content at some length, showing that exclusion of the items common to both measures does not provide a satisfactory solution to this problem, as they usually reflect overlap in the definition of the constructs. Such a problem seems to be the inevitable consequence of an atheoretical and ad hoc approach to defining and assessing marital quality.

Finally, it is critical to note that with rare exceptions, marital quality is assessed via self-report. Ironically, even behaviorally oriented psychologists who rejected the utility of self-report when they began to study marriage systematically in the 1970s used self-reports of marital quality as a criterion variable in their studies. Indeed, a primary goal was to account for variability in such reports of marital quality. This feature of the marital quality literature is important when one considers the two dominant approaches to studying marital quality over the last 20 years. One approach has been to view marital quality as a characteristic of the relationship between spouses instead of, or in addition to, the spouses' feelings about the marriage. This approach favored use of such terms as "adjustment" and was particularly dominant in the 1970s (Spanier & Lewis, 1980). However, it is questionable whether spouses are the best, or even good, reporters of relationship properties. It is clear that spouses often do not agree even on such basic issues as how often they have sex.[1] Self-report seems better suited to the second major approach to marital quality, which focuses on how married persons feel about their marriages. This approach has used such terms as "marital satisfaction" and "marital happiness," and became more widespread in the 1980s.

Although the picture painted thus far appears somewhat gloomy, it need not necessarily be viewed in this way. On the contrary, there has been considerable progress over the last 20 years in explaining variance in marital quality, and especially in the psychometric sophistication of measures of marital quality (for a review, see Fincham, Fernandes,

& Humphreys, 1993). Indeed, some scholars have concluded that the "psychometric foundation is reasonably solid and need not be redone" (Gottman & Levenson, 1984, p. 71). The basis for such a conclusion appears to be the fact that different measures of marital quality inter-correlate highly, suggesting that differences in item content across measures are relatively unimportant (e.g., Heyman et al., 1994). In fact, "different operations designed to measure marital satisfaction converge and form one dimension" (Gottman, 1979, p. 5).

Such conclusions are quite reasonable for some research purposes. For instance, they suffice if the goal is to select "happy" or "satisfied" versus "unhappy" or "dissatisfied" spouses, as is often done in clinical research on marriage. Here the exact content of the measure used to select groups is less important than its ability to identify correctly the groups of interest. However, to the extent that one's goal is to develop theory for advancing understanding of marital quality or to devise conceptually sound measures of marital quality, these conclusions are less appropriate.

Accepting that current conceptions and operationalizations of marital quality are adequate for all purposes is based on an assumption that constructs related at the empirical level are equivalent at the conceptual level. This can lead to a problem that is demonstrated by considering the example of height and weight. These two dimensions correlate to about the same degree as many measures of marital quality, yet much is gained by keeping height and weight separate. Imagine designing a door frame on the basis of only a composite measure of the users' "bigness" and not their height! Keeping empirical and conceptual levels of analysis separate has the advantage of forcing researchers to articulate the nature of the construct and the domain of observables to which it relates before developing measures of the construct. Such practices are likely to facilitate theoretical development and the construction of more easily interpreted measures of marital quality. In addition, careful conceptualization of the construct of marital quality creates an opportunity to develop theoretically based and empirically robust dimensions of marital quality that may meet the need for identifying "subtypes" of couples.[2]

In sum, the concept of marital quality has received a great deal of attention from social scientists. Although researchers have made considerable progress in measuring and explaining variability in marital quality, they have failed to specify adequately the subject of their inquiries, while at the same time proceeding as though the referent for the construct were clear. It can be argued that at the level of measurement the referent *is* clear, owing to the widespread use of a limited number of instruments (most often the MAT and the DAS). However, the interpretation of scores obtained from these measures is far from clear. We therefore offer a new conception of marital quality in the remainder of this chapter.

MARITAL QUALITY: TOWARD A MORE COMPLETE ACCOUNT

In this section we outline an approach to marital quality that is theoretically simple, can be easily operationalized, and yet can accommodate the richness of clinical and everyday observations made about marital quality. We first review prior attempts to respond to the state of affairs outlined in the preceding section before outlining our approach as it builds on one of these responses.

Attempts to Clarify the Construct of Marital Quality

There have been two major responses to the lack of clarity about marital quality. One response has been the attempt to develop multidimensional measures of the construct (Snyder, 1979). This response is consistent with Beach and O'Leary's (1985) call for work recognizing "that marital quality may not be a unitary construct and will not be accurately reflected by a single-outcome measure of marital happiness" (p. 1063). Perhaps the best-developed of these measures is the Marital Satisfaction Inventory (Snyder, 1981). This measure includes a scale which attempts to provide a control for socially desirable responses (Conventionalization); a scale comprising items that tap the individual's overall dissatisfaction with the marriage (Global Distress); and nine scales assessing different dimensions of marital interaction (e.g., time together, disagreement about finances, sexual dissatisfaction). The Marital Satisfaction Inventory is a psychometrically sophisticated instrument that offers a profile of marital quality much as the Minneapolis Multiphasic Personality Inventory (MMPI) offers a profile of individual functioning, and, like the MMPI, it offers actuarial data to assist in its interpretation. It represents an important advance in research on marital quality. Unfortunately, however, the potential it offers for providing a more comprehensive picture of the marriage through profile analysis has not been adequately explored.

Even though it provides a multidimensional picture of marriage, the Marital Satisfaction Inventory accords one of the dimensions a special status. Specifically, the Global Distress scale occupies a special status, as it is a criterion against which the remaining dimensions are validated. Hence items that tap overall evaluations of the respondent's marriage are used to interpret the validity of items that assess various domains of the marriage. This is consistent with a pervasive tendency in the literature to favor global evaluations of a marriage—a preference that is not often explicitly discussed. Thus, for example, a single item in the MAT that assesses "marital happiness" is heavily weighted so that it accounts for 22% of the total possible test score. However, if all the items in the test were weighted equally, it would account for only 6.6% of the total possible score.

Not surprisingly, a second response to the circumstances described earlier has been to define marital quality as the spouses' subjective, global evaluations of the relationship (e.g., Fincham & Bradbury, 1987; Norton, 1983). The strength of this approach is its conceptual simplicity, as it avoids the problem of interpretation that arises in many omnibus measures of marital quality. Because it has a clear-cut interpretation, this approach allows the antecedents, correlates, and consequences of marital quality to be examined in a straightforward manner. Crosby (1991) argues that such a view of marital quality is the most accurate and useful from the perspective of clinical practice—a viewpoint supported by Jacobson's (1985) observation that overall evaluations of the marriage represent the final common pathway through which marital dysfunction is expressed. This viewpoint has given rise to such measures as the Quality of Marriage Index (Norton, 1983) and the Kansas Marital Satisfaction Scale (Schumm et al., 1986). Fincham and Bradbury (1987) have argued that this view of marital quality reflects the evaluative dimension of the semantic differential (Osgood, Suci, & Tannenbaum, 1957). The semantic differential is used to assess the connative meaning of concepts and consists of a series of bipolar adjective rating scales (e.g., "good–bad," "pleasant–unpleasant"). Numerous studies by Osgood and colleagues have shown that three dimensions underlie the meaning of concepts, namely evaluative, potency, and activity dimensions. Because the evaluative dimension usually accounted for the largest amount of variability among scale items, Osgood and colleagues viewed it as equivalent to a person's attitude. Thus, Fincham and Bradbury (1987) have argued that ratings of the marriage on bipolar adjective scales can be used to yield a parsimonious operationalization of marital quality (three items are usually sufficient to assess dimensions of a concept; see Osgood et al., 1957).

One criticism of this approach is the view that unidimensional, global scales "often do not provide much information beyond the fact that a couple is distressed" (Fowers, 1990, p. 370). However, the same is true of the most widely used scales of marital quality, the MAT and the DAS. Both the MAT and the DAS are typically used to provide a summary, overall measure of marital quality. Although Spanier (1976) found evidence for four factors in the DAS—Dyadic Satisfaction, Dyadic Cohesion, Dyadic Consensus, and Affectional Expression—these factors have not always been replicated (e.g., Sharpley & Cross, 1982), and both the disproportionate sampling and differing item formats across factors suggest that the factors are artifactual (see Norton, 1983).

Notwithstanding these observations about the MAT and DAS, they remain the most widely used measures of marital quality. Indeed, measures reflecting the multidimensional and unidimensional responses outlined above have had a limited impact. For example, the Marital Satisfaction Inventory and the Kansas Marital Satisfaction Scale have been used relatively infrequently compared to the MAT and DAS (e.g., the article describing the Kansas Marital Satisfaction Scale has been cited 70 times, and citations for the Marital Satisfaction Inventory number 77). In contrast, articles reporting traditional measures of marital quality have been cited much more frequently (769 times for the MAT, 918 times for the DAS; Social Sciences Citation Index, 1981–1995).

It therefore appears that any attempt to advance understanding of marital quality in the empirical literature will have to offer a significant advantage over MAT and DAS scores in order to overcome the inertia that has developed concerning these two measures. After all, there is a large data base relating to these measures (e.g., within 12 years of its development, the DAS had been used in over 1,000 studies). In the remainder of the chapter, we outline an approach to understanding and measuring marital quality that represents such an advance.

A New Conception of Marital Quality: Step 1

Our approach builds on the theoretically straightforward conception of marital quality as the spouses' global, evaluative judgments of the marriage (Fincham & Bradbury, 1987). This conception is expanded to reflect the complexities found in discussions of marital quality and in the reality of everyday life. For example, clinical observation suggests that a spouse's marital behavior is not always driven by a single undifferentiated view of his or her marriage; some spouses can show great tenderness toward their partners, followed by acutely negative affect toward the partners moments later. Ideally, a measure of marital quality should accommodate such phenomena.

Measures of marital quality should also capture important differences between couples. Consider Sue and Saul, who report a rollercoaster relationship. Both list great sex and having a lot of fun together as some of the good things in their relationship. However, they have concerns about the physical fights they get into and the frequent yelling that occurs in the front of the children. In contrast, Pam and Paul report a very steady but uneventful life together. They tend always to agree on things, and nothing particularly positive or negative ever happens between them. Each spouse wonders whether this is all marriage has to offer. Both couples may report a similar level of overall marital quality, but a single, summary index of marital quality—whether it represents evaluative judgments of the marriage or the score on a traditional test such as the MAT or the DAS—seems to mask important differences between them.

The first step toward addressing such complexity is to conceive of evaluative judgments of the marriage as multidimensional, comprising positive marital quality (PMQ) and negative marital quality (NMQ) dimensions. Although simple, this conception has profound implications. For example, it alerts us to an important assumption in much of the psychological literature, including the marital literature. This assumption is reflected in the pervasive use of scales anchored by positive (e.g., "happy") and negative ("unhappy") endpoints that do not allow positive and negative dimensions to be expressed independently. In this regard, the marital literature is no different, for example, from the literature on attitudes, where "social scientists typically assess people's attitudes by placing them on a bipolar evaluative continuum" (Eagly & Chaiken, 1993, p. 90). In fact, attitudes "are largely treated as unidimensional summary statements" even though they may in principle be considered multidimensional (Thompson, Zanna, & Griffin, 1995, p. 362). There is growing awareness in the attitude literature that this practice is not optimal, and, where appropriate, we draw on this literature in developing our conception of marital quality.

Another implication of this two-dimensional approach is that it has the potential to provide a more differentiated view of those who are neither high nor low in marital quality. This is important, because it is unclear how to interpret responses that fall at the midpoint of a bipolar scale. Do such responses reflect the irrelevance of both poles (e.g., neither satisfied nor dissatisfied), or do they reflect some agreement with each pole (e.g., equally satisfied and dissatisfied)? That is, one can distinguish between "indifference," or caring about neither of the two endpoints, and "ambivalence," or caring strongly about both. From everyday observation it is quite easy to recognize spouses who are not engaged in their marriage and yet are neither happy nor unhappy with it (such as Pam and Paul, described earlier). Similarly, ambivalent spouses whose behavior often vacillates between positive and negative extremes are also recognizable (such as Sue and Saul, described earlier). Although such groupings have not been discussed in marital research, they can be hypothesized to exhibit avoidant and ambivalent attachment styles, and thereby to have indirectly received attention in recent research. Our analysis has the advantage of clearly identifying such spouses and allows the relation to attachment style to be empirically evaluated.

The implications of our two-dimensional approach to marital quality are illustrated in Figure 11.1. The two dimensions, PMQ and NMQ, can be crossed to produce a fourfold typology of couples that can be distinguished in terms of important characteristics of their marriages. Two of the categories are already identified through established measures. Those high on PMQ and low on NMQ seem to fit the traditional understanding of "happy" or "satisfied" spouses, just as those high on NMQ and low on PMQ fit the traditional understanding of "distressed" spouses. The two other categories of spouses (high PMQ–high NMQ and low PMQ–low NMQ), however, are not currently distinguished in most measures of marital quality and correspond to our distinction between "ambivalent" and "indifferent" spouses. In such a typology, ambivalent and indifferent spouses should not differ in scores on traditional, unidimensional measures of marital quality, but should have significantly lower scores than happy spouses and significantly higher scores than distressed spouses on such measures. The utility of this typology should be further supported to the extent that ambivalent and indifferent spouses are found to differ on variables that have been shown to be related to marital quality.

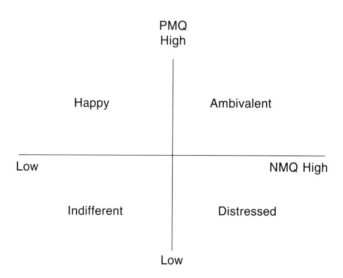

FIGURE 11.1. Typology of couples derived from a two-dimensional conception of marital quality. PMQ, positive marital quality; NMQ, negative marital quality.

What evidence exists to support the analysis offered thus far? In answering this question, we begin by noting that analogous two-dimensional analyses have emerged in other areas of research and advanced understanding in those areas. For example, a two-dimensional assessment is used in the study of affect, although the axes are often rotated to yield positive and negative dimensions. Summarizing such work, Watson, Clark, and Tellegen (1988) conclude that even though positive and negative affect are often assumed to be strongly negatively correlated, "they have in fact emerged as highly distinctive dimensions that can be meaningfully represented as orthogonal dimensions in factor analytic studies of affect" (p. 1063). Elsewhere, we (Beach & Fincham, 1994) have already offered an analysis of marriage that is based on a two-dimensional structure of affect. The present research supplements this analysis by exploring the more general question of whether assessment of marital quality can be enhanced by including both positive and negative components.

Similarly, positive and negative dimensions have been identified in attitude research, in an attempt to examine ambivalence as a property of attitudes. To collect positive and negative dimensions of attitudes, Kaplan (1972) divided the semantic differential into positive and negative components. Kaplan's research, and subsequent work (see Thompson et al., 1995), have shown that respondents have no difficulty in responding to the two components and that the responses do not provide redundant information. In fact, the positive and negative dimensions are remarkably independent, with mean correlations in the range of – .05 (Kaplan, 1972) to – .40 (Thompson et al., 1995).

Although surprisingly little attention has been given to the possibility that marital quality may comprise separate positive and negative dimensions, there is some evidence to support this viewpoint. Orden and Bradburn (1968) presented an early multidimensional approach to the assessment of marriages that points toward such a possibility. Based on self-report of behaviors, they found three factors that they labeled Sociability, Companionship, and Tensions. This behavioral type of assessment has not been followed extensively, "in part because spouses seem to disagree over the occurrence of daily behaviors in their relationship" (O'Leary & Smith, 1991, p. 198), although interest in behavior (especially as a dependent measure) has continued. Still, their approach includes a positive dimension made up of two factors (Sociability and Companionship) and a negative dimension (Tensions).

Soon thereafter, Rollins and Feldman (1970) distinguished companionship with the spouse, which they viewed as positive, from negative feelings derived from interaction with the spouse. Their approach was also used in Gilford and Bengtson's (1979) attempt to analyze positive and negative dimensions of marital satisfaction. Following Orden and Bradburn's (1968) lead, Marini (1976) attempted to relate positive and negative dimensions of marriage to general positive and negative affect. Outside of the marital field, Rodin (1978) similarly argued that liking and disliking are separate judgments. More recently, Johnson, White, Edwards, and Booth (1986) also found two main dimensions, which they note are positive and negative, when they analyzed responses in five areas of marriage. There is thus some evidence that satisfaction and dissatisfaction within personal relationships are not polar opposites.

In regard to global evaluations of a marriage, the first question is whether responses can be obtained on positive and negative dimensions that yield relatively independent dimensions of marital quality. Our initial attempts to examine this issue were crude and simply involved asking spouses to rate independently the extent to which each end-point of the bipolar adjectives typically used in semantic differential scales (e.g., "good–bad") characterized their marriage. This procedure yielded responses that were highly negatively correlated (correlations ranged from − .70 to − .85). This was somewhat puzzling, in view of the much lower correlations found in the attitude ambivalence literature. However, Kaplan's (1972) decomposition of the semantic differential contained an important element missing from our own—namely, the instruction to consider only positive (negative) qualities when making a rating of positivity (negativity), *and to ignore negative (positive) qualities.*

Consequently, in our most recent study (see Fincham & Linfield, in press), we explicitly instructed approximately 120 couples to evaluate one dimension at a time in three marital areas (feelings about the marriage, feelings about one's spouse, and qualities of one's spouse). Thus, for example, spouses rated the item "Considering only good feelings you have about your marriage, and ignoring the bad ones, evaluate how good these feelings are." The response scale, which ranged from 0 to 10, was anchored by "not at all good" (0) and "extremely good" (10).

The consistency of responses to items assessing PMQ and NMQ was high (alpha coefficients for husbands, .87 and .91, and for wives, .90 and .89, for PMQ and NMQ, respectively). More importantly, the correlations between PMQ and NMQ scores were comparable to those found between positive and negative dimensions of attitudes in social-psychological research (− .41 and − .39 for husbands and wives, respectively). These results were encouraging, but it was nonetheless possible that the positive and negative items reflected a single underlying dimension of marital quality.

To examine this possibility, a confirmatory factor analysis was conducted. When all six items were used as indicators of a single latent measure of marital quality, a poor fit was found between the model and the obtained data. However, when a two-factor model was posited in which positive and negative items were hypothesized to load on separate, yet correlated, dimensions of marital quality, a much better fit was obtained for both spouses. To determine whether a two-factor model is more appropriate than a single-factor model, the models were compared statistically. The two-factor model showed a significantly better fit. Thus, the data obtained for marital quality items were best accounted for by a two-dimensional model in which positive and negative items defined separate, but related, factors.[3]

A concern that arises is whether this two-dimensional structure is a function of general affective style. As noted earlier, affect has a two-dimensional structure, and responses to PMQ and NMQ questions may simply reflect an individual's general level of affectivity. We found an association between affectivity and PMQ and NMQ scores, but the magnitude of the associations (ranging from .32 to .49) shows that only a small portion (less than 25%) of the variance is shared. Thus marital quality scores do not simply reflect affectivity. However, in view of the association documented, it is still important to demonstrate that affectivity does not account for any associations established for this approach to marital quality.

Although important, the documentation of a nonspurious, two-dimensional structure for evaluative judgments pertaining to marriage is a necessary but not sufficient step for establishing its utility. An important question that now arises is whether a two-dimensional approach accounts for variance in constructs known to be related to marital quality. If so, is this variance unique, or does it simply reflect variance that would be captured by a traditional, unidimensional measure of marital quality? To answer this question, Fincham and Linfield (in press) examined two well-established correlates of marital quality: behavior and attributions. In each case, both a traditional marital quality measure (the MAT) and PMQ and NMQ dimensions were used to predict reports of partner behaviors over the past week and attributions for negative partner behaviors (as assessed by the Relationship Attribution Measure; Fincham & Bradbury, 1992).

Table 11.1 shows that PMQ and NMQ accounted for unique variance in both spouses' reported behavior (ratio of positive to negative behaviors reported) and in wives' attributions. Interestingly, the MAT also accounted for unique variance. These findings were not an artifact of general affective style, as they all remained significant when general spousal affectivity (as assessed by the Positive and Negative Affect Schedule; Watson et al., 1988) was included in the prediction of behaviors and attributions.

Earlier, we have argued that a two-dimensional view of marital qual-

TABLE 11.1. Unique Variance in Behavior and Attributions Explained by Measures of Marital Quality

	MAT		PMQ and NMQ	
	ΔR^2	F	ΔR^2	F
	Husbands			
Partner behavior	.074	14.66***	.070	6.93**
Causal attributions	.102	16.82***	.016	1.29
Responsibility attributions	.040	5.86*	.039	2.85
	Wives			
Partner behavior	.031	5.86*	.097	9.23***
Causal attributions	.028	4.30*	.075	5.85**
Responsibility attributions	.006	0.72	.060	3.74*

Note. MAT, Marital Adjustment Test; PMQ, positive marital quality; NMQ, negative marital quality. $*p < .05.$ $**p < .01.$ $***p < .001.$ ΔR^2 represents the amount of variability in behavior and attribution that is uniquely associated with each marital quality measure. F is used to test whether ΔR^2 is statistically significant.

ity allows distinctions that are not afforded by unidimensional measures. Specifically, Figure 11.1 shows a typology of spouses that not only distinguishes happy from distressed spouses, but also identifies ambivalent and indifferent spouses. Thus, it can be argued that (1) the MAT scores of these two groups would fall between those of happy and of distressed spouses, and (2) ambivalent and indifferent spouses should display different characteristics.

To examine these hypotheses, Fincham and Linfield (in press) formed four groups of spouses, using median scores on the PMQ and NMQ dimensions. Those scoring above the median were classed as high on that dimension, and those scoring below the median were classed as low on the dimension. The MAT scores of ambivalent and indifferent spouses were significantly lower than those of happy spouses and significantly higher than those of distressed spouses. However, in keeping with our earlier analysis, ambivalent and indifferent the groups did not differ from each other in overall marital quality (MAT scores), despite differences between them on the correlates of marital quality. That is, ambivalent and indifferent wives differed in reports of behavior and in attributions. Ambivalent wives attributed significantly more cause and responsibility to their partners for negative events, and reported higher ratios of negative to positive partner behaviors. In contrast, ambivalent and indifferent husbands did not differ significantly in attributions or in reports of behavior.

It is important to note that NMQ and PMQ are continuous dimensions, and therefore that the primary value of the typology presented is heuristic. There is ongoing research to examine how best to combine positive and negative attitude dimensions to yield a continuous measure (see Thompson et al., 1995). For example, the multiplicative effect of PMQ and NMQ (the interaction term) has served as a measure of ambivalence in Katz's research (Katz & Hass, 1988; Hass, Katz, Rizzo, Bailey, & Eisenstadt, 1991). As Hass et al. (1991) point out, however, ambivalence should reflect similarity of responses on positive and negative dimensions, as well as their extremity. A multiplicative combination of dimension scores violates this view, as it produces greater (rather than less) ambivalence as the dissimilarity in scores increases. Thompson et al. (1995) compare various combinations. They recommend one (number of response options − |positive − negative| + [positive + negative]/2) that yields component measures of similarity (number of response options − |positive − negative|) and intensity ([positive + negative]/2). This allows examination of the relative roles of each component in associations between ambivalence and other variables.

In sum, there is preliminary evidence to support a two-dimensional view of marital quality comprising positive and negative evaluations. This approach has several advantages in addition to its conceptual clarity. First, it provides a clear link with research on attitudes in social psychology, and thus creates the potential for research on marital quality to inform and be informed by theoretical and methodological developments in this broader literature. Second, it opens up new areas for marital quality research. For example, change in marriage is currently under intense research. However, unidimensional measures of marital quality can only provide a global index of change, whereas the analysis offered here suggests that changes in marital quality may follow several different paths. For instance, it will be theoretically important if happily married spouses first increase negative evaluations only (became ambivalent) before then decreasing positive evaluations and becoming distressed, as compared to a progression in which negative evaluations increase and positive evaluations decrease at the same time. Such progressions may in turn differ in important ways from one where there is simply a decline in positive evaluations over time. Documenting the existence of different avenues of change in marital quality, examining their determinants, and exploring their consequences suggests a program of research that may do much to advance our understanding of how marriages succeed and fail.

A New Conception of Marital Quality: Step 2

Up to this point, we have concentrated on showing that spouses can have both positive and negative evaluations of their marriage. This is important, but it does not go far enough, in that we do not know when these different evaluations will affect behavior. Consider the observation made earlier that a spouse can treat his or her partner very tenderly one moment and then quite negatively the next. For example, in the case of Sue and Saul, why do they experience passion toward each other at one moment in time and experience intense anger toward each other at a different moment in time? A second step can be taken toward answering this question by considering the broader literature on cognition–behavior relations.

The relation between cognition and behavior has been the subject of psychological inquiry throughout the 20th century, and the advent of the human information-processing metaphor in psychology has stimulated advances in this area. This can again be illustrated by reference to the attitude literature. As the second element of our approach builds on this literature, we offer a fairly detailed account of this illustration.

Influenced by theory and research on memory as a network of associated elements, Fazio (1990, 1995) has defined an "attitude" as an association between an object and a summary evaluation of the object. This association can vary in strength, such that for some objects (e.g., "spider" for spider phobics) their mere mention or presentation activates an evaluation automatically, whereas for others (e.g., "spoon") an evaluative association is weak or nonexistent. Fazio argues that the strength of this association is critical in understanding the relation between attitudes and behaviors. This is because the strength of the association determines whether the attitude is available when the person acts in relation to the attitude object. When the attitude is highly accessible, it is likely to affect subsequent behavior. By using the latency of an evaluative response to the attitude as an index of associative strength, Fazio has been able to examine these ideas empirically.

For example, Fazio and Williams (1986) measured attitudes toward the 1984 U.S. presidential candidates and the accessibility of the attitudes. At each level of response on the attitude scale, the sample was divided into two groups: a high-accessibility group (those who responded relatively quickly) and a low-accessibility group (those who responded relatively more slowly). This procedure ensured that the distribution of attitudes was equivalent in the two accessibility groups—an important consideration, as accessibility tends to correlate with attitude extremity. The researchers showed that attitudes were more predictive of voting behavior 4 months later in the high-accessibility group (.89) than in the low-accessibility group (.66). Similar findings have been obtained for response latencies obtained via computer-assisted telephone interviews during the 1990 Ontario provincial election (Bassili, 1993). The role of accessible attitudes in moderating attitude–behavior relations has also been demonstrated in experimental studies (e.g., Fazio, Powell, & Williams, 1989).

It is important to note that attitude accessibility has a number of other consequences. For instance, it influences the processing of information about the attitude object. Thus, the Fazio and Williams (1986) study showed that the speed with which people made evaluative judgments about President Reagan moderated the relation between their attitudes toward Reagan and their judgments about the 1984 presidential debates; for fast responders, the correlation between their attitude towards Reagan and their judgment of the impressiveness of the Republican's performance was significantly higher (.738) than that for slow responders (.404). In a similar vein, accessible attitudes ease decision making, enhance the quality of decisions, and orient attention (Blascovich et al., 1993; Roskos-Ewoldsen & Fazio, 1992).

How is all this relevant to marital quality? In answering this question, it is useful to specify the level at which we conceptualize responses to self-report inventories concerning marital quality. Following Dahlstrom's (1969) distinctions (outlined earlier), we view such responses as reflections of attitudes; in our case, these attitudes concern global, evaluative judgments. Following Fazio, we hypothesize that the importance of these judgments for understanding marital interaction will be influenced by their accessibility. Marital interaction often unfolds in a relatively quick and seemingly mindless manner—the very circumstance under which accessible attitudes are considered to be most powerful.[4]

The implications of this view for understanding marriage are quite profound. Take, for example, the "sentiment override" hypothesis described in the marital literature (Weiss, 1980). According to this hypothesis, a spouse responds to questions about the partner or marriage in terms of his or her dominant sentiment about the marriage, rather than in terms of the specific question asked. That is, the spouse responds noncontingently. If this hypothesis is correct, it has important implications for research. In its strongest form, it poses a threat to the validity of self-report studies on marriage. Specifically, if dimensions of marriage assessed via self-report simply reflect sentiment toward the marriage, they will necessarily be correlated if the range of marital satisfaction sampled is not restricted.

However, sentiment override can be conceptualized as "top-down" or theory-driven processing. Viewed in this way, marital quality is a concept that can influence the processing of spouse- and marriage-relevant information, can affect behavior, and so on. This means that the strength of the association in memory between the representation of the partner and the spouse's sentiment (evaluation) about the partner will determine whether the sentiment is called to mind when questions are asked about the partner or marriage. One of the most robust findings in the social cognition literature is that concepts made available through situational manipulations (e.g., priming) or naturally occurring states (e.g., depression) can influence the encoding of new information (see Wyer & Srull, 1989). Such encoding in turn tends to influence retrieval of material from memory. Concepts easily accessed from memory can therefore have a pervasive impact on spouses' behavior. However, as reflected in Fazio's definition of "attitude," not all concepts are equally accessible or brought to mind with equal ease. In fact, the importance of individual differences in concept accessibility is well documented (Markus & Smith, 1981). Thus, even if marital quality is chronically accessible to all spouses, individual differences in accessibility may still exist. Once we allow for this, the sentiment override hypothesis becomes more complex and may only apply to a certain group of spouses (those with accessible attitudes).

Is there any evidence to support this element of our analysis of marital quality? Fincham, Garnier, Gano-Phillips, and Osborne (1995) measured the accessibility of spouses' evaluative judgments via two procedures. The first involved a binary choice (positive–negative) when various items, including marriage-relevant items (e.g., "your wife"), served as stimuli. The second concerned answers to questions about the marriage (e.g., "The relationship I have with my husband is satisfying") given on 5-point rating scales (ranging from "strongly disagree" to "strongly agree"). In each case response latencies were timed. Latencies were adjusted for differences in baseline speed of responding, and fast and slow groups were formed that did not differ in marital quality (e.g., for the rating task, groups were formed at each response point on the scale). For both husbands and wives, fast responders showed a higher correlation between MAT scores and judgments of partner contributions to negative marital events ($-.52$ and $-.51$ for husbands and wives, respectively) than slow responders ($-.09$ and $.24$ for husbands and wives, respectively). For husbands, accessibility also moderated the relation between MAT scores and anticipated wife behavior in an upcoming interaction (fast group $= .70$, slow group $= .37$). The same results were found when latencies derived from the rating scale task were used.

Similar results were found in a more recently completed study with the choice reaction time task. Accessibility again moderated the relation between MAT scores and anticipated partner behavior (but this time for wives only; fast group $= .72$, slow group $= .38$). In addition, accessibility moderated the relation between two measures of marital quality in husbands. The correlation between the MAT score and the Quality Marriage Index (Norton, 1993), an index reflecting the global evaluation conception of marital quality, was higher (.90) in the high-accessibility group than in the low-accessibility group (.52). There is therefore initial evidence to support the value of including accessibility in our analysis of marital quality.

Although the relevance of these findings for understanding marriage has been questioned (see Baucom, 1995), they have important implications. For example, because spouses whose marital quality is highly accessible are likely to process information about their partners in terms of marital quality, we can hypothesize that, relative to spouses whose marital quality is not as highly accessible, their marital quality will remain stable over time. We have some evidence to support this hypothesis. Using the choice reaction time task to form the two accessibility groups, we examined correlations among current MAT scores, corresponding scores collected 12 months earlier and collected 18 months earlier. Table 11.2 shows the correlations obtained for the two groups. For both husbands and wives, corresponding test–retest correlations differed significantly in the two groups. Given the noise in reaction time data and the use of only four partner stimuli to form fast and slow groups, we find these results quite compelling.

Perhaps the most important implication of this element of our analysis is that the vast literature on the correlates of marital quality needs to be reworked. The overall correlation between marital quality and other variables may be misleading if the magnitude of the association turns out to be higher for one category of spouses (fast responders) and lower for another (slow responders). Previously nonsignificant correlations may turn out to be significant, at least for one group of spouses, and some correlates of marital quality may prove to be more important than previously thought. The incorporation of accessibility or associative strength into research on marital quality and its correlates is analogous to the refinement of a diagnostic category in a psychiatric nosology into several subcategories. It is not that the original broad category (or set of correlates) is wrong, but rather that it is crude. The more homogeneous subcategories allow a more precise picture to emerge that includes differential correlates for subcategories, new correlates, and so on.

In sum, this element of our analysis also has the potential to further our understanding of marital quality; it shows how marital quality may influence information processing, judgments, decision making, and behavior in marriage. Thus, for example, just as the accessibility of constructs that characterize the self influences information processing (e.g., Markus & Smith, 1981), constructs relevant to relationships are also likely to influence information processing. This influence most likely reflects the fact that much cognitive processing in close relationships

TABLE 11.2. Correlations between Marital Adjustment Test (MAT) Scores over Time for High-Accessibility (above Diagonal) and Low-Accessibility (below Diagonal) Groups

	1	2	3
		Husbands	
1. Current MAT score		.93*	.87*
2. MAT score 12 months earlier	.82		.89*
3. MAT score 18 months earlier	.62	.64	
		Wives	
1. Current MAT score		.79*	.67*
2. MAT score 12 months earlier	.52		.85
3. MAT score 18 months earlier	.29	.76	

Note. Asterisks (*) indicate significantly higher correlation compared to corresponding correlation below diagonal.

is automatic and occurs outside of conscious awareness (Fincham, Bradbury, & Scott, 1990). Spouses therefore need not engage in controlled or conscious, effortful processing for accessibility effects to operate. However, in our research spouses have had the opportunity to engage in deliberative processing, and yet we have still found accessibility effects. An important task in future research is not only to explore the potential impact of accessibility effects, but to determine the conditions under which they operate in marriage. Again, it should be noted that our analysis provides a clear link with a broader literature on attitudes and opens new areas of inquiry in the marital field.

A New Conception of Marital Quality: Step 3

The final element of our analysis is to link the preceding two steps. This element is somewhat more speculative, as we have not collected data on it. Nonetheless, it seems reasonable to argue that the PMQ and NMQ dimensions can each be studied in terms of their accessibility. That is, the cognitive representation of the partner is hypothesized to be associated with a negative evaluation node and with a positive evaluation node.

In principle it should be possible, in most cases, to prime positive and negative partner evaluations. If demonstrated, such priming effects would allow us to explain the clinical observation with which we have begun our reanalysis—namely, that a spouse can show tenderness toward the partner, followed rapidly by negative behavior toward the partner.

In such a case, the switch from positive to negative spouse behavior can be explained by a change in the accessibility of the NMQ dimension. For example, the partner, in responding to the spouse's tenderness, may do or say something that fires the spouse's association between the partner and negative evaluation node. Alternatively, this association may be activated internally by the spouse when he or she accesses a thought that triggers this association.

Again, however, clinical observation suggests that matters may not be this simple. Most clinicians will be familiar with the type of couple in which it is almost impossible to get a spouse to acknowledge anything positive about his or her partner. Similarly, at the other extreme, we have encountered in our research spouses who cannot see or acknowledge anything negative about their partners. In such cases, the asymmetry in partner associations with positive and negative evaluations is likely to be maximal, with one of the associations approximating 0. The relative strength of each association may therefore be important in understanding the impact of marital quality on information processing, behavior, and so on.

Presumably, the analysis of ambivalence offered in relation to ratings of PMQ and NMQ (and of attitudes more generally) can be applied also to the accessibility of the dimensions. Thus, for example, the extent to which each association is similar in magnitude, and the extent to which the absolute magnitude is high, will predict inconsistency in marital behavior, in the processing of partner behavior, and so on. This is because the marital quality dimensions are most easily primed under such conditions, and PMQ and NMQ would, on average, have an equal probability of being primed.

Although we have not specifically investigated these ideas, we do have some relevant data. For example, we have data that bear on an important assumption in integrating the two-dimensional and accessibility components of our analysis—namely, that the accessibility of PMQ and NMQ evaluations are relatively independent. Spouses were asked to evaluate partner behaviors that included target items clearly designed to be either negative or positive. This was done to ensure that spouses would give both types of evaluations. We calculated latency scores for these two sets of targets, taking into account respondents' baseline speed of responding. The correlation between speeds of responding to the two types of events was then computed. Although they were related (husbands $= .30$, wives $= .35$), the magnitude of the correlation was sufficiently low to suggest that speed of responding in making positive and negative evaluations is relatively independent.[5]

Given our analysis, an issue that arises is how PMQ and NMQ are combined when a spouse provides a single, global evaluation of the partner or marriage. This is particularly important because a summary global evaluation of the marriage, rather than a particular behavior or set of behaviors, represents the final common pathway through which marital dysfunction is expressed when, for example, spouses seek professional help (Jacobson, 1985). Moreover, there is a large literature on this topic, and it behooves us to maintain continuity with that literature in building a cumulative body of knowledge on marriage. Is there a threshold for negative sentiment about the marriage that, once crossed, leads a spouse to express marital dysfunction regardless of any positive feelings? If so, this suggests the need to focus on determinants of negative evaluations. Or does the magnitude of the discrepancy between positive and negative evaluations drive the expression of marital distress? In this case, one can focus on the determinants of positive *and* negative evaluations.

Again, we have some very preliminary data that relate indirectly to this question. It follows from our two-dimensional analysis of marital quality that spouses will differ in the ease with which they can make a single, summary judgment of the partner. As spouses make more similar ratings on the two dimensions and these ratings increase in magnitude (i.e., they experience ambivalence), they should have greater difficulty making a summary judgment. To examine this possibility we computed two ambivalence scores, following the procedure used by Katz and Hass (1988) and the one recommended by Thompson et al. (1995), and examined their association with speed of making evaluative judgments of the partner. The two procedures produced indices that correlated significantly ($p < .01$) and similarly with speed of making summary judgments (husbands = .35 and .34; wives = .47 and .41, for Katz & Thompson et al. measures, respectively). Thus, the exact procedure used to calculate ambivalence did not influence the correlates found for this property of attitudes. Overall, the positive correlations obtained provide indirect support for the view that positive and negative dimensions are integrated in reaching a summary judgment.

APPLICATIONS AND LIMITATIONS

We have attempted throughout the chapter to spell out the implications of our analysis for understanding marriage. In this section we focus on the more practical implications of our analysis for helping couples. In doing so, however, we must add two important cautions regarding practical application. First, there is the need for a solid foundation of research to support theory before it is applied. Second, supportive research is not sufficient for application; the application itself needs to be empirically evaluated. As neither condition has been met in the present case, the following applications are necessarily speculative.

Perhaps the most important application stems from the recognition that much information processing in marriage occurs automatically or without conscious awareness. Up to now, though, the advice given by most therapists working with couples focuses on modifying the contents of conscious thoughts (e.g., clients' specific beliefs, assumptions), providing missing information in clients' knowledge base, and helping clients to make decisions (e.g., Baucom & Epstein, 1990). Although extremely valuable, the focus on conscious judgments has virtually excluded consideration of automatic processing in the marital literature. Indeed, many of the conscious judgments a spouse makes about the marriage may reflect post hoc rationalizations for actions that resulted from automatic processing of the partner's behavior—processing that is beyond the spouse's awareness.

Does this omission matter in helping couples? Yes and no. It is possible to view cognitive interventions in marital therapy as addressing automatic processing. That is, simply getting spouses to think about their behavior, explore alternative interpretations of the behavior, and so on can disrupt, automatic processing. In other words, the therapist makes more accessible alternative concepts and this alters automatic processing. However, few therapists are aware of this possible impact on automatic processing, and fewer still use knowledge of automatic and controlled processing to maximize the impact of their interventions. Attention to automatic processes can lead to important changes in a therapist's behavior. For example, consider a therapist who is aware of the fact that a spouse processing the partner's behavior stores in memory a summary judgment about the behavior, and that this summary judgment is more likely to influence subsequent processing than is retrieval of the behavior itself. Knowing also that people tend to process information in terms of concepts currently available in short-term memory, such a therapist might behave subtly to make salient particular positively valenced concepts, which might then influence processing of the behavior. Such interventions might result in important changes over time in the accessibility of the PMQ and NMQ dimensions.

Spouses might themselves use knowledge of these automatic processing effects to alter their marital quality. At the simplest level, we know that the frequency and recency of concept use influence its accessibility. Therefore, simply by making a point of thinking about the positive dimension of the marriage every day (or more frequently if necessary), a spouse can influence the accessibility of the PMQ dimension. This increased accessibility may then have cumulative or "snowball" effects, as it might influence the way he or she views certain partner behaviors, and so on. At a slightly more complex level, when they find themselves feeling negative about their partners, spouses might ask themselves what they are calling to mind. Is this recalled material the whole story, or have the positive elements been overlooked? Even when a negative feeling is entirely warranted (as sometimes occurs in every marriage), a spouse can minimize the impact by not engaging in repeated mental rehearsal of the event. Such rehearsal will strengthen the accessibility of negative associations relating to the partner or marriage, and may in turn have snowball effects.

Our analysis also suggests clinical practices that have been avoided by some therapists. For example, behaviorally oriented marital therapists have tended to avoid having spouses engage in conflict during therapy sessions. But we suggest the exact opposite. For example, nonconscious memories can influence automatic processing and trigger reactions to particular partner behaviors or conflict situations that are quite inappropriate. Thus, unless contraindicated, we allow spouses to engage in overt conflict during a therapy session. This permits us to interrupt the conflict and inquire about cognitions and affects that may only be accessible to a spouse when he or she is engaged in the conflict. It also allows us to observe conflict behavior directly and to identify possible thoughts and feelings of which the spouse is unaware but that appear to underlie his or her behavior. Because conflict during therapy sessions can undermine progress, it is important that this procedure be implemented with considerable care. However, it does allow us, for example, to identify the automatic triggering of nonconscious memories from past relationships in the present marriage. Steps can then be taken to avoid such occurrences.

Although it is extremely difficult to do without professional guidance, spouses might try to implement the procedure described above. That is, they can try to take a "time out" during the heat of marital conflict and write down exactly what they are thinking and feeling. More importantly, they should try to specify what kinds of thoughts a person thinking, feeling, and behaving like them would be assumed to have (even if they do not consciously experience having such thoughts and feelings). If these thoughts and feelings can be identified, the spouses can then ask themselves whether they really mean to behave in accordance with such thoughts and feelings. In some cases, spouses can be quite surprised when they stop and do this, as they realize that their behavior is based on thoughts and feelings that they do not feel are really justified.

In sum, our analysis has important practical implications. Therapists and spouses who wish to explore these further should consult a self-help text specifically written for that purpose (Fincham et al., 1993). This text begins by helping spouses decide whether self-help is advisable or whether they need professional help. Again, we caution our readers as to the speculative nature of the applications described here, and we add the further caution that self-help is not always a good idea.

CONCLUSION

We have begun this chapter with several observations about current work regarding marital quality. These observations have led us to offer a new analysis of marital quality. The analysis defines marital quality in terms of global, evaluative judgments and documents that these judgments reflect positive and negative dimensions. Understanding the role of these dimensions in marriage requires consideration of the concept of accessibility, and we have argued that the accessibility of each of these dimensions will determine their impact.

Our analysis has many advantages. It is conceptually simple and allows clear interpretation of measures derived from it. Because it does not include heterogeneous content, it also avoids the problem of content overlap between measures of marital quality and measures of correlated concepts (e.g., communication)—a problem that is pervasive in research on the correlates of marital quality. The level at which to interpret responses to questions about marital quality is clearly specified, and because the concept refers only to evaluative judgments, it is more likely to be transportable across cultures than most existing measures. A further advantage is that it not only suggests refinement in current knowledge of marital quality (e.g., regarding accessibility of marital quality and its correlates), but also identifies new areas of inquiry in the marital literature (e.g., the study of ambivalence). Finally, our analysis clearly situates the study of marital quality in a broader psychological literature that offers much to marital researchers and that may itself be enriched by marital research.

ACKNOWLEDGMENTS

Frank D. Fincham was supported in the preparation of this chapter by a grant from the Economic and Social Research Council of Great Britain, and Steven R. H. Beach was supported by a grant from the National Science Foundation. We would like to thank Emma Lycett, Gordon Harold, Samantha Watson, Rachel Frost, and Anne-Marie Ruan for their helpful comments on an earlier draft of the chapter.

NOTES

1. Clearly, reports on some properties of the relationship can only be obtained from spouses (e.g., frequency of intercourse), but other properties may be beyond the awareness of all but the most psychologically sophisticated (e.g., the pattern of interaction during conflict).

2. In support of this theoretical position is some emerging evidence that global, evaluative items are also empirically distinct from other types of items in the DAS. For example, Heyman, Weiss, and Eddy (1991) found that responses to items assessing disagreement in various areas differed significantly from items assessing satisfaction in these areas. In a similar vein, Whisman and Jacobson (1992) found that couples showed less improvement following treatment on a satisfaction measure than the DAS.

3. As it can be argued that the PMQ and NMQ dimensions emerged because of the wording of the questions used to assess them, Fincham and Linfield (in press) report similar results using spouses' ratings of the extent to which affective adjectives (see Watson, Clark, & Tellegen, 1988) described their feelings about the marriage. Scores for positive and negative adjective ratings, like PMQ and NMQ, were moderately and negatively correlated (husbands = .42; wives = − .39). Moreover, the magnitude of the correlations between the PMQ score and positive affective adjectives (husbands = .52; wives = .47) and the NMQ score and negative affective adjectives (husbands = .38; wives = .57) suggests that the dimensions assessed by the PMQ and NMQ do not simply reflect affective ratings of the marriage.

4. To the extent that persons are motivated and have the opportunity to reflect on their behavior, attitude accessibility should be less important, as deliberative, controlled processing will dominate (Fazio, 1990).

5. In general, positive responses occur much faster than negative responses in choice reaction time tasks. However, we were not interested in the magnitude of responses, but rather in their rank-ordering across positive and negative dimensions.

REFERENCES

Banmen, J., & Vogel, N.A. (1985). The relationship between marital quality and interpersonal sexual communication. *Family Therapy, 12,* 45–58.

Bassili, J. N. (1993). Response latency versus certainty as indices of the strength of voting intentions in a CATI survey. *Public Opinion Quarterly, 57,* 54–61.

Baucom, D. H. (1995). A new look at sentiment override–Let's not get carried away yet: Comment on Fincham et al. (1995). *Journal of Family Psychology, 9,* 15–18.

Baucom, D. H., & Epstein, N. (1990). *Cognitive-behavioral marital therapy.* New York: Brunner/Mazel.

Beach, S. R. H., & Fincham, F. D. (1994). Toward an integrated model of negative affectivity in marriage. In S. M. Johnson & L. S. Greenberg (Eds.), *The heart of the matter: Perspective on emotion in marital therapy* (pp. 257–287). New York: Brunner/Mazel.

Beach, S. R. H., & O'Leary, K. D. (1985). Current status of outcome research in marital therapy. In L. L'Abate (Ed.), *Handbook of family psychology and therapy* (Vol. 2, pp. 1035–1072). Homewood, IL: Dorsey Press.

Bienvenu, M. J. (1970). Measurement of marital communication. *Family Coordinator, 19,* 26–31.

Blascovich, J., Ernst, J. M., Tomaka, J., Kelsy, R. M., Salomon, K. L., & Fazio, R. H. (1993). Attitude accessibility as a moderator of autonomic reactivity during decision making. *Journal of Personality and Social Psychology, 64,* 165–176.

Bollen, K. A. (1980). Issues in the comparative measurement of political democracy. *American Sociological Review, 45,* 370–390.

Burman, B., & Margolin, G. (1992). Analysis of the association between marital relationships and health problems: An interactional perspective. *Psychological Bulletin, 112,* 39–63.

Crosby, J. F. (1991). Cybernetics of cybernetics in assessment of marital quality. *Contemporary Family Therapy, 13,* 3–15.

Dahlstrom, W. G. (1969). Recurrent issues in the development of the MMPI. In J. M. Butcher (Ed.), *Research developments and clinical applications* (pp. 1–40). New York: McGraw-Hill.

Eagly, A. H., & Chaiken, S. (1993). *The psychology of attitudes.* Orlando, FL: Harcourt Brace Jovanovich.

Fazio, R. H. (1990). Multiple processes by which attitudes guide behavior: The MODE model as an integrative framework. In M. P. Zanna (Ed.), *Advances in experimental social psychology* (Vol. 11, pp. 74–97). Newbury Park, CA: Sage.

Fazio, R. H. (1995). Attitudes as object–evaluation associations: Determinants, consequences, and correlates of attitude accessibility. In R. E. Petty & J. A. Krosnick (Eds.), *Attitude strength: Antecedents and consequences* (pp. 247–282). Hillsdale, NJ: Erlbaum.

Fazio, R. H., Powell, M. C., & Williams, C. J. (1989). The role of attitude accessibility in the attitude-to-behavior process. *Journal of Consumer Research, 16,* 280–288.

Fazio, R. H., & Williams, C. J. (1986). Attitude accessibility as a moderator of the attitude–perception and attitude–behavior relations: An investigation of the 1984 presidential election. *Journal of Personality and Social Psychology, 51,* 505–514.

Fincham, F. D. (in press). Marital quality. In E. A. Blechman & K. D. Brownell (Eds.), *Behavioral medicine and women: A comprehensive handbook.* New York: Guilford Press.

Fincham, F. D., & Bradbury, T. N. (1987). The assessment of marital quality: A reevaluation. *Journal of Marriage and the Family, 49,* 797–809.

Fincham, F. D., & Bradbury, T. N. (1992). Assessing attributions in marriage: The Relationship Attribution Measure. *Journal of Personality and Social Psychology, 62,* 457–468.

Fincham, F. D., Bradbury, T. N., & Scott, C. K. (1990). Cognition in marriage. In F. D. Fincham & T. N. Bradbury (Eds.), *The psychology of marriage: Basic issues and applications* (pp. 118–149). New York: Guilford Press.

Fincham, F. D., Fernandes, L. O., & Humphreys, K. (1993). *Communicating in relationships: A guide for couples and professionals*. Champaign, IL: Research Press.

Fincham, F. D., Garnier, P. C., Gano-Phillips, S., & Osborne, L. N. (1995). Pre-interaction expectations, marital satisfaction and accessibility: A new look at sentiment override. *Journal of Family Psychology, 9*, 3–14.

Fincham, F. D., & Linfield, K. (in press). A new look at marital quality: Can spouses be positive and negative about their marriage? *Journal of Family Psychology*.

Fowers, B. J. (1990). An interactional approach to standardized marital assessment: A literature review. *Family Relations, 39*, 368–377.

Gilford, R., & Bengtson, V. (1979). Measuring marital satisfaction in three generations: Positive and negative dimensions. *Journal of Marriage and the Family, 41*, 387–394.

Glenn, N. D. (1990). Quantitative research on marital quality in the 1980s: A critical review. *Journal of Marriage and the Family, 52*, 818–831.

Gotlib, I. H., & McCabe, S. B. (1990). Marriage and psychopathology. In F. D. Fincham & T. N. Bradbury (Eds.), *The psychology of marriage: Basic issues and applications* (pp. 226–257). New York: Guilford Press.

Gottman, J. M. (1979). *Marital interaction: Experimental investigations*. New York: Academic Press.

Gottman, J. M., & Levenson, R. W. (1984). Why marriages fail: Affective and physiological patterns in marital interaction. In J. C. Masters & K. Yarkin-Levin (Eds.), *Boundary areas in social and developmental psychology* (pp. 67–106). New York: Academic Press.

Hass, R. G., Katz, I., Rizzo, N., Bailey, J., & Eisenstadt, D. (1991). Cross-racial appraisal as related to attitude ambivalence and cognitive complexity. *Personality and Social Psychology Bulletin, 17*, 83–92.

Heyman, R. E., Sayers, S. L., & Bellack, A. S. (1994). Global marital satisfaction versus marital adjustment: An empirical comparison of three measures. *Journal of Family Psychology, 8*, 432–446.

Heyman, R. E., Weiss, R. L., & Eddy, J. M. (1991). *Dissatisfaction with marital satisfaction: Toward a more useful clinical measure of marital functioning*. Unpublished manuscript, University of Oregon.

Jacobson, N. S. (1985). The role of observation measures in marital therapy outcome research. *Behavioral Assessment, 7*, 287–308.

Johnson, D. R., White, L. K., Edwards, J. N., & Booth, A. (1986). Dimensions of marital quality: Toward methodological and conceptual refinement. *Journal of Family Issues, 7*, 31–49.

Kaplan, K. J. (1972). On the ambivalence–indifferent problem in attitude theory and measurement: A suggested modification of the semantic differential technique. *Psychological Bulletin, 77*, 361–372.

Katz, I., & Hass, R. G. (1988). Racial ambivalence and American value conflict: Correlational and priming studies of dual cognitive structures. *Journal of Personality and Social Psychology, 55*, 893–905.

Lively, E. L. (1969). Toward conceptual clarification: The case of marital interaction. *Journal of Marriage and the Family, 31*, 108–114.

Locke, H. J., & Wallace, K. M. (1959). Short marital adjustment prediction tests: Their reliability and validity. *Marriage and Family Living, 21*, 251–255.

Marini, M. M. (1976). Dimensions of marital happiness: A research note. *Journal of Marriage and the Family, 38*, 443–448.

Markus, H., & Smith, J. (1981). The influence of self-schemata on the perception of others. In N. Cantor & J. F. Kihlstrom (Eds.), *Personality, cognition, and social interaction* (pp. 233–262). Hillsdale, NJ: Erlbaum.

Norton, R. (1983). Measuring marital quality: A critical look at the dependent variable. *Journal of Marriage and the Family, 45*, 141–151.

Nye, F. I., & MacDougall, E. (1959). The dependent variable in marital research. *Pacific Sociological Review, 12*, 67–70.

O'Leary, K. D., & Smith, D. A. (1991). Marital interactions. *Annual Review of Psychology, 42*, 191–212.

Orden, S. R., & Bradburn, N. M. (1968). Dimensions of marriage happiness. *American Journal of Sociology, 73*, 715–731.

Osgood, C. E., Suci, E. J., & Tannenbaum, P. H. (1957). *The measurement of meaning.* Urbana: University of Illinois Press.

Rodin, M. J. (1978). Liking and disliking: Sketch of an alternative view. *Personality and Social Psychology Bulletin, 4*, 473–478.

Rollins, B., & Feldman, H. (1970). Marital satisfaction over the family life cycle. *Journal of Marriage and the Family, 32*, 20–28.

Roskos-Ewoldsen, D. R., & Fazio, R. H. (1992). On the orienting role of attitudes: Attitude accessibility as a determinant of an object's attraction of visual attention. *Journal of Personality and Social Psychology, 63*, 198–211.

Schumm, W. R., Paff-Bergen, L. A., Hatch, R. C., Obiorah, F. C., Copeland, J. M., Meens, L. D., & Bugaighis, M. A. (1986). Concurrent and discriminant validity of the Kansas Marital Satisfaction Scale. *Journal of Marriage and the Family, 48*, 381–387.

Sharpley, C. F., & Cross, D. G. (1982). A psychometric evaluation of the Spanier Dyadic Adjustment Scale. *Journal of Marriage and the Family, 44*, 739–741.

Snyder, D. K. (1979). Multidimensional assessment of marital satisfaction. *Journal of Marriage and the Family, 41*, 813–823.

Snyder, D. K. (1981). *Marital Satisfaction Inventory.* Los Angeles: Western Psychological Association.

Snyder, D. K. (1982). Advances in marital assessment: Behavioral, communications, and psychometric approaches. In C. D. Spielberger & J. N. Butcher (Eds.), *Advances in personality assessment* (Vol. 1, pp. 169–201). Hillsdale, NJ: Erlbaum.

Spanier, G. B. (1976). Measuring dyadic adjustment: New scales for assessing the quality of marriage and similar dyads. *Journal of Marriage and the Family, 38*, 15–28.

Spanier, G. B., & Lewis, R. A. (1980). Marital quality: A review of the seventies. *Journal of Marriage and the Family, 42*, 825–839.

Thompson, M. M., Zanna, M. P., & Griffin, D. W. (1995). Let's not be indifferent about (attitudinal) ambivalence. In R. E. Petty & J. A. Krosnick

(Eds.), *Attitude strength: Antecedents and consequences* (pp. 361–386). Hillsdale, NJ: Erlbaum.

Trost, J. E. (1985). Abandon adjustment! *Journal of Marriage and the Family, 47,* 1072–1073.

Veroff, J., Kulka, R. A., & Douvan, E. (1981). *Mental health in America: Patterns of help seeking from 1957 to 1976.* New York: Basic Books.

Watson, D., Clark, L. A., & Tellegen, A. (1988). Development and validation of brief measures of positive and negative affect: The PANAS scales. *Journal of Personality and Social Psychology, 54,* 1063–1070.

Weiss, R. L. (1980). Strategic behavioral marital therapy: Toward a model for assessment and intervention. In J. P. Vincent (Ed.), *Advances in family intervention, assessment and theory* (Vol. 1, pp. 229–271). Greenwich, CT: JAI Press.

Whisman, M. A., & Jacobson, N. S. (1992). Change in marital adjustment following marital therapy: A comparison of two outcome measures. *Psychological Assessment, 4,* 219–223.

Wyer, R. S., & Srull, T. K. (1989). *Memory and cognition in its social context.* Hillsdale, NJ: Erlbaum.

PART 4

PSYCHOTHERAPY AND
SATISFACTION IN
CLOSE RELATIONSHIPS

CHAPTER 12

Acceptance in Couple Therapy and Its Implications for the Treatment of Depression

JAMES V. CORDOVA
NEIL S. JACOBSON

Depression frequently affects and is affected by intimate relationships. Long-standing problems within an intimate relationship can often set the stage for depression in at least one partner (Beach, Whisman, & O'Leary, 1994; Beach & Nelson, 1990; Beach & O'Leary, 1993; Brown, Adler, & Bifulco, 1988; Brown, Andrews, Harris, Adler, & Bridge, 1986; Brown & Harris, 1978; Brown, Lemryre, & Bifulco, 1992; Markman, Duncan, Storaasli, & Howes, 1987; Monroe, Bromet, Connell, & Steiner, 1986; O'Leary, Riso, & Beach, 1990; Paykel, 1979; Schaefer & Burnett, 1987; Waltz, Badura, Pfaff, & Schott, 1988). And even if the relationship itself is not the cause of depression, depression invariably has a major effect on the quality of a couple's relationship (Billings, Cronkite, & Moos, 1983; Birtchnell, 1988; Horwitz & White, 1991; O'Leary, Christian, & Mendell, 1994; Schuster, Kessler, & Aseltine, 1990; Weiss & Aved, 1978; Weissman, 1987). In either case, addressing depression as an issue for the couple is often the best way to deal with both the couple's distress and the individual's depression.

In this chapter we discuss the evolution of our thinking about couple therapy from a tradition focused exclusively on change toward one that strives for a balance between change and acceptance. We also discuss what we mean by "acceptance" and how the principles of acceptance can be used both in and outside of therapy. In particular, we discuss depression as a couple issue and highlight the implications of the principles of acceptance for addressing depression in couple therapy.

RESEARCH ON COUPLE THERAPY AS A TREATMENT FOR DEPRESSION

Because depression more often than not occurs within the context of an intimate relationship, treating depression with couple therapy has been studied several times (Beach & O'Leary, 1992; Jacobson, Dobson, Fruzzetti, Schmaling, & Salusky, 1991; Foley, Rounsaville, Weissman, Sholomaskas, & Chevron, 1989). Two of these studies focused on traditional behavioral couple therapy (TBCT; Beach & O'Leary, 1992; Jacobson et al., 1991), and one focused on interpersonal psychotherapy for couples (Foley et al., 1989). The literature to date supports the following conclusions. First, TBCT has been shown to be an effective treatment for depression if a depressed person reports that marital distress is the cause of his or her depression. In other words, if a person presents with major depression *and* believes that he or she is depressed because of problems in his or her relationship, then TBCT is as effective in ameliorating depression as is cognitive therapy directed specifically at the symptoms of depression. In addition, in unhappy marriages with a depressed spouse, only TBCT had an effect on the quality of the marriage (as opposed to cognitive therapy), with approximately 40% of couples no longer distressed at the end of therapy (O'Leary & Beach, 1990, 1992). Therefore, although cognitive therapy might be just as effective a treatment for depression as TBCT, it does not address the co-occurring problem of relationship distress. In other words, TBCT appears to help alleviate the symptoms of depression *and* improve the quality of the relationship. Note, however, that the major qualifier for TBCT's success is that the depressed person attributes his or her depression to problems in the relationship. TBCT was not found to be as successful with couples in which the depressed individual did not blame his or her depression on the relationship. It is our contention that integrating the principles of acceptance into change-oriented TBCT creates a more effective treatment of depression, regardless of whether the depression is attributed to the relationship or to factors outside the relationship.

FROM TRADITIONAL TO INTEGRATIVE BEHAVIORAL COUPLE THERAPY

Behavioral marital therapy (Jacobson & Margolin, 1979)—or TBCT, as we are calling it in this chapter—has consistently been shown to be an effective treatment for couple distress (Baucom & Hoffman, 1986; Gurman, Kniskern, & Pinsof, 1986; Jacobson, 1978, 1984). TBCT has focused almost exclusively on trying to help partners achieve any and all changes they request from each other in therapy. Although this approach has been very successful in general, improving the relationships of between half and two-thirds of couples presenting for therapy (Jacobson, Schmaling, & Holtzworth-Munroe, 1987), concern remained for those couples that were not improving. Research had shown that these couples were not simply treatment-resistant, but that they were generally less able to change the problems from which they suffered. On average, the members of these couples were more severely distressed, older, and more emotionally disengaged (Baucom & Hoffman, 1986; Hahlweg, Schindler, Revenstorf, & Brengelmann, 1984), as well as more polarized on basic issues (Jacobson, Follette, & Pagel, 1986). Partners with these characteristics were less capable of being as collaborative and compromising as TBCT required. Those things that TBCT tried to help these couples change were, for all intents and purposes, unchangeable. Because of this, TBCT was mostly ineffective with these couples. In order to help such couples improve their relationships, it became apparent that therapy would have to help them come to terms with those things about their relationships that were unlikely to change. In other words, these couples had to learn to accept some unchangeable aspects of their relationships. The pursuit of this goal led to the development of integrative behavioral couple therapy (IBCT; Christensen, Jacobson, & Babcock, 1995; Jacobson, 1992; Jacobson & Christensen, 1996; Cordova & Jacobson, 1993). IBCT aims to integrate the traditional emphasis on promoting change with a new emphasis on promoting emotional acceptance.

WHAT DO WE MEAN BY "ACCEPTANCE"?

What exactly do we mean by "acceptance"? Acceptance has recently received a great deal of attention from behavioral psychologists and behavior therapists (see Hayes, Jacobson, Follette, & Dougher, 1994). Although the concept is not new to psychotherapy, it has only recently been given serious attention by more behaviorally oriented theorists. Traditionally, behavioral therapies have focused exclusively on promoting overt behavioral change. Recently, however, behavior therapists have begun to recognize the importance of promoting emotional acceptance when more overt change is unlikely. This shift in emphasis has occurred only recently, perhaps because behavior therapists have been extremely successful in treating a wide range of problems using specifically change-oriented techniques, and have spent a great deal of time refining these techniques and testing their efficacy empirically. This type of work takes time and dedication, and this may be why therapists have only recently begun to focus on the limits of their change-promoting technologies. However, such limits do exist. Not all situations are amenable to overt change. Many of the problems that people struggle with are simply immutable. Very often, the healthiest response in such cases is to accept that those circumstances will not change and give up the struggle to change them. Acceptance, however, can mean many different things, and we want to be as clear as possible about what we mean when we use the term.

As noted above, acceptance is often the healthiest response to situations that are unlikely to change; therefore, acceptance is promoted in the context of the unalterable. Given a situation that is essentially unalterable, a person can respond in two different ways. One way is to struggle relentlessly to change the situation. This is often a reasonable response, given that so many situations can actually be changed for the better. However, when a situation cannot be changed, struggling to change it is not only ineffective, but exhausting, distracting, and eventually depressing. Ineffective, relentless struggle is often the option that has been chosen by people who present for psychotherapy riddled with anxiety, guilt, hopelessness, and depression. Obviously, struggling to change something unchangeable is a waste of time and energy, and it is definitely not what we mean by acceptance. Another response to the unchangeable is simply to resign oneself to the hopelessness of the situation and resolve to suffer in bitter silence. This is also not what we mean by acceptance. Hopeless resignation is often the hallmark of clinical depression and the usual end result of desperately engaging an unwinnable struggle. The healthiest type of acceptance is one that comes to terms with the unchangeable situation in a way that allows the person to disengage from the unwinnable struggle, gain a broader perspective on the situation, and once again begin the pursuit of meaningful activities.

Aspects of Acceptance: Toward a Definition

Our definition of acceptance has several interdependent parts. The first involves giving up the struggle to change that which cannot be changed.

Often it is the struggle to change the unchangeable that causes the most pain and suffering. Giving up the struggle involves people's identifying how they are struggling and learning to respond differently. It is a coming to terms with those situations in which efforts are wasted or destructive. It is the process of stopping, and thus freeing the time and energy to reevaluate.

Take, for example, the case of Bill and Nancy. Nancy's previous marriage ended when she discovered her first husband's infidelity. As a result, within her current marriage to Bill, she is constantly worried that Bill might cheat on her. She calls him several times a day and becomes upset if she doesn't know where he has been. She shows a great deal of jealousy and is frequently hurt and angry. Bill in turn is miserable. He feels punished for the previous husband's infidelity, and he resents not being trusted despite the fact that he has done nothing to earn Nancy's suspicion.

This situation can be characterized as resulting from the struggle on Nancy's part to change something essentially unchangeable—the fact that being in a relationship means being vulnerable. The unchangeable situation in this example is that Nancy has been hurt badly in the past and is now made vulnerable to similar pain by loving and trusting her current husband. She struggles against her own vulnerability by expending a great deal of time and energy worrying about Bill and trying to keep track of his whereabouts. As a result of her struggle, she, Bill, and the relationship suffer. Giving up the struggle in this example requires both Nancy and Bill to see the pattern that they are stuck in from a neutral perspective and to regard it as something for which neither of them is directly to blame. From this nonblaming perspective, they are in a better position to understand what is happening in their relationship without necessarily reacting to it. Nancy may at times feel vulnerable and insecure, but she can have those feelings and share them without entering into a relationship-damaging pattern. This giving up of the struggle against vulnerability necessarily suggests another aspect of acceptance: sitting still with that which will not change.

Sitting still with that which will not change means finding a way to tolerate whatever the aversive situation is, without engaging in the same efforts to change it and without running away. It comes from developing a new perspective from which to reevaluate the situation. Once one has given up the struggle to change something, one necessarily has to learn what to do instead. This can be hard, given that despite its ineffectiveness, the person has often become quite used to struggling. Furthermore, these types of behaviors are usually negatively reinforced (meaning that reinforcement is derived by avoiding some aspect of the aversive situation). In our example, although Nancy's attempts to be invulnerable cause both her and Bill a great deal of distress, Nancy is reinforced to continue them because of a derived relationship between her hypervigilance and his not having an affair. In other words, Nancy may believe that despite the destructive effects of her jealousy, at least it is working to keep Bill faithful. If she can give up her attempts to defeat her own vulnerability within the relationship, then she must learn how to live with that vulnerability. This is the process of learning to tolerate aversive emotions without hiding from them or denying them (see Cordova & Kohlenberg, 1994). IBCT has incorporated several very useful methods for learning to tolerate negative circumstances.

A third aspect of acceptance is the process of moving beyond sitting still with the unchangeable and toward embracing it. In other words, real acceptance moves beyond simply tolerating and toward discovering those aspects of the situation that can be appreciated. For example, existential theorists, when discussing accepting one's own mortality, point to the power death has to imbue each moment of one's life with significance. Similarly, within our example, as Nancy comes to terms with her inherent vulnerability within an intimate relationship, she can begin to appreciate that those feelings of vulnerability are simply one necessary aspect of her love for Bill. To the degree that she avoids contact with her vulnerability, she also avoids contact with her strong positive emotions and true intimacy. In learning to embrace her vulnerability, she makes it possible for herself to experience the positive aspects of her relationship more fully. IBCT frequently works with couples in this respect to help them identify the positive aspects of negative circumstances.

The final aspect of our definition of acceptance involves seeking active, healthy responses in the face of an unchangeable situation. This may be the most important aspect of acceptance in terms of its beneficial effects on depression. Giving up the struggle frees all of the time and energy previously devoted to escape and avoidance for the pursuit of more healthy behavior (see Hayes, 1987; Dougher, 1994; Dougher & Hackbert, 1994). Hayes (1987) gives the example of an agoraphobic woman's giving up the struggle not to be anxious and going out to shop despite her anxiety. In our example, as Nancy gives up her struggle with vulnerability and learns to sit still with and embrace it, she places herself in a better position to do healthy things both for herself and for her relationship. Although Nancy cannot change the fact that she is vulnerable in her relationship, there are things she can do despite the anxiety that vulnerability creates. For example, she and Bill can both talk about their feelings of vulnerability and the fear and love underlying these feelings, as a means of building greater intimacy between them. Promoting such expressions of "softer" emotions is an essential component of the acceptance work of IBCT.

In summary, acceptance is a complex process, and our definition attempts to account for that complexity by elucidating four essential components of acceptance. We therefore define acceptance as a process of (1) giving up the struggle to change the unchangeable, (2) sitting still with and (3) embracing both the negative and positive aspects of the situation, and (4) actively engaging in healthy behavior despite that which cannot be changed.

What Acceptance Is Not

Given the definition of acceptance above, we believe it is equally important to point out what acceptance is not. As we have noted earlier, acceptance is not hopeless resignation. Hopeless resignation is one of the hallmarks of depression, and our approach to acceptance assumes an active engagement in life despite those things that cannot be changed. Acceptance also does not mean tolerating the status quo. As we enter the 21st century, men and women are continuing to negotiate their shared roles in the family, moving often toward more egalitarian relationships. By promoting acceptance in intimate relationships as a means of treating and preventing depression, we are not advocating that men and women accept unhealthy power differences within their relationships. Some things can be changed; some things can be accepted. As the well-known "Serenity Prayer" indicates, wisdom lies in knowing the difference.

TECHNIQUES FOR PROMOTING ACCEPTANCE

The acceptance techniques of IBCT fall into four broad categories: (1) empathic joining around the problem, (2) unified detachment from the problem, (3) developing tolerance for negative behavior, and (4) developing skills in self-care. We give a brief description of each technique here, and will provide more detailed descriptions when we discuss their application in the treatment of depression. Note that although traditional change techniques such as behavior exchange, communication training, and problem-solving training remain an integral part of IBCT, we are focusing here exclusively on the implications of the acceptance techniques for the treatment of depression within a couple therapy context. A full description of all components of IBCT is provided in other sources (Christensen et al., 1995; Jacobson, 1992; Jacobson & Christensen, 1996; Cordova & Jacobson, 1993).

Empathic Joining around the Problem

Empathic joining around the problem is one of the primary means toward emotional acceptance. "Empathic joining" refers to an increased emotional understanding between partners; it provides a means of lessening the probability that the partners will become polarized, by increasing their capacity to understand each other. A distressed couple often enters therapy hurt and angry, and therefore the partners blame each other for the relationship's problems. Blame and defensiveness are the hallmarks of polarization and indicate that the partners have taken opposite sides on some contentious issues in their relationship. The goal with such partners is to help them approach their difficult problems as opportunities to draw closer emotionally and work collaboratively. Toward this end, each partner is encouraged to clearly communicate the softer emotions underlying the usual expressions of "hard" emotions, which put one partner in the role of the accuser and the other in the role of the accused. Hard emotions include anger, resentment, contempt, and righteous indignation. The most likely responses to hard emotional expressions are defensiveness and counteraggression. More often than not, expressions of hard emotions lead to escalating hostilities rather than to satisfactory resolutions.

"Soft" emotions, on the other hand, include such feelings as sadness, loneliness, insecurity, fear, and love. The expression of these emotions reveals a person's vulnerability within the relationship and is more likely to elicit empathy from the partner than defensiveness and anger. IBCT therapists assert that all expressions of hard emotions have softer emotions underlying them. Furthermore, developing a fuller understanding of each other's softer emotions helps intimate partners feel close to each other despite their common problems. This is because each partner is able to empathize with the sadness or fear the other person is experiencing, rather than making contact solely with the other person's anger. Generally people respond to expressions of soft emotions by drawing closer and providing comfort, rather than by feeling blamed and fighting back. As the partners become more open with their softer feelings, particularly about unchangeable situations, they are better able to create further intimacy within their relationship rather than further destruction.

Unified Detachment from the Problem

In conjunction with empathic joining around the problem, emotional acceptance is fostered by developing what we call "unified detachment from the problem." The goal of unified detachment is to help the couple develop a perspective from which both partners can come together as a team around a common problem without blaming each other. Instead of regarding each other as opponents, the partners are shown how they might approach common problems as a couple. Toward this end, the partners are taught to recognize the common patterns they fall into in response to their problems. More often than not, distressed couples repeat one or two interaction patterns across a majority of their conflicts. For example, one of the most common is the "demand–withdraw" pattern, in which one partner approaches the other demanding some change, and the other simply withdraws either by leaving or by refusing to talk about it. In therapy, the members of a couple identify and talk about the common problematic themes that characterize their relationship. The therapist, in turn, points out that these themes are neither partner's fault and can be regarded as events that they can work together to oppose (if something can be changed) or to support each other through (if something is unlikely to change). The underlying message is that often it is not necessarily the particular issue that is causing problems, but the way in which the couple interacts around that issue.

Developing Tolerance for Negative Behavior

Perhaps one of the most important aspects of promoting acceptance is learning to tolerate those things in the relationship that cause distress but are unlikely to change. IBCT has several ways of promoting emotional tolerance for negative behavior. The first is the highlighting of understandable reasons—that is, emphasizing the historical or other motivations for each partner's behavior. This helps each partner to see that the other's behavior is not motivated solely by maliciousness, but is a reasonable response, given who the person is and where he or she comes from. It is generally easier to tolerate irritating or distressing behavior that is understandable and reasonable rather than malicious or mysterious.

The second method highlights the positive features of negative behavior. Both partners are helped to appreciate that their unresolvable problems may also have positive features that contribute to the health of their relationship. For example, if one partner is a spendthrift and the other is a skinflint, this difference may cause a great deal of conflict and distress in the relationship. However, it may also be true that these differences complement each other. In other words, the skinflint may assure that they as a couple save money well and spend wisely, whereas the spendthrift may assure that they enjoy some of what they have more often.

The third method for promoting tolerance involves preparing a couple for easily foreseeable slip-ups. The therapist and couple work together to anticipate problems the couple may encounter in the future, and prepare to deal with them in advance. For example, the patterns that have been identified in the relationship may very well continue to occur throughout the course of the relationship. Given that this can be predicted, the couple can prepare for those inevitabilities. In general, it is simply easier to tolerate those things that can be predicted.

Developing Self-Care Skills

"Self-care" refers to the process of encouraging each partner to take personal responsibility for himself or herself as well as for the health of the relationship. It is particularly important during destructive interactions for each partner to take personal responsibility for his or her own well-being. Encouraging both partners to take personal responsibility for their own needs and the needs of the relationship changes the usual response to dissatisfaction from blaming to active coping.

APPLYING ACCEPTANCE TO TREATING DEPRESSION IN COUPLE THERAPY

The goal of IBCT with a couple that includes a depressed partner is to create a context in which both partners begin engaging in more active and effective behaviors in their relationship. This is accomplished by helping the couple create a positive balance between change and acceptance. One of the primary strengths of IBCT is the flexibility it allows the therapist to tailor treatment to the unique needs of each couple. Flexibility is particularly important in the treatment of depression, because within the context of an intimate relationship the onset of depression may occur through two different pathways, each affecting therapy in a different way. For some people, depression may result from a long history of distress in their relationships. For others, depression may result from circumstances outside of their relationships and may have little to do with how satisfied the persons were with their relationships prior to becoming depressed. In either type of case, however, the onset of depression has implications for a couple's relationship. In the first type, depression may compound existing problems in the relationship. In the second type, depression may create problems that were previously nonexistent.

Often the members of a couple may experience problems in their relationship for a long time before one partner begins manifesting the symptoms of depression (Ilfeld, 1976). Usually in such cases, the depressed partner openly identifies the problems in the relationship as the cause of his or her depression. When this is the case, IBCT works directly on the causes of the couple's distress, and depression can be regarded as a side effect of that distress. In such cases it is assumed that the depression will lift when the distress is alleviated. This initial treatment formulation may be altered, however, if over the course of therapy it becomes obvious that relationship distress is not the sole variable controlling the depression.

When, on the other hand, one partner's depression precedes the couple's distress, IBCT adjusts its focus to work directly on the depression and its effect on the couple's relationship. In general, the structure of therapy will be geared more heavily toward acceptance. Depression, simply given its nature, is not amenable to isolated relationship change strategies. The research bears out this assumption, in that people who do not attribute their depression to problems in their relationships are not usually helped by TBCT (Beach & O'Leary, 1992; Jacobson et al., 1991).

DEPRESSION:
THE ABSENCE OF EFFECTIVE BEHAVIOR

When a therapist is treating a couple with a depressed member, it is important for the therapist to assess the presence and severity of the depression, based on the standard conceptualization in the *Diagnostic and Statistical Manual of Mental Disorders*, fourth edition (American Psychiatric Association, 1994). However, once depression has been diagnosed, we advocate a conceptualization of depression that is much less focused on the symptoms and much more focused on the depressed person's lack of active engagement.

Although there are many ways of conceptualizing depression, our view is that depression is best understood in terms of what a person *is not* doing, rather than in terms of what he or she *is* doing (see Ferster, 1973). In other words, we believe the most striking fact about the behavior of depressed individuals is that there simply isn't that much of it. In particular, depressed people do not do very many things that result in positive consequences. In fact, depression can be described as a deterioration in the active pursuit of positive consequences. The treatment of a depressed person, then, should focus on what has led to this deterioration. In fact, when depression occurs in the context of an intimate relationship, what has led to this deterioration determines a great deal about the optimal structure and course of treatment.

Other definitions of depression tend to focus exclusively on the symptoms of depression. These symptoms include making self-denigrating comments, focusing on the negative aspects of life, excessive crying, complaining, compulsive talking, excessive sleeping, excessive worrying or ruminating, thoughts of suicide, an inability to experience pleasure, and generalized feelings of sadness. Our view is that a more effective approach to treating depression focuses not so much on removing the symptoms of depression as on replacing them with more active and positively reinforceable behaviors.

In addition to the fact that depressed people engage in very little behavior that results in positive consequences, much of the behavior they do engage in serves primarily primitive escape and avoidance functions (see Ferster, 1973). In other words, a great deal of a depressed person's behavior is in the service of decreasing contact with the aversive aspects of his or her life. These attempts at escape and avoidance are considered "primitive" because many of them only occur in the absence of more effective means of dealing with aversive situations or obtaining positive consequences. In other words, many of the symptoms of depression only occur because the depressed individual does not have more active and effective behavior available. Thus, in answering the question "What is depression?", our view is that depression is often what is left in the absence of more effective behavior.

In terms of treating depression within a couple therapy context, we believe it is most effective to focus on what has led to the stripping of the depressed person's repertoire and what is maintaining the absence of active engagement. In other words, what is it about the interaction between the person and his or her environment that has made the person vulnerable to depression? Briefly, we define a person's "repertoire" as all of the behavior available to that person within a specific context. Ferster (1973) identifies three ways in which a behavioral repertoire can increase a person's vulnerability to depression by decreasing the amount of effective behavior available. According to Ferster, depressogenic repertoires are (1) a rigid repertoire, (2) a repertoire that ineffectively avoids aversive situations, and (3) a repertoire that does not include sufficient exploratory behaviors. In short, a behavioral repertoire that is limited in its breadth, flexibility, or effectiveness increases a person's susceptibility to depression. In addition, such limitations necessarily increase a relationship's susceptibility to distress. We go over each of these vulnerabilities in turn, provide clinical case examples, and discuss how IBCT addresses these vulnerabilities.

A Rigid Repertoire

A rigid repertoire is basically one that does not adapt well to a changing environment. In other words, when things change, the person with a rigid repertoire does not change and/or responds by engaging in ineffective behaviors such as complaining and sulking. Although a rigid repertoire may work well within the appropriate circumstances, any change in those circumstances can drastically reduce the effectiveness of the available behavior. For example, consider a young man who has grown up in a small town, but suddenly moves to New York to attend a university. Much of what he has learned about how to get along in the world—including how to meet people, where to go to have fun, and even how to get around—is suddenly no longer effective. Such a dramatic decrease in this person's repertoire of effective behavior greatly increases the likelihood that he will become depressed, especially if he is unable to work actively to acquire new behavior. His repertoire can be thought of as relatively rigid, in that it works well within a circumscribed environment, but when that environment changes dramatically he simply cannot adapt.

A person with a rigid repertoire is necessarily more vulnerable to depression, because the nature of circumstances, particularly in relationships, is change. Over the course of any relationship, both partners are likely to change in both subtle and dramatic ways. What each partner does for a living may change (frequently more than once in today's economy). What each likes to do for entertainment may change. In addition, politics, physical health, psychological health, financial health, habits, tendencies, predilections, and priorities all are subject to various degrees of change over time. A person with a repertoire devoid of the behaviors necessary to adapt to these changes is extremely susceptible to relationship distress and depression.

The key to addressing this type of deficit is for the depressed person to begin to accept a certain lack of predictability in relationships, while at the same time learning specific skills for negotiating new ways of dealing with those changes that do occur. In general, the goal with a rigid repertoire is to foster flexibility. In other words, a person must increase the number of options he or she has for interacting with a changing environment. Within couple therapy, promoting emotional acceptance creates a more flexible emotional repertoire and sets the stage for more effective behavior in general.

For example, consider the case of Jack and Jill. When Jack and Jill initially presented for therapy, they were severely distressed and were beginning to consider separating. In addition, Jill was suffering several symptoms of depression that had been gradually worsening over the previous 6 months. Jack and Jill had met and married 6 years earlier in San Diego, following Jack's discharge from the Navy. They both described the first few years of their relationship in very positive terms. However, approximately a year and a half prior to their presenting for therapy, they had moved from San Diego to Seattle for Jack's job. Jill, who had been born and raised in San Diego, never seemed to adjust to the move. She complained of being alone most of the time, and she resented the fact that Jack's schedule required him to work during the evenings. She felt abandoned by him and convinced that she wasn't an important part of his life. In response, she was often angry with him and felt irritable and depressed. She longed for San Diego and was beginning to consider leaving Jack and moving back home.

Jack, in turn, complained about their constant arguing. He felt he was constantly "walking on eggshells" around Jill, for fear of starting an argument or hurting her feelings. He complained that they spent little time together because they had few common interests, and recently because she was asleep or withdrawn most of the time he was home. He felt helpless in the face of her dissatisfaction and depression, was angry at her for "falling apart," and was beginning to think he might be better off without her.

Jill's slip into depression can be understood as resulting from what we are calling a rigid repertoire. She had been born and raised in the same house and the same neighborhood in San Diego. All of her friends were people she had either grown up with or gone to school with. The things she did for fun revolved primarily around the proximity of a warm ocean coast and an active night life. When she and Jack moved to Seattle, her repertoire of effective behaviors was devastated. She left her friends and family in San Diego, and since it seemed she had always simply had friends, she had never really learned how to go about making new friends. The work she had done had been within her father's business; thus, in addition, she had never had to actively pursue work. Jack's job required him to work a shift starting in the early afternoon and ending in the late evening. He had recently become involved in backpacking and had always been an avid skier, neither of which Jill particularly enjoyed. Thus Jill rather suddenly found herself without friends, without a job, and with a husband who spent most of his time at work and in the mountains. This drastic environmental change was exacerbated by the fact that Jill simply did not have within her repertoire the skills necessary to adapt to the change.

Although Jill's depression was not the sole focus of therapy, couple therapy was able to address it as a problem around which Jack and Jill could come together as a couple. Specifically, couple therapy addressed how they could come to terms with and begin to address the rigidity of Jill's repertoire. As a first step toward this goal, work was done in therapy to increase Jack and Jill's empathy for each other by helping them express their softer feelings. As noted above, they were both frustrated and quite angry with each other when first presenting for therapy. As a result, their in-session discussions were blaming, defensive, and righteously indignant. Work in therapy focused on helping each of them understand that indeed softer emotions were underlying their anger, blame, and defensiveness. Jack was able to talk to Jill about feeling guilty that he had dragged her away from her home and feeling responsible for her suffering. Because he felt guilty, he reacted defensively whenever she complained about Seattle or said how much she missed San Diego. He was also able to talk about how helpless he felt to make things better for her, and how these feelings of helplessness made him frustrated, angry, and eventually withdrawn. They were also able to appreciate that these feelings of frustration and anger were ultimately rooted in how much he loved and cared about Jill. After all, if he didn't love her, why would he care that she suffered?

Jill, on the other hand, was able to talk about how frightened she was of her own depression and how helpless she felt to "snap out of it." She expressed feelings of guilt about her depression, about not having been able to get a job, and about the state of their relationship. She talked about how much she missed spending time with Jack, and she became able to see that her feelings of resentment and irritation were rooted in her desire to be closer to him. Most importantly, both Jack and Jill were able to express their compassion and caring toward one another.

In general, when the partners are talking about the depression, it is helpful for each partner to talk about the softer feelings elicited by the depression. It is important in terms of fostering acceptance for each person to understand clearly that a bout with depression is going to be hard on both individuals within the relationship, as well as on the relationship itself. Couple therapy works with the couple to bring to light the soft emotions underlying any anger and resentment, as well as any unspoken soft emotions elicited by the depression. Over the course of therapy, the partners work with the therapist to communicate and begin to deal with their feelings about the depression, including the loneliness, sadness, apprehension, hopelessness, and frustration that each of them may feel. The therapist also helps underscore the positive feelings often left unspoken, such as love, tenderness, compassion, empathy, caring, respect, and desire. As the partners begin to contact each other's softer emotions, they usually begin feeling closer to each other and more willing to join together in dealing with occurrences of depression.

In Jack and Jill's case, promoting greater empathy defused the anger and hurtfulness that they both brought into therapy; it also began to increase the flexibility of Jill's emotional repertoire. Given some emotional softening on their part, the therapist could begin to help them build their tolerance toward their recent history and toward the rigidity of Jill's repertoire. Because tolerance has its roots in understanding, it was fostered by highlighting the understandable reasons for both Jack and Jill's recent behavior, as well as for Jill's difficulty in adapting to the move. It became obvious that Jill had simply been ill prepared by her experiences in San Diego to do the things that would have been necessary for her to adapt well to any move (e.g., actively pursuing work, friendships, and other positive experiences). By discussing these issues, Jack and Jill were able to appreciate that there were indeed understandable reasons both for their current predicament and for Jill's difficulty in adapting. The goal was to help Jack and Jill begin to remove some of the blame from each other and place it instead on the understandable circumstances. Understanding the roots of a person's rigid repertoire can in and of itself be therapeutic, because it prepares the couple for how to deal with its repercussions in the future.

In this particular example, as Jack and Jill became more collaborative with each other, they were able to begin to work together toward changing some of the problematic aspects of their relationship. The specific goal in regard to Jill's rigid repertoire became to broaden her repertoire slowly to include those things that would make her more effective in her current environment. Once Jack and Jill were able to observe and talk about Jill's difficulty in adapting, they were able to derive and implement several possible solutions. Jill began to try new activities and explore new interests. She also began to look into classes to brush up on her job-hunting skills and to make herself more marketable. In addition, Jack began to cooperate with Jill on increasing their socializing as a couple, so that they both could form larger social networks.

Finally, as a couple, they prepared for the fact that Jill might continue at times to have difficulty in adapting to new or changing situations. Time was spent predicting the changes they could anticipate and thinking about how they might work together to adapt more smoothly to changes in the future. This is called "preparing for slip-ups" and builds tolerance toward relationship difficulties that are likely to recur (such as difficulty in adapting to changing circumstances). As partners learn to tolerate future occurrences of common problems, those problems become less able to create severe distress. Furthermore, by definition, preparing for slip-ups helps creates a repertoire for responding flexibly to future problems, thus decreasing a person's vulnerability to depression.

An Ineffectively Avoidant Repertoire

A repertoire that ineffectively avoids or deals with aversive situations also increases a person's vulnerability to depression. It is simply the case that some means of dealing with unpleasant circumstances are more effective than others. Some people's capacity to deal with aversive situations is seriously limited. For example, a person growing up with a violent or alcoholic parent can learn that there is virtually nothing he or she can do to escape or deal with the family's problems. Studies on learned helplessness have shown that when aversive situations cannot be avoided, the most likely response is simply to stop trying (Miller & Seligman, 1975). In addition, a person's capacity to learn better ways of coping is limited by the distraction of unrelenting emotional agitation. Within the context of an intimate relationship, a person with a limited repertoire for dealing with aversive situations may simply resign himself or herself to problems that could be easily ameliorated, or, alternatively, may continue utilizing ineffective strategies in an unwinnable struggle. Under such circumstances, a person may learn to reduce contact with problems in the relationship through emotional withdrawal or through withdrawal into other areas of life such as work. These strategies may work to reduce contact with aversive situations, but are certainly not optimally effective. On the other hand, a person may perpetuate problems within the relationship by persistently engaging in those ineffective strategies that are available. With no repertoire for healthy acceptance, an entire category of effective strategies for managing conflict is simply unavailable. The ultimate result is that problems within the relationship are either perpetuated or left unresolved, and the person's chances of becoming depressed as a result are greatly increased.

Couple therapy addresses an ineffectively avoidant repertoire by helping the couple learn how to deal actively and effectively with all types of aversive situations, whether these are amenable to negotiated change or not. Take, for example, the case of Chuck and Diane. Chuck and Diane had developed a particularly destructive pattern of interaction around making day-to-day purchases. Chuck complained that Diane rarely consulted him and often spent too much money on things they simply didn't need. He complained that her spending was out of control and that she threw money away without thinking. He was especially angry that she didn't seem to take his concerns about their money seriously. This particular issue was a source of almost daily conflict between the two of them.

In turn, Diane complained that Chuck was completely obsessed with money, that he was tight-fisted, and that if it were up to him she would never spend money on anything. She said that she didn't consult him about purchases, because if she did he always said "no." She felt there was no point in talking with him about purchases, because it always led to an argument. She also complained that he had a double standard, because he bought the things he wanted and she never complained.

Chuck and Diane described an incident that exemplified their arguments in regard to this issue. Diane owned a tropical fish tank that both she and Chuck enjoyed. Stopping at the pet store on the way home for fish food, she decided to buy a new fish for the tank. She reported in the session that she knew buying the fish was going to cause an argument, and that knowing this made her both anxious and angry. She said, "I can't believe I have to go through this for every little thing I want to buy. He has no right to tell me what I can and cannot buy, and I shouldn't have to beg him to buy a little $8 fish." She decided to buy the fish despite fully anticipating the blow-up that would result. When she arrived home, she showed the fish to Chuck, and he immediately became extremely angry. Chuck reported saying, "I'm sick and tired of you doing this. We can't afford to be throwing money away on all these animals. I should just kill them all and be done with it." Chuck was embarrassed to report that he had said this, and added that it was exactly like something his father would have said. Diane, in response, yelled that he wasn't going to lay a hand on her animals, and then began to call him every name she could think of. He responded by saying "Forget it" and withdrawing to the living room. Diane in turn withdrew to the bedroom and slammed the door. They spent the rest of the evening apart, and hard feelings continued through the next day.

When this incident was reviewed in therapy, it became apparent that it was a perfect example of a common theme. Since Diane felt sure Chuck would say "no" to anything she wanted to buy, she simply bought what she wanted anyway. She knew that this led to painful arguments, but she was willing to pay that price in exchange for the freedom to exercise her own best judgment about purchases. In turn, Chuck felt that he had so little control over Diane's spending that he had to take advantage of any chance to stop her from buying something. Therefore, any time she asked first before buying, he felt compelled to say "no." Chuck felt helpless, anxious about their money, and resentful that she seemed not to care. Diane felt stuck because she believed the only way she could ever get what she wanted was to tolerate these destructive arguments as a necessary evil.

This is a good example of what we mean by an ineffectively avoidant repertoire, because it illustrates the ultimate result of poorly managing aversive situations. Diane and Chuck remained in almost constant contact with the aversiveness of these destructive arguments because they had only one ineffective way of resolving their dilemma. Continual exposure to anger, resentment, and bitterness contributed greatly to Diane's feelings of depression. In addition, Chuck and Diane were actively avoiding each other, and therefore had completely eliminated any opportunities they might have had to learn better ways of solving this problem.

Couple therapy initially focused on fostering greater empathy between Chuck and Diane, because their interactions around this issue had become almost exclusively hostile. This work consisted of acknowledging the pain each partner was in as a result of their constant conflict, as well as the love and caring that still remained within the relationship. The therapist also explained that Chuck and Diane were stuck in a mutual trap. This trap was created by each of their understandable attempts to resolve the problem. The fact that Chuck felt the only way he could exert any control over Diane's spending was always to say "no" only made it more likely that she would not consult him in the future. This in turn made it more likely that he would continue to feel pressured to say "no" and struggle against her financial equality.

By discussing their mutual trap, partners become able to gain some perspective on their common problem. This is essentially the primary goal of unified detachment from the problem. Discussing Chuck and Diane's mutual trap as a common problem from which they both suffered and for which neither of them was specifically to blame created a context within which they could join together to commiserate about it, instead of simply blaming each other and feeling victimized. It furthermore provided for them an avenue through which they could talk about this problematic pattern without engaging in it. Finally, discussion of their mutual trap allowed the therapist to highlight for the couple that both partners had perfectly understandable reasons for the roles they played in this destructive pattern.

Often each member of a couple presenting for therapy is convinced that the other person is acting maliciously and is deliberately trying to hurt or anger him or her. Uncovering nonhostile reasons for the other's actions helps create a context for greater intimacy by decreasing blaming and counteraggression. Often the reasons for a partner's actions derive from his or her personal history. For example, Chuck's relentless concern about money resulted from his having been raised in a family that was constantly struggling to make ends meet and in which being financially conservative had been a matter of survival. Reasons other than historical ones may also exist. For example, Diane's failure to consult Chuck resulted from her feeling that this was the only way she could maintain any independence or power within the relationship. The main point of uncovering the understandable reasons for each person's behavior is to provide for each partner a more complete understanding of the other, thus fostering empathy.

In addition, the positive features of this difference between Chuck and Diane were highlighted, to counterbalance their exclusive focus on the more obvious negative features. Distressed partners often focus exclusively on the negative aspects of their relationship. However, fundamental differences within the relationship may have both negative and positive connotations. When the positive connotations are highlighted, the couple gains a more complete picture of the relationship. For example, despite the fact that Chuck and Diane argued a great deal about her being a "spendthrift" and his being a "skinflint," these differences also provided a nice balance for them as a couple. Chuck's focus on saving money assured that both he and Diane would have the money they needed for emergencies, retirements, and large investments. In turn, Diane's willingness to spend money assured that both she and Chuck would be able to enjoy some of their money on a day-to-day basis. Highlighting the positive features of a couple's situation helps create tolerance by balancing out the negative aspects of that situation. As Chuck and Diane began to appreciate that their differences were neither maliciously motivated nor wholly negative, they became better able to tolerate the tensions these differences created.

Note that three of the four IBCT acceptance techniques were used to foster emotional acceptance around this issue. Efforts were made to promote empathic joining around the problem, unified detachment from the problem, and tolerance for the part each partner played in the problem (highlighting of understandable reasons, as well as appreciation of the problem's positive features). This emphasizes the fact that couple therapy interventions are not wholly independent components administered one at a time, but are instead used in different combinations, depending on the unique nature of the couple's problems.

Fostering emotional acceptance between Chuck and Diane in regard to their financial issues allowed them to see clearly how ineffectively they were dealing with this source of aversiveness within their relationship. It also allowed them to see that they were both suffering and that this mutual suffering contributed to Diane's depressive symptoms. Increased emotional acceptance allowed them to give up the unwinnable struggle to change each other, and thus freed up that time and energy for exploring other more effective ways of addressing their concerns. Emotional acceptance, in other words, created a context in which Chuck and Diane were able to collaborate on resolving this problem together. The therapist did not ask them to change the pattern they had developed. However, once they were able to identify and talk about this problematic pattern, they suggested their own strategy for changing it. In consultation with their therapist, they began regularly reviewing their finances as a couple, so that responsibilities could be shared and handling finances could remain independent of individual blame. Over the course of therapy, they reported that these meetings were going well and that each had a fuller understanding of the other's concerns.

A Limited Exploratory Repertoire

Still another type of repertoire that increases a person's vulnerability to depression is one that inhibits the normal exploration of the environment. Limited exploration necessarily stunts the growth of a person's repertoire, and a small repertoire is less effective, less adaptive, and less capable of dealing with aversive situations. Ferster (1973) points out that a nonexploratory repertoire may result from a history in which a child's primary caretaker is frequently unresponsive. If the child's early actions have little or no effect on the primary caretaker, then the child does not learn what to do or what to pay attention to in order to get his or her needs met. This stunted perceptual capacity limits the effectiveness of the environment to stimulate exploratory behavior. The less exploration there is, the less a person learns about how to behave effectively, and the greater his or her vulnerability to depression.

A limited exploratory repertoire may also influence intimate relationships, in that couples, like individuals, may be less susceptible to distress and depression if they continue to explore their environment for new shared activities and experiences. Unfortunately, if they cannot free themselves from their unwinnable struggles, then little time, energy, and motivation will be left for actively broadening their capacity for positive experiences. Consider again the case of Jack and Jill. As noted earlier, they argued frequently and had taken to spending less and less time with each other. In addition, the two of them enjoyed different things and had few common interests. Jack enjoyed outdoor activities like backpacking, skiing, and kayaking. Jill, on the other hand, enjoyed more urban activities such as nightclubs, plays, and dinner out. Jack was willing to engage in his interests on his own, but Jill was reluctant to go out without Jack. This situation contributed to Jill's depression by further limiting her opportunities to engage in positive activities. Her depression was also compounded by their mutual withdrawal, in that pleasant interactions between the two of them were becoming increasingly rare. It could be said that both Jill as an individual and Jack and Jill as a couple had limited exploratory repertoires, and that these limitations contributed both to Jill's depression and to the couple's distress. Jill as an individual was not actively exploring her environment for new enjoyable activities she might engage in. This was true in terms not only of things she might do socially, but of things she might do vocationally. Her repertoire was limited to things that were either currently impossible or unlikely. Therefore, as noted earlier, this necessarily smaller repertoire increased her susceptibility to depressive symptoms.

As a couple, Jack and Jill were no longer exploring their environment for new activities they could pursue together. Their mutual with-drawal and different interests had devastated their repertoire for shared activities. The fact that their repertoire of shared activities was small and by no means growing any larger was a major contributor to their distress as a couple. In general, they shared few pleasant activities, and their interactions consisted mostly of "walking on eggshells" and arguing.

Couple therapy approached the issue of Jack and Jill's mutual with-drawal by simply illuminating it as a recognizable pattern within their relationship. Each time they discussed an incident that resulted in their mutual withdrawal, it was discussed as an example of a common pat-tern. These patterns or themes were discussed in a nonblaming way; the therapist emphasized only that they should come to recognize the theme, and not that they necessarily had to change it. The theme was discussed as something that they could understand as a couple and com-miserate about. Jack and Jill were thus able to gain some perspective on their pattern of mutual withdrawal and to recognize some of the negative side effects it was having on their relationship.

Couple therapy also highlighted for Jack and Jill that their differ-ent interests had positive as well as negative implications for their rela-tionship. The negative implications were that having different interests resulted in their spending even less "quality time" together. Jack en-gaged in his outdoor activities alone, and Jill and he rarely if ever did the things she enjoyed. The untapped positive feature of this difference was that it provided more options from which they could choose in searching for things the two of them could do together. It had yet to be fully determined which of Jack's outdoor activities Jill might also enjoy. Jill had for the most part simply assumed that she would not like any of Jack's outdoor interests. In addition, they had not thoroughly explored Jill's interests for things they might enjoy together. Jack had also assumed that he would not like activities he had not yet even tried.

Along these same lines, couple therapy worked to help Jill under-stand the importance of pursuing her own self-care regarding the size of her effective repertoire. It also helped Jack to realize the importance of more active exploration of the environment, both for Jill as an in-dividual and for the two of them as a couple. For Jill, taking respons-ibility for her own self-care entailed actively seeking out new sources of positive experience, as well as finding ways to resume engaging in those activities she enjoyed but was currently ignoring. Jack was en-couraged to support her in this and to do what he could to facilitate her efforts to broaden her repertoire.

Promoting active self-care—the fourth IBCT acceptance technique—is often an important part of couple therapy, because it makes clear how important it is that each individual within the relationship take personal responsibility for his or her own welfare as well as for the welfare of the relationship. Emphasizing self-care helps to shift the burden for each individual's emotional well-being from his or her partner directly to the individual. This promotes within each partner a more active approach toward his or her own happiness; thus, it works to increase active exploration of the environment and to decrease the likelihood of unproductive cross-blaming.

Our view of acceptance as promoting healthy behavior despite negative circumstances fits well with viewing depression as resulting from a scarcity of effective behavior. Because of this, we believe that IBCT, with its emphasis on fostering emotional acceptance, may very well be a great deal more effective in terms of treating depression within a couple therapy context than previous behavioral couple therapies have been. IBCT creates a context in which partners can deal effectively with the problems within their relationship that may be unchangeable. Oftentimes working toward emotional acceptance is the most effective response a couple can make to circumstances that are unlikely to change. Because a broad repertoire of effective behavior may very well be the best defense against the recurrence of depression, fostering a capacity for emotional acceptance may contribute greatly to treating depression within a couple context. Chuck and Diane, for example, will probably continue to have different attitudes toward money. Struggling to try to change this difference will be not only ineffective, but ultimately quite destructive. For Chuck and Diane, the most effective response to this difference will be to learn how to tolerate it and appreciate it as an aspect of their relationship with both positive and negative features. The theory underlying IBCT posits that effective behavior is the key to ameliorating both a couple's distress and an individual's depression, and that a truly effective repertoire is capable of both change and acceptance.

IMPLICATIONS AND CONCLUSIONS

What are the implications of this approach for maintaining relationship satisfaction when one partner is depressed? The primary implication is that satisfaction depends heavily on a healthy balance of acceptance and change. In order to arrive at this balance a couple must learn how to distinguish problems that can be resolved through negotiated change from those that are unchangeable. Although this distinction may differ from couple to couple, there are some general guidelines that can be followed.

First, efforts at change should be limited to the types of problems that are amenable to negotiation and compromise. In a very real sense, these are the only situations that can, in any sense, be changed. Part-ners can easily rip an otherwise meaningful relationship to shreds through ill-fated attempts to force a type of change that cannot be negotiated. For example, the partners cannot negotiate away emotional vulnera-bility, or differences between them in desires or beliefs. However, they can negotiate about what each partner does in the relationship and what they do together as a couple. For example, they can negotiate shared responsibilities for finances, household chores, and child care.

Those aspects of a relationship that are unlikely to change tend to fall into three broad categories. The first includes all those things that happen inside a person and cannot be consciously controlled, such as thoughts, feelings, predispositions, beliefs, perspectives, and natural tendencies. The second includes those things that could theoretically be changed, but only at the expense of diminishing one partner or the other. These include aspirations, independence, habits, hobbies, pastimes, and friendships. The third includes those existential truths about relating and intimacy that are often avoided or ignored. An ex-ample of such an existential truth is that intimate relationships are in-herently dangerous. True intimacy necessarily involves the risk of loss, hurt, rejection, and disappointment. Intimate relationships are at times unavoidably painful. The closer two people are, the easier it is for them to hurt each other even unintentionally. As partners come to accept that they will sometimes hurt each other and that they are capable of recovering from such times, they in turn will become able to stay more open and less guarded within the relationship. Thus they will remain more open to genuine intimacy, despite the occasional hurt.

Another example of a truth in the third category is that relation-ships are inevitably imperfect, unknowable, impermanent, and com-plex. Striving for acceptance in intimate relationships helps couples deal with their inevitable imperfections. It helps partners realize that they *will* miscommunicate and misunderstand each other on occasion, and that they cannot always know each other's thoughts and feelings. Satisfaction is also fostered through coming to terms with the existen-tial fact that even the best relationships end, through either divorce or death. Openly embracing intimacy's impermanence can deepen the partners' appreciation of each other immeasurably. Finally, maintain-ing a satisfying relationship with another human being is a complex and complicated enterprise. This, together with the other existential unchangeables, is the unavoidable price of admission to a genuinely satisfying and meaningful relationship.

A healthy balance of change and acceptance is particularly impor-tant when one member of a couple is depressed. In such cases, "change" may refer to those things each partner can do to cope actively with the depression. For example, there may be specific things the depressed spouse can do to care actively for himself or herself when depressed, including seeking help early. In turn, the nondepressed spouse may need to foster a social support network to help him or her cope with the stress of nurturing a depressed spouse.

In terms of working toward healthy acceptance, it seems essential that the members of the couple learn to join together around the fact that one partner's depression is inevitably difficult for both. Actively preparing in advance for such times may reduce the stress on the relationship considerably. Although an episode of depression is difficult for both partners, relationship satisfaction can be maintained despite the depression. Maintaining satisfaction during such times may depend on nurturing compassion for each other through fully understanding the effects of depression, both on each person and on the relationship. Working together as a couple to cope with the depression fosters intimacy and removes blame. Finally, it is essential that the partners prepare in advance for future episodes of depression by discussing how they will cope with it as a couple.

REFERENCES

American Psychiatric Association. (1994). *Diagnostic and statistical manual of mental disorders* (4th ed.). Washington, DC: Author.

Baucom, D. H., & Hoffman, J. A. (1986). The effectiveness of marital therapy: Current status and applications to the clinical setting. In N. S. Jacobson & A. S. Gurman (Eds.), *Clinical handbook of marital therapy* (pp. 597–620). New York: Guilford Press.

Beach, S. R. H., & Nelson, G. M. (1990). Pursuing research on major psychopathology from a contextual perspective: The example of depression and marital discord. In G. Brody & I. E. Siegel (Eds.), *Family research* (Vol. 2, pp. 227–259). Hillsdale, NJ: Erlbaum.

Beach, S. R. H., & O'Leary, K. D. (1992). Treating depression in the context of marital discord: Outcome and predictors of response for marital therapy vs. cognitive therapy. *Behavior Therapy, 23,* 507–528.

Beach, S. R. H., & O'Leary, K. D. (1993). Marital discord and dysphoria: For whom does the marital relationship predict depressive symptoms? *Journal of Social and Personal Relationships, 10,* 405–420.

Beach, S. R. H., Whisman, M. A., & O'Leary, K. D. (1994). Marital therapy for depression: Theoretical foundation, current status, and future directions. *Behavior Therapy, 25,* 345–371.

Billings, A. G., Cronkite, R. C., & Moos, R. H. (1983). Social environmental factors in unipolar depression: Comparisons of depressed patients and controls. *Journal of Abnormal Psychology, 92,* 119–133.

Birtchnell, J. (1988). Depression and family relationships: A study of young, married women on a London housing estate. *British Journal of Psychiatry, 153,* 758–769.

Brown, G. W., Adler, Z., & Bifulco, A. (1988). Life events and recovery from chronic depression. *British Journal of Psychiatry, 152,* 487–498.

Brown, G. W., Andrews, B., Harris, T., Adler, Z., & Bridge, L. (1986). Social support, self-esteem and depression. *Psychological Medicine, 16,* 813–831.

Brown, G. W., & Harris, T. (1978). *Social origins of depression: A study of psychiatric disorders in women.* New York: Free Press.

Brown, G. W., Lemryre, L., & Bifulco, A. (1992). Social factors and recovery from anxiety and depressive disorders: A test of specificity. *British Journal of Psychiatry, 161,* 44–54.

Christensen, A., Jacobson, N. S., & Babcock, J. C. (1995). Integrative behavioral couple therapy. In N. S. Jacobson & A. S. Gurman (Eds.), *Clinical handbook of couple therapy* (pp. 31–64). New York: Guilford Press.

Cordova, J. V., & Jacobson, N. S. (1993). Couples distress. In D. H. Barlow (Ed.), *Clinical handbook of psychological disorders: A step-by-step treatment manual* (2nd ed., pp. 481–512). New York: Guilford Press.

Cordova, J. V., & Kohlenberg, R. J. (1994). Acceptance and the therapeutic relationship. In S. C. Hayes, N. S. Jacobson, V. M. Follette, & M. J. Dougher (Eds.), *Acceptance and change: Content and context in psychotherapy* (pp. 125–142). Reno, NV: Context Press.

Dougher, M. J. (1994). The act of acceptance. In S. C. Hayes, N. S. Jacobson, V. M. Follette, & M. J. Dougher (Eds.), *Acceptance and change: Content and context in psychotherapy* (pp. 125–142). Reno, NV: Context Press.

Dougher, M. J., & Hackbert, L. (1994). A behavior-analytic account of depression and a case report using acceptance-based procedures. *The Behavior Analyst, 17,* 321–334.

Ferster, C. B. (1973). A functional analysis of depression. *American Psychologist, 28,* 857–869.

Foley, S. H., Rounsaville, B. J., Weissman, M. M., Sholomaskas, D., & Chevron, E. (1989). Individual versus conjoint interpersonal therapy for depressed patients with marital disputes. *International Journal of Family Psychiatry, 10,* 29–42.

Gurman, A. S., Kniskern, D. P., & Pinsof, W. M. (1986). Research on the process and outcome of marital and family therapy. In S. L. Garfield & A. E. Bergin (Eds.), *Handbook of psychotherapy and behavior change* (3rd ed., pp. 565–624). New York: Wiley.

Hahlweg, K., Schindler, L., Revenstorf, D., & Brengelmann, J. C. (1984). The Munich marital therapy study. In K. Hahlweg & N. S. Jacobson (Eds.), *Marital interaction: Analysis and modification* (pp. 3–26). New York: Guilford Press.

Hayes, S. C. (1987). A contextual approach to therapeutic change. In N. S. Jacobson (Ed.), *Psychotherapists in clinical practice: Cognitive and behavioral perspectives* (pp. 327–387). New York: Guilford Press.

Hayes, S. C., Jacobson, N. S., Follette, V. M., & Dougher, M. J. (Eds.). (1994). *Acceptance and change: Content and context in psychotherapy.* Reno, NV: Context Press.

Horwitz, A. V., & White, H. R. (1991). Becoming married, depression, and alcohol problems among young adults. *Journal of Health and Social Behavior, 32,* 221–237.

Ilfeld, F. W., Jr. (1977). Current social stressors and symptoms of depression. *American Journal of Psychiatry, 134,* 161–166.

Jacobson, N. S. (1978). A review of the research on the effectiveness of marital therapy. In T. J. Paolino & B. S. McCrady (Eds.), *Marriage and marital therapy: Psychoanalytic, behavioral, and systems theory perspectives* (pp. 395–444). New York: Brunner/Mazel.

Jacobson, N. S. (1984). A component analysis of behavioral marital therapy: The relative effectiveness of behavior exchange and problem solving training. *Journal of Consulting and Clinical Psychology, 52,* 295–305.

Jacobson, N. S. (1992). Behavioral couple therapy: A new beginning. *Behavior Therapy, 23,* 493–506.

Jacobson, N. S., & Christensen, A. (1996). *Integrative couple therapy: Promoting acceptance and change.* New York: Norton.

Jacobson, N. S., Dobson, K., Fruzzetti, A. E., Schmaling, K. B., & Salusky, S. (1991). Marital therapy and a treatment for depression. *Journal of Consulting and Clinical Psychology, 59,* 547–557.

Jacobson, N. S., Follette, W. C., & Pagel, M. (1986). Predicting who will benefit from behavioral marital therapy. *Journal of Consulting and Clinical Psychology, 54,* 518–522.

Jacobson, N. S., & Margolin, G. (1979). *Marital therapy: Strategies based on social learning and behavior exchange principles.* New York: Brunner/Mazel.

Jacobson, N. S., Schmaling, K. B., & Holtzworth-Munroe, A. (1987). Component analysis of behavioral marital therapy: Two-year follow-up and prediction of relapse. *Journal of Marital and Family Therapy, 13,* 187–195.

Markman, H. J., Duncan, S. W., Storaasli, R. D., & Howes, P. W. (1987). The prediction of marital distress: A longitudinal investigation. In K. Hahlweg & M. Goldstein (Eds.), *Understanding major mental disorder: The contribution of family interaction research* (pp. 266–289). New York: Family Process Press.

Miller, W. R., & Seligman, M. E. (1975). Depression and learned helplessness in man. *Journal of Abnormal Psychology, 84,* 228–238.

Monroe, S. M., Bromet, E. J., Connell, M. M., & Steiner, S. C. (1986). Social support, life events, and depressive symptoms: A one year prospective study. *Journal of Consulting and Clinical Psychology, 54,* 424–431.

O'Leary, K. D., & Beach, S. R. H. (1990). Marital therapy: A viable treatment for depression and marital discord. *American Journal of Psychiatry, 147,* 183–186.

O'Leary, K. D., Christian, J. L., & Mendell, N. R. (1994). A closer look at the link between marital discord and depressive symptomatology. *Journal of Social and Clinical Psychology, 14,* 1–9.

O'Leary, K. D., Riso, L. P., & Beach, S. R. H. (1990). Attributions about the marital discord/depression link and therapy outcome. *Behavior Therapy, 21,* 413–422.

Paykel, E. S. (1979). Recent life events in the development of the depressive disorders. In R. A. Depue (Ed.), *The psychology of the depressive disor-*

ders: Implications for the effects of stress (pp. 245–262). New York: Academic Press.

Schaefer, E. S., & Burnett, C. K. (1987). Stability and predictability of quality of women's marital relationships and demoralization. Journal of Personality and Social Psychology, 53, 1129–1136.

Schuster, T. L., Kessler, R. C., & Aseltine, R. H. (1990). Supportive interactions, negative interactions and depressed mood. American Journal of Community Psychology, 18, 423–438.

Waltz, M., Badura, B., Pfaff, H., & Schott, T. (1988). Marriage and the psychological consequences of a heart attack: A longitudinal study of adaptation to chronic illness after 3 years. Social Science and Medicine, 27, 149–158.

Weiss, R. L., & Aved, B. M. (1978). Marital satisfaction and depression as predictors of physical health status. Journal of Consulting and Clinical Psychology, 46, 1379–1384.

Weissman, M. M. (1987). Advances in psychiatric epidemiology: Rates and risks for major depression. American Journal of Public Health, 77, 445–451.

CHAPTER 13

The Erosion of Marital Satisfaction over Time and How to Prevent It

MARI L. CLEMENTS
ALLAN D. CORDOVA
HOWARD J. MARKMAN
JEAN-PHILIPPE LAURENCEAU

Many individuals have an intense need for love, support, and acceptance, but find themselves disappointed and dissatisfied in relationships. The love and satisfaction that they seek from their partners appear elusive. Many theories have been advanced regarding why people so desperately crave and vigorously pursue companionship and connection. Yet for most of us, the question "Why do people want romantic relationships?" is not a particularly interesting one. Instead, we simply take it on faith that human beings need to feel cared for, to feel important, and (as adolescents and adults) to be romantically tied to a significant other. The most important question for most people is "Why is it so hard for relationships to work out?"

We are thus faced with a bit of a paradox: Human beings need love and romantic affiliation. Yet if this is a normal part of the human experience, why are romantic relationships often so difficult to maintain? Why do relationships that start with great hopes and high satisfaction begin to disintegrate and bring pain and suffering to both partners? The goal of this chapter is to answer this age-old question—the answer to which has for years eluded researchers in psychology, sociology, and personal relationships. To answer this question, we consider the nature of marital satisfaction, gender differences in satisfaction, and the role of family transitions in satisfaction. We then present a theory to explain the erosion of satisfaction over time.

WHY SATISFACTION?

One need only casually scan the magazines in a supermarket checkout line to confirm the fact that the United States as a nation is hyperaware of marital satisfaction and always on the lookout for ways to improve it. People seem to know intuitively that when marital satisfaction is high, spouses and their children are happier and healthier. As marital satisfaction erodes, rates of personal, work, and family problems increase, leading to high rates of divorce or to stable but unhappy families (Barnett & Gotlib, 1988; Jacobson, 1985; Veroff, Kulka, & Douvan, 1981; Waring & Patton, 1984). Clearly, understanding marital satisfaction—and its erosion—has meaningful implications for individual spouses, marriages, families, and society as a whole.

Researchers, too, have realized the importance of marital satisfaction. In the next few sections, we take a brief look at how researchers have defined and studied satisfaction, and at what their work has revealed.

THE DEFINITION OF SATISFACTION

Examining the existing literature on marriage, we find that the most commonly investigated construct is "satisfaction." This research has an extensive history, with its roots in the field of sociology. Initially, investigators studied the role of sexuality in marital success or satisfaction (e.g., Davis, 1929; Hamilton, 1929). As the field began to grow, researchers turned their attention to developing questionnaires and measures that would allow them both to assess and to predict marital adjustment (e.g., Burgess & Cottrell, 1939; Locke & Wallace, 1959; Spanier, 1976; Terman & Wallin, 1949). This tradition of measuring satisfaction, and of predicting how satisfied couples will be in the future, provides the basis for much of present-day marital research.

"Marital satisfaction" has been defined as an attitude concerning the quality of a marital relationship and has been described as a process that is susceptible to changes over time. Other terms used to denote such satisfaction include "marital quality," "marital adjustment," and "marital success" (Fincham & Bradbury, 1987; Spanier & Lewis, 1980). For our purposes, we consider marital satisfaction to be the person's overall evaluation of his or her marriage. Virtually all measures of satisfaction include an assessment of this overall evaluation. As we explain in the next section, men and women may have somewhat different bases for their answers to this question.

ARE THERE GENDER DIFFERENCES IN MARITAL SATISFACTION?

Do the images of married men and women that are prevalent in popular culture have a basis in reality? Is the vision of the henpecked husband escaping from his wife to the corner bar for a drink, or of the beleaguered and overworked wife who grudgingly tolerates her bumbling husband, supported by research? Certainly we can find instances that support these stereotypes of how men's and women's attitudes toward marriage and their spouses differ. Still, when we look at the research, the picture is far from clear.

Some researchers do in fact suggest that gender may exert an important influence on marital satisfaction. For example, wives seem to be more responsive to their husbands' support than husbands are to their wives' support (Acitelli & Antonucci, 1994; Julien & Markman, 1991). In other words, husbands' supportive behaviors increase wives' satisfaction to a greater extent than wives' supportive behaviors increase husbands' satisfaction. Thus, husbands' supportive behaviors may shape the development and outcome of the marital relationship more than wives' supportive behaviors do (Acitelli & Antonucci, 1994).

Along these same lines, a study of more than 7,000 couples in the United States revealed that men are somewhat more satisfied with their marriages than women are (Fowers, 1991). The author of this study also noted that, consistent with the idea that men are more satisfied with marriage, married men have lower rates of mental illness than their single counterparts, whereas married women have higher rates than single women. These findings are not without controversy, however. In a review of 56 studies, marriage was associated with greater well-being for both men and women (Wood, Rhodes, & Whelan, 1989).

So what does research tell us about men and women in marriage? Do women get the short end of the marital stick? The answer is "No, not exactly." More complex explanations seem better able to account for differences in men's and women's marital satisfaction. We base these explanations on our research with 100 married couples whom we have followed for nearly 15 years. For our Denver Family Development Study, we began studying men and women who were just planning marriage. These couples completed a series of self-report forms, and then we videotaped them talking about a major problem area in their relationship. We have continued to track these families at approximately 1- to 1½-year intervals as they married, had children, divorced, became unhappy, or stayed happy over time.

In looking at these couples, we found different levels of marital satisfaction for husbands and wives. In contrast to some previous research, however, we found that wives consistently reported higher levels of satisfaction than did husbands across the marriage (Markman, Duncan, Storaasli, & Howes, 1987; Markman & Hahlweg, 1993). Although this finding is surprising and stands in contrast to popular lore and some previous research, it is consistent with some more recent research. A number of recent studies have found wives' satisfaction to be equal to or even higher than that of their husbands (Aron & Henkemeyer, 1995; Huston & Vangelisti, 1991; Karney, Bradbury, Fincham, & Sullivan, 1994; Karney & Bradbury, 1995; MacDermid, Huston, & McHale, 1990; Tucker & Aron, 1993). This shift in research findings may reflect societal changes that have increasingly favored women and have given wives more options.

One additional potential explanation for these differences could be that satisfaction differs in some way for wives and husbands. It could be that husbands and wives evaluate their relationships in different ways. To examine this interpretation of our findings, we took a closer look at the actual satisfaction questionnaires that the partners completed, and we think that there may be some support for this kind of explanation.

Marital satisfaction measures often consist of several questions assessing areas such as happiness, levels of agreement, and regrets in the relationship. When we examined the patterns of answers that husbands and wives gave to these questions, we found some interesting differences. For husbands, all of the questions seemed to be tapping one underlying dimension. Their perceptions of marital satisfaction were fairly uniform and were best captured by questions about their overall happiness in marriage, lack of regrets in marrying, and the amount of agreement between themselves and their wives on the issues of displays of affection and sex. This dimension was found at all time points, from before marriage to many years after marriage.

On the other hand, wives' marital satisfaction seemed to reflect two underlying components. The first component was the same as the one found for their husbands. A second component, however, reflected the wives' evaluation of the relationship in the context of other relationships. For wives, marital satisfaction seemed to reflect not only the quality of their personal relationships with their husbands, but also the way the couples interacted with other people. This dimension was best captured by questions about agreement between wives and husbands in the areas of proper behavior, philosophy of life, dealing with in-laws, and friends. Both of these components seemed important in explaining wives' satisfaction from the engagement period to many years into the marriage.

Taken together, these findings suggest that marital satisfaction may mean one "thing" for husbands and two "things" for wives. The overall dimension of general marital happiness is equally important for both partners, but for wives there appears to be an additional important component. The existence of this second component is consistent with the view that women are more oriented than men to relationships, with more reliance on social connectedness and social support (Gilligan, 1982). Furthermore, this difference may be reflecting real changes in relationships, such as men's participating more in events and life within the home, and women's participating more actively and consistently outside the home. This leads us to focus on how satisfaction changes over time.

RELATIONSHIP SATISFACTION OVER TIME

What happens to couples' levels of satisfaction over time? Does marriage improve with time like a good wine? Is there an inexorable slide toward aggravation and disharmony? Or, as some researchers have argued, does satisfaction over time resemble a "U," with satisfaction highest during the early and later years and lowest in the middle period (Anderson, Russell, & Schumm, 1983; Rollins & Cannon, 1974)?

Some researchers have presented evidence that satisfaction steadily decreases over time (Johnson, Amoloza, & Booth, 1992). For example, as part of a 40-year study on college men and their wives, Vaillant and Vaillant (1993) found that marital satisfaction steadily declined over time. However, when these same couples were asked to think back and report on their satisfaction over time, the U-shaped pattern best described their responses.

In our research, we have found that marital satisfaction declined across the early years of the couples' relationships. Spouses were happier and more satisfied in the premarital and early years of marriage than at points later in their relationships (Markman & Hahlweg, 1993). This decline has been seen for both husbands and wives. This finding is consistent with work by other researchers, and at first glance may suggest no hint of optimism for couples. However, although the couples showed a definite decline in their ratings of satisfaction over time, they have remained happy in their marriages. Perhaps even more importantly, the declines seemed to level off. After being married for several years, the couples reached a level of satisfaction that appears (thus far) to be relatively stable. Findings regarding patterns of change in marital satisfaction have prompted exploration of the underlying causes of such changes over time.

For example, in recent years, researchers and the popular press alike have focused on family transitions to help explain why marital satisfaction declines over time. The transition to parenthood has been central in this research (Belsky, Lang, & Huston, 1986; Cowan et al., 1985; Ruble, Fleming, Hackel, & Stangor, 1988). After the birth of the first child, parents have reported declines in marital satisfaction, positive interactions, and romantic love, while also reporting increases in marital conflict and relationship problems. In short, nearly everything positive in the partners' relationship with each other is expected to decrease after the birth of the first child, while nearly everything negative is expected to increase.

Books and articles written for expectant parents caution them to expect changes in their marriage. These changes may be given a positive spin in some such works, but they seem primarily aimed at educating future parents about the difficulties in their relationship that the birth of a child will bring. With all these negative effects attributed to children, one might wonder why couples would choose to have children at all.

On the other hand, there is a strong societal bias toward having children. More than 90% of U.S. couples have at least one child (Houseknecht, 1987), and many have more than one. If children cause problems in marriage, why would couples choose to repeat this "mistake"? At least as common as the conceptualization of the child as a tiny marriage wrecker is the idea of the child as a bundle of joy or a blessed event. Having a child "to save our marriage" is a widely recognized (if ill-advised) strategy taken by some unhappy couples. If children cause declines in marriage, one might wonder why such views would be in favor.

Our research, along with that of other researchers, has shed some interesting light on the role of children in the development of marital distress. Although early studies almost universally showed difficulties in marriage after the birth of the first child, several recent studies (Huston, McHale, & Crouter, 1986; Kurdek, 1993) have shown that declines in marital functioning in this developmental period may not be entirely attributable to children.

Some of the couples in our study had children and some did not. When we looked at the relationships of parents before and after the birth of the first child, we found that marital satisfaction declined after children were born (Clements & Markman, 1997). Furthermore, we found that these declines fit in the overall picture of the couples' marriages. Satisfaction was at its highest at the beginning of the study, when couples were planning marriage, and began to wane almost immediately. Although couples were generally still quite happy after the birth of the first child, their satisfaction levels began to decline noticeably very early in their relationships. In other words, marital satisfaction did not begin its decline with the birth of the first child, but rather with the exchanging of the marriage vows!

Even more important than the detection of this pattern for parents were our findings with childless couples. Couples that had been married the same length of time but had not had children also experienced equivalent declines in satisfaction. Whether couples had children or not did not appear to matter; all of the couples experienced declines in marital satisfaction over the early years of marriage.

Thus, both parents and childless couples experienced declines in marital satisfaction. The fact that these declines were essentially identical in size and timing has led us to believe that although having children may influence partners in many ways, children do not cause difficulties in marriage or declines in marital satisfaction per se.

Nonetheless, marital satisfaction clearly declines over time. Since family transitions such as the birth of children cannot adequately account for these changes, we are left with this question: Why does marital satisfaction decline over time? Although these declines may coincide with particular periods in the family life cycle, it has been suggested that marital satisfaction is better explained by the way spouses interact than by family transitions (Clements & Markman, 1997; Huston & Vangelisti, 1991).

THE EROSION THEORY OF SATISFACTION

Most theories of why marriages fail, including those held both by professionals and by the couples themselves, fall into one of three categories: The spouses either made the wrong choice, fell out of love, or grew apart. The first type of explanation suggests that couples are swept up in the excitement and romance of courtship. Members of these couples may have committed themselves prematurely to marriage without having built a sturdy foundation of friendship or without realizing that they are fundamentally different (e.g., they have different basic values or outlooks on life). The second perspective suggests that although the spouses were once truly in love, the "spark" originally fueling their marriage has somehow been extinguished. The third perspective suggests that partners who were once close have changed over time, so that the connection that once bound them close together has weakened and stretched, leaving two separate people who no longer feel a bond with each other.

We assert that the data from our longitudinal research, as well as clinical experience, suggest that this conventional wisdom—though perhaps capturing elements of individuals' relationship experiences—is wrong. Instead, we present a theory of relationship distress that we call "erosion theory."

Our conceptualization of erosion theory assumes that couples begin their relationships with relatively high degrees of positive factors, such as attraction, love, commitment, trust, friendship, and intimacy. In cultures where marital choice is based primarily upon these factors, premarital couples generally report very high levels of positive factors, although each partner's level can vary. In cultures in which marital choice is constrained by arranged marriages or rigid social hierarchy, the level of positive factors present premaritally may also differ. Positive relationship factors can be thought of as forming a "relationship bank account" (RBA; Notarius & Markman, 1993). Satisfaction can be thought of as the "balance" of each partner's RBA. This balance may vary on a day-to-day, week-to-week, and year-to-year basis.

As relationships continue, all couples experience disagreements and conflicts. Storaasli and Markman (1990) found that the top three areas of conflict for young couples were money, communication, and sex. Other typical problem areas included in-laws, chores, careers, drinking and drugs, children, and recreation. The number and type of conflict areas, however, are less important than how couples handle these conflicts in predicting the future of the relationship (Clements, Stanley, & Markman, 1997).

Research has revealed key destructive ways of handling conflict. These patterns have been found to be gender-linked and to involve cycles of escalation and withdrawal (Christensen & Heavey, 1990; Heavey, Layne, & Christensen, 1993). In couples that develop relationship problems, males tend to withdraw from conflicts, while females tend to pursue. Furthermore, the seeds of these patterns have been found even in dating couples (Markman, Silvern, Clements, & Kraft-Hanak, 1993).

In general, our research has shown couples with dysfunctional premarital interaction patterns—especially a tendency to approach discussions of relationship issues with invalidation, negative affect, and withdrawal—to be at risk for marital distress and divorce (Markman, Stanley, & Blumberg, 1994). Happy couples have not typically shown these difficulties to the same degree. Instead, spouses in satisfied couples have been more successful in regulating their anger, displeasure, and frustration toward their partners.

To illustrate what we mean by "successfully regulating" negative emotions, consider the following example: A husband who is angry with his wife for coming home late without having called may respond by saying, "I felt worried about you when you were late. I really wish you'd call next time," rather than by angrily snapping, "You're always late! Can't you be considerate of me once in a while?" In the first scenario, the husband is managing his anger and worry in a way that is likely to promote a constructive discussion, ultimately leading to increased intimacy and trust in the relationship. In the second scenario, the husband initiates a negative escalation cycle: His negativity will probably be followed by invalidation from his spouse, to which he in turn will respond negatively.

The destructive patterns of handling conflict actively erode the positive factors that bring partners together and fuel relationship satisfaction. Although precise estimates are difficult to make, it has been estimated that one destructive act can erase 5, 10, or even 20 positive acts of kindness (Gottman, 1994; Notarius & Markman, 1993). Research has revealed that the presence of negative behaviors predicts future problems much more strongly than the absence of positive behaviors does (Notarius & Markman, 1993). Thus, erosion theory asserts that destructive fights actively erode the positive factors in relationships, depleting the balance of each partner's RBA, and lowering relationship satisfaction.

Positive acts (e.g., making love, having an intimate talk, going to a baseball game, preparing a meal together) are clearly important as deposits to the RBA. However, the deposit value of a positive act generally does not equal the withdrawal value of a negative act. Partners who closely monitor satisfaction, or "keep score," and make decisions about investing in their marriage based on their current level of satisfaction are like stock market investors who try to time the market; both strategies are doomed to failure.

WHAT PREDICTS DISTRESS AND DIVORCE?

One of the burning questions that we have been addressing in our research over the last 15 years is why the vast majority of couples experience substantial happiness in their relationships in the beginning, but are unable to sustain these positive circumstances over time. Over 50% of these couples eventually divorce, and a sizable number of others become chronically distressed but do not divorce.

Our research has enabled us to address this question by examining the factors that predict future distress and divorce. Here we report the results of a series of analyses on what predicts divorce and distress; these analyses are presented in detail in a forthcoming paper (Clements et al., 1997).

The most striking finding is that the factors that most people think predict divorce and distress—how much in love a couple is, how similar or different the partners are, how good their sex lives are, how attracted they are to each other, and how satisfied they are with their relationship before marriage—are *not* able to predict the future of a relationship. Other studies have shown that these factors do seem to predict who marries whom, but it is important to note that these factors will not predict the probability of success of the relationship over time.

In contrast, what *does* seem to predict the future of a relationship is how a couple handles differences when these emerge, because for virtually all couples, differences and conflicts are inevitable. Couples must decide where to live, how to divide household chores, whose career is going to be more important, whether or not to have children (and if so, when), how to spend their money, how to balance their friends and families, what to do in their "free" time, and so on. It is not the decisions spouses make about these everyday issues that are important; it is *how* those decisions are made that seems to forecast the future of a relationship. Partners who handle conflict by engaging in destructive tactics before they are married are at risk for a stormy relationship.

In the 13th year of our longitudinal study of marriage, we divided couples into one of two groups. Those couples that remained happy with their relationships over time were placed in the "happy" group. Next, we combined those couples that had separated or divorced, or had been unhappy with their relationships for several years, and placed them in the "unhappy" group.

We then went back to the first time we saw these couples, while they were still just planning marriage. We systematically examined the premarital characteristics that would predict in which group each couple would land. The results revealed that couples that became unhappy, separated, or divorced tended to deal with disagreements before marriage more destructively than those couples that remained happy over time. Interestingly, the variables reflecting more positive ways of communicating had little predictive power.

Before we describe the implications of these findings, readers can take the following test to assess the degree to which their own relationships or the relationships of couples with which they are working may be at risk for future problems. This questionnaire was based on our research and developed by Stanley and Markman (1996) for use in a national poll on marriage in the United States.

DANGER SIGNS FROM NATIONAL SURVEY
(Stanley & Markman, 1996)
PREP, Inc.

Indicate whether each of the following statements is true or false:

1. Little arguments escalate into ugly fights with accusations, criticisms, name calling, or bringing up past hurts.
2. My partner criticizes or belittles my opinions, feelings, or desires.
3. My partner seems to view my words or actions more negatively than I mean them to be.
4. When we have a problem to solve, it is like we are on opposite teams.
5. I hold back from telling my partner what I really think and feel.
6. I think seriously about what it would be like to date or marry someone else.
7. I feel lonely in this relationship.
8. When we argue, one of us withdraws . . . that is, doesn't want to talk about it any more, or leaves the scene.

Although members of many couples can occasionally answer "yes" to one or two of these questions, a repeated pattern of these kinds of interactions spells trouble for a relationship. For readers whose relationships (or those of their clients) are not reflected in the questions above, the outlook for such relationships is probably quite good. Nevertheless, there are things that spouses can do now to preserve and strengthen even good relationships and help prevent difficulties from arising. On the other hand, if one or more questions really seemed to capture a relationship, it is likely that the relationship is at risk for significant problems, either now or in the future. However, there are steps that the partners can take to address these potential problems.

In considering these suggestions, readers should keep in mind that they can be used to make a good relationship even better, as well as to improve one that is beginning to emit distress signals. Often couples do not consider the value of preventive steps that protect and strengthen the special qualities of their unions. Yet, although a person one wouldn't embark on a camping trip without first consulting the weather forecast, or head out into a downpour without galoshes and a rain slicker, people very often do just this in relationship terms. That is, they overlook the often simple, fail-safe measures that they can take that will make their relationship journey much more comfortable and fulfilling.

Our research on what predicts the development of distress suggests that the danger signs outlined above can be very detrimental to couples' relationships (Markman et al., 1994). Our research and clinical experience suggest that three critical interaction patterns in particular create difficulties for couples: "escalation," "withdrawal," and "invalidation."

"Escalation" refers to the tendency for a couple to allow negative interactions to "snowball." When angry or upset, one person may say something that the partner perceives as negative. The partner then responds with something negative, and the discussion tends to escalate into a fight. All too often these fights end in verbal or physical abuse.

"Withdrawal" refers to the tendency for one or both members of a couple to deal with relationship conflicts by withdrawing or avoiding the confrontation. They may even use other creative ways not to deal with a problem. We have found that men tend to withdraw more from conflict than women (Stanley & Markman, 1996). When men withdraw, it is a stronger predictor of future problems than when women withdraw.

These findings have added to the rich literature on the differences between men and women in relationships. However—in contrast to conventional wisdom and the complaints by many women who go to marital therapy that men are not good at intimacy or that men are not interested in communication—our findings suggest that the major difference between men and women is not in the area of intimacy, but in terms of how conflict is handled. Simply put, men tend to withdraw in the face of conflict, while women seem to be more comfortable handling it. On the other hand, when men and women feel safe from conflict early in their relationships, their communication in terms of intimacy tends to be equivalent. (See Markman et al., 1994, for details.)

Finally, the third danger sign, "invalidation," refers to the tendency of one or both members of a couple, when angry, to criticize or attack the partner(s) personally. In earlier work, Gottman, Notarius, Gonso, and Markman (1976) called these behavioral patterns "character assassinations." More recently, Notarius and Markman (1993) designated these types of behavior as "zingers."

When escalation, withdrawal, and/or invalidation accumulate over time, they actively erode the positive elements of relationships that bring people together in the first place and leave them feeling increasingly unhappy, sad, and lonely. These interactional tendencies or danger signs, as well as some of their attitudinal consequences, are reflected in questionnaire presented earlier.

It is very important to note—particularly in a book about satisfaction in close relationships—that early levels of premarital satisfaction do not adequately predict future levels of marital satisfaction. Just as a meteorologist cannot predict today's high temperature from last week's temperature, how happy a couple is before marriage is not the best predictor of how happy the couple is going to be years later. Furthermore, what does predict future satisfaction has to do with how couples communicate and, in particular, how they handle conflict. These are the elements that can erode the high levels of satisfaction with which most couples begin their relationships. The good news is that, just as there are tools to prevent erosion in the natural world, when it comes to the relationship world there are tools that couples can learn and use to prevent erosion of the elements of fun, friendship, sensuality, attraction, and so forth. These skills can "shore up" relationships, protecting them from the winds and waves of conflict that may threaten couples' happiness. A sampling of these tools is presented later in the chapter.

Finally, we want to note that these danger signs or predictors of future problems are not static properties in relationships that are impossible to change. They reflect interactional patterns that have probably been learned from the families in which individuals were raised, and can therefore be unlearned and replaced with more constructive ways of handling conflict.

We have found in our research that young couples are just as committed to having successful relationships as their parents and grandparents were. They realize that divorce is not a successful solution for relationship problems. However, young couples may be at more of a disadvantage than were their parents before them, because many people marrying today either are children of divorce or conflict themselves, or are marrying persons who are. Thus, they may be lacking positive modeling and the protective umbrella of tools needed to construct a successful relationship and maintain high levels of satisfaction over time. However, the good news is that these couples seem to be very motivated to discover the skills to which we have been referring, in order to give their relationships the maximum opportunity to succeed.

STRATEGIES TO PREVENT EROSION OF SATISFACTION AND TO ENHANCE SATISFACTION

Given that satisfaction is highest in the early stages of marital relationships and tends to erode over time, we have focused in our work on reaching couples in the premarital stage. However, the tools we have developed to help couples prevent the erosion of satisfaction have also been used with couples making the transition to parenthood (Heavey, 1995; Jordan, 1995), with couples attempting to save failing marriages (Notarius & Markman, 1993), and with couples whose members would simply like to enhance their relationship satisfaction.

These tools involve teaching couples a set of communication and conflict management skills, as well as ways to protect and preserve the positive factors in their relationships. We have developed a program called the Prevention and Relationship Enhancement Program (PREP; Markman & Floyd, 1980) that systematically covers the following topics for couples: basic communication skills, destructive communication patterns, expressing criticism constructively, expectations, hidden issues, fun, problem solving, friendship, commitment, spiritual and religious beliefs, sensual/sexual enhancement, and ground rules for communication. The development of PREP grew out of earlier work (e.g., Gottman, Markman, & Notarius, 1977), which clearly discriminated between the communication quality of distressed and nondistressed couples. The conceptual underpinnings of PREP are based on a cognitive-behavioral model, with roots in the theory, research, and clinical practice of behavioral marital therapy; research and clinical advances in understanding the role of cognitive factors in marital relationships; and social competence and social exchange theories (e.g., Markman, Floyd, Stanley, & Jamieson, 1984). The primary goal of PREP is to provide an educational experience for couples that will enable them to increase their communication and problem-solving skills—skills associated with effective marital functioning and the prevention of marital distress.

The premarital stage, when couples' satisfaction is likely to be at its peak, is an ideal time for teaching couples skills to carry with them into marriage. To this end, current efforts in our laboratory are focused on investigating the effectiveness of PREP, compared to that of other premarital interventions, with couples planning marriage within various religious organizations. Specifically, in our investigation, couples are being randomly assigned to one of three treatment conditions: PREP administered by our research staff, PREP administered by clergy we have trained, and a control group in which couples receive the premarital intervention normally delivered by their religious organization. The inclusion of the clergy-administered PREP condition is designed to yield information about the possibilities for disseminating premarital skills training in community settings.

Evidence is available on the efficacy of prevention approaches for couples in general (Behrens & Sanders, 1994; Hahlweg & Markman, 1988) and that of the PREP program in particular (Markman, Floyd, Stanley, & Storaasli, 1988; Markman, Renick, Floyd, Stanley, & Clements, 1993; Renick, Blumberg, & Markman, 1992), as well as on the effects of cognitive-behavioral approaches to marital therapy (Dunn & Schwebel, 1995; Sher, Baucom, & Larus, 1990). Therefore, we focus here on describing some of the tools that we have found most useful for helping prevent erosion of satisfaction and for enhancing satisfaction. However, we do want to highlight one major finding from our work: The effects of the PREP program on satisfaction are significant in the early years of marriage, but these effects are attenuated over time.

This highlights the need for "booster" sessions of PREP—follow-up intervention sessions that review the specific tools. In our current investigation, a subset of couples in the two PREP conditions is being invited to attend booster sessions at yearly intervals. Couples in the booster session condition will participate in 2-hour sessions similar in format to regular PREP sessions. Leaders will present short "lecturettes" reviewing major points from the program, and couples will be asked to review and practice the skills in the context of recent life changes and problems. Drawing on our RBA model, we can think of couples' using skills both to prevent withdrawals and to increase deposits. Given our findings on what predicts distress and divorce (i.e., negative relationship factors are more predictive than positive factors), we place more emphasis on decreasing withdrawals than on increasing deposits, though both are featured.

Preventing Withdrawals (Erosion Protection)

A key PREP tool designed to prevent withdrawals is the speaker–listener technique. This is a highly structured discussion format used to ensure that each partner is able both to express thoughts and feelings fully and to hear the other partner accurately. The discussion begins with one partner as the speaker and the other as the listener. The partners change roles, often several times, during the discussion. The speaker literally has the floor, which is a small piece of cardboard labeled "the floor," signaling the person's ability to speak without interruption. Speakers talk from their own points of view, using "I" statements (e.g., "I think . . . ," "I feel . . . " rather than "You feel . . . ," "You say . . . "). The listener is not allowed to interrupt the speaker and summarizes the speaker at 20- to 30-second intervals to ensure understanding. The speaker is encouraged to communicate nonverbally in a way that enhances the listener's understanding (e.g., speaking with a positive voice tone, showing a neutral or positive facial expression), while the listener is encouraged to inhibit responses that will invalidate the speaker (e.g., rolling eyes, shaking head).

Furthermore, in PREP couples are taught to separate the process of problem discussion from problem solution. A couple is taught to solve problems only after both partners have thoroughly voiced their feelings and thoughts by means of the speaker–listener technique. We have found that the need to agree on an issue often fades away in a validating conversation.

In addition, several other tools and guidelines are used in PREP to decrease withdrawals. One such guideline is for a couple to make a date to discuss a particular relationship issue. Thus, the problem is to some extent encapsulated from the rest of the relationship, such that the couple can lay it aside with the knowledge that there will be a set time for addressing it later.

Another discussion skill is to focus on the problem through face-to-face interaction without distractions (e.g., television, music, children). When discussions are not going well or the talk is getting too "hot," a couple is encouraged to call a time out. At that point, the couple agrees to stop talking and to pick up the discussion within 24 hours. This allows either partner to leave the discussion without incurring resentment or anger.

Finally, PREP teaches couples to deal with any obstacles that prevent them from engaging in a fruitful discussion. If one partner is unwilling to talk about an issue, he or she should discuss why he or she does not want to talk. Often the reluctant partner is afraid that any discussion will erupt into conflict. The safety and structure of the speaker–listener technique are designed to help allay such concerns.

Increasing Deposits

Like any good financial management strategy, the PREP approach seeks not only to minimize withdrawals but to maximize deposits. Thus, several PREP modules focus on enhancing the positive elements of romantic relationships. This goal is achieved by program leaders' overarching emphasis that the program is designed to "make a good thing better," as well as through specific exercises and activities.

One example of these tasks is the "fun deck." This activity involves a couple's brainstorming a list of fun activities, and each partner's individually picking three favorite activities. Then the partners exchange their lists of top three activities, and select at least one of each partner's activities that they will make sure happens in the following week. Couples usually enjoy this homework assignment and are encouraged to continue using their fun decks after PREP ends.

Another example of an enhancement task is the "friendship talk." In this activity, spouses set aside a block of time outside the PREP session to "talk like friends." During the friendship talk, problem discussion is prohibited; the talk revolves around sharing hopes, goals, or feelings and thoughts about personal, not couple, issues. The friendship talk is not only a way for the partners to experience nonjudgmental, supportive sharing, but to enhance their intimacy and trust with each other. A strong sense of intimacy and trust is the cornerstone for one of the most important characteristics of strong relationships: commitment.

Increasing Commitment

Greater levels of self-disclosure and less conflict about marital issues have both been associated with higher levels of personal-dedication commitment (Markman et al., 1994). "Personal-dedication commitment" is the intrinsic desire to maintain and improve the quality of the relationship. This type of commitment is very different from "constraint commitment," which refers to how difficult it would be to leave the relationship (see Markman et al., 1994, for a discussion of this issue). We have identified the following as factors that are consistent with personal-dedication commitment in relationships: desiring the long-term success of the relationship, maintaining high priority for the relationship, having a team orientation as opposed to an orientation toward oneself alone, valuing sacrificing for the partner, and avoiding monitoring of alternatives.

"Monitoring of alternatives" refers to seriously entertaining notions of affairs or relationships with individuals other than the partner. Individuals with less dedication monitor alternative romantic partners to a greater degree than do more dedicated partners. In addition, less dedicated couples engage more in "score keeping," or monitoring the flux of the partners' respective contributions to the relationship. This short-run view is diametrically opposed to the long-term outlook that satisfied couples maintain.

In PREP, we normalize the vagaries of day-to-day marital satisfaction, and build on our financial metaphor by emphasizing the value of thinking of marriage as a long-term investment. Our work suggests that the relationship between personal-dedication commitment and satisfaction is reciprocal: Satisfied couples are those that are higher in personal dedication, and deeper dedication grows out of a history of marital satisfaction. Thus, personal-dedication commitment is a significant and important concept in understanding and preventing the erosion of marital satisfaction.

CONCLUSION

In summary, the tools we have presented from PREP (and, indeed, all of PREP itself) are designed to help couples develop the skills and gain the insights needed to maintain high levels of relationship satisfaction over time and to prevent the lessening of satisfaction—something that seems inevitable in most marriages. However, we want to highlight the fact that this lessening is not a passive diminishing of the positive factors that draw people together, but an active *erosion* of these positive elements as a result of destructive interaction, communication, and conflict management. Again, we repeat that the positive factors that draw people together—love, attraction, perceived and actual similarities, trust, and commitment—are indicative of marital choice, but not marital success. Instead, how couples handle differences is the critical factor. When differences are not handled well, the positive elements in a relationship erode over time. In this chapter we have presented our initial version of erosion theory, along with empirical data from a longitudinal study that led us to this theory. We have found that nearly everyone wants to maintain high levels of satisfaction in a relationship and is very motivated to have a long-term love and friendship relationship with one partner. These types of relationships not only are valued, but also are positive influences on individuals' mental and physical health and on the health of society at large.

REFERENCES

Acitelli, L. K., & Antonucci, T. C. (1994). Gender differences in the link between marital support and satisfaction in older couples. *Journal of Personality and Social Psychology, 67,* 688–698.

Anderson, S. A., Russell, C. S., & Schumm, W. R. (1983). Perceived marital quality and family life-cycle categories: A further analysis. *Journal of Marriage and the Family, 45,* 127–139.

Aron, A., & Henkemeyer, L. (1995). Marital satisfaction and passionate love. *Journal of Social and Personal Relationships, 12,* 139–146.

Barnett, P. A., & Gotlib, I. H. (1988). Psychosocial functioning and depression: Distinguishing among antecedents, concomitants, and consequences. *Psychological Bulletin, 104,* 97–126.

Behrens, B. C., & Sanders, M. R. (1994). Prevention of marital distress: Current issues in programming and research. *Behaviour Change, 11,* 82–93.

Belsky, J., Lang, M., & Huston, T. L. (1986). Sex typing and division of labor as determinants of marital change across the transition to parenthood. *Journal of Personality and Social Psychology, 50,* 517–522.

Burgess, E. W., & Cottrell, L. S. (1939). *Predicting success or failure in marriage.* New York: Prentice-Hall.

Christensen, A., & Heavey, C. L. (1990). Gender and social structure in the demand/withdraw pattern of marital conflict. *Journal of Personality and Social Psychology, 59,* 73–81.

Clements, M. L., & Markman, H. J. (1997). *Declines in marital functioning over the transition to parenthood: Blame the marriage and not the child.* Manuscript in preparation.

Clements, M. L., Stanley, S. M., & Markman, H. J. (1997). *Prediction of marital distress and divorce: A discriminant analysis.* Manuscript in preparation.

Cowan, C. P., Cowan, P. A., Heming, G., Garret, E., Coysh, W. S., Curtis Boles, H., & Boles, A. J. (1985). Transitions to parenthood: His, hers, theirs. *Journal of Family Issues, 6,* 451–481.

Davis, K. B. (1929). *Factors in the sex life of twenty-two hundred women.* New York: Harper.

Dunn, R. L., & Schwebel, A. I. (1995). Meta-analytic review of marital therapy outcome research. *Journal of Family Psychology, 9,* 58–68.

Fincham, F. D., & Bradbury, T. N. (1987). The assessment of marital quality: A reevaluation. *Journal of Marriage and the Family, 49,* 797–809.

Fowers, B. J. (1991). His and her marriage: A multivariate study of gender and marital satisfaction. *Sex Roles, 24,* 209–221.

Gilligan, C. (1982). *In a different voice: Psychological theory and women's development.* Cambridge, MA: Harvard University Press.

Gottman, J. M. (1994). *Why marriages succeed or fail.* New York: Simon & Schuster.

Gottman, J. M., Markman, H. J., & Notarius, C. I. (1977). The topography of marital conflict: A sequential analysis of verbal and nonverbal behavior. *Journal of Marriage and the Family, 39,* 461–478.

Gottman, J. M., Notarius, C. I., Gonso, J., & Markman, H. (1976). *A couple's guide to communication.* Champaign, IL: Research Press.

Hahlweg, K., & Markman, H. J. (1988). Effectiveness of behavioral marital therapy: Empirical status of behavioral techniques in preventing and alleviating marital distress. *Journal of Consulting and Clinical Psychology, 56,* 440–447.

Hamilton, G. V. (1929). *A research in marriage.* New York: Boni.

Heavey, C. L. (1995). Promoting the marital adjustment of first time parents: A pilot test of PREP. In C. L. Heavey (Chair), *Marital adjustment during the transition to parenthood.* Symposium conducted at the annual meeting of the Association for Advancement of Behavior Therapy, Washington, DC.

Heavey, C. L., Layne, C., & Christensen, A. (1993). Gender and conflict structure in marital interaction: A replication and extension. *Journal of Consulting and Clinical Psychology, 61,* 16–27.

Houseknecht, S. K. (1987). Voluntary childlessness. In M. B. Sussman & S. K. Steinmetz (Eds.), *Handbook of marriage and the family* (pp. 369–395). New York: Plenum Press.

Huston, T. L., McHale, S., & Crouter, A. (1986). When the honeymoon's over: Changes in the marital relationship over the first year. In R. Gilmour & S. Duck (Eds.), *The emerging field of personal relationships* (pp. 109–132). Hillsdale, NJ: Erlbaum.

Huston, T. L., & Vangelisti, A. L. (1991). Socioemotional behavior and satisfaction in marital relationships: A longitudinal study. *Journal of Personality and Social Psychology, 61,* 721–733.

Jacobson, N. S. (1985). The role of observational measures in behavior therapy outcome research. *Behavioral Assessment, 7,* 297–308.

Johnson, D. R., Amoloza, T. O., & Booth, A. (1992). Stability and developmental change in marital quality: A three-wave panel analysis. *Journal of Marriage and the Family, 54,* 582–594.

Jordan, P. L. (1995). PREP Pilot: Transition to parenthood. In C. L. Heavey (Chair), *Marital adjustment during the transition to parenthood*. Symposium conducted at the annual meeting of the Association for Advancement of Behavior Therapy, Washington, DC.

Julien, D., & Markman, H. J. (1991). Social support and social networks as determinants of individual and marital outcomes. *Journal of Social and Personal Relationships, 8*, 549–568.

Karney, B. R., & Bradbury, T. N. (1995). *Measuring the trajectory of marital quality in newlyweds*. Poster presented at the annual meeting of the Association for Advancement of Behavior Therapy, Washington, DC.

Karney, B. R., Bradbury, T. N., Fincham, F. F., & Sullivan, K. T. (1994). The role of negative affectivity in the association between attributions and marital satisfaction. *Journal of Personality and Social Psychology, 66*, 413–424.

Kurdek, L. A. (1993). Nature and prediction of changes in marital quality for first-time parent and nonparent husbands and wives. *Journal of Family Psychology, 6*, 255–265.

Locke, H. J., & Wallace, K. M. (1959). Short marital adjustment and prediction tests. Their reliability and validity. *Marriage and Family Living, 21*, 251–255.

MacDermid, S. M., Huston, T. L., & McHale, S. M. (1990). Changes in marriage associated with the transition to parenthood: Individual differences as a function of sex-role attitudes and changes in the division of household labor. *Journal of Marriage and the Family, 52*, 475–486.

Markman, H. J., Duncan, S. W., Storaasli, R. D., & Howes, P. W. (1987). The prediction and prevention of marital distress: A longitudinal investigation. In K. Hahlweg & M. Goldstein (Eds.), *Understanding major mental disorders: The contribution of family interaction research* (pp. 266–289). New York: Family Process Press.

Markman, H. J., & Floyd, F. (1980). Possibilities for the prevention of marital discord: A behavioral perspective. *American Journal of Family Therapy, 8*, 29–48.

Markman, H. J., Floyd, F. J., Stanley, S. M., & Jamieson, K. (1984). A cognitive/behavioral program for the prevention of marital and family distress: Issues in program development and delivery. In K. Hahlweg & N. S. Jacobson (Eds.), *Marital interaction: Analysis and modification* (pp. 396–428). New York: Guilford Press.

Markman, H. J., Floyd, F., Stanley, S. M., & Storaasli, R. (1988). The prevention of marital distress: A longitudinal investigation. *Journal of Consulting and Clinical Psychology, 56*, 210–217.

Markman, H. J., & Hahlweg, K. (1993). The prediction and prevention of marital distress: An international perspective. *Clinical Psychology Review, 13*, 29–43.

Markman, H. J., Renick, M. J., Floyd, F. J., Stanley, S. M., & Clements, M. (1993). Preventing marital distress through communication and conflict management training: A 4- and 5-year follow-up. *Journal of Consulting and Clinical Psychology, 61*, 70–77.

Markman, H. J., Silvern, L., Clements, M., & Kraft-Hanak, S. (1993). Men and women dealing with conflict in heterosexual relationships. *Journal of Social Issues, 49*(3), 107–126.

Markman, H. J., Stanley, S. M., & Blumberg, S. L. (1994). *Fighting for your marriage: Positive steps for preventing divorce and preserving a lasting love.* San Francisco: Jossey-Bass.

Notarius, C. I., & Markman, H. J. (1993). *We can work it out: Making sense of marital conflict.* New York: Putnam.

Renick, M. J., Blumberg, S. L., & Markman, H. J. (1992). The Prevention and Relationship Enhancement Program (PREP): An empirically based preventive intervention program for couples. *Family Relations, 41,* 141–147.

Rollins, B. C., & Cannon, K. L. (1974). Marital satisfaction over the family life cycle: A re-evaluation. *Journal of Marriage and the Family, 36,* 271–283.

Ruble, D. N., Fleming, A. S., Hackel, L. S., & Stangor, C. (1988). Changes in the marital relationship during the transition to first time motherhood: Effects of violated expectations concerning division of household labor. *Journal of Personality and Social Psychology, 55,* 78–87.

Sher, T. G., Baucom, D. H., & Larus, J. M. (1990). Communication patterns and response to treatment among depressed and nondepressed maritally distressed couples. *Journal of Family Psychology, 4,* 63–79.

Spanier, G. B. (1976). Measuring dyadic adjustment: New scales for assessing the quality of marriage and similar dyads. *Journal of Marriage and the Family, 38,* 15–38.

Spanier, G. B., & Lewis, R. A. (1980). Marital quality: A review of the seventies. *Journal of Marriage and the Family, 42,* 825–839.

Stanley, S. M., & Markman, H. J. (1996). *A national survey of marriage.* Unpublished manuscript, PREP, Inc., Denver, CO.

Storaasli, R. D., & Markman, H. J. (1990). Relationship problems in the early stages of marriage: A longitudinal investigation. *Journal of Family Psychology, 4,* 80–98.

Terman, L. M., & Wallin, P. (1949). The validity of marriage prediction and marital adjustment tests. *American Sociological Review, 14,* 497–504.

Tucker, P., & Aron, A. (1993). Passionate love and marital satisfaction at key transition points in the family life cycle. *Journal of Social and Clinical Psychology, 12,* 135–147.

Vaillant, C. O., & Vaillant, G. E. (1993). Is the U-curve of marital satisfaction an illusion? A 40-year study of marriage. *Journal of Marriage and the Family, 55,* 230–239.

Veroff, J., Kulka, R. A., & Douvan, E. (1981). *Mental health in America: Patterns of help seeking from 1957 to 1976.* New York: Basic Books.

Waring, E. M., & Patton, D. (1984). Marital intimacy and depression. *British Journal of Psychiatry, 145,* 641–644.

Wood, W., Rhodes, N., & Whelan, M. (1989). Sex differences in positive well-being: A consideration of emotional style and marital satisfaction. *Psychological Bulletin, 106,* 249–264.

CHAPTER 14

A Schema-Focused Perspective on Satisfaction in Close Relationships

JEFFREY YOUNG
VICKI GLUHOSKI

Schema-focused therapy was developed by Young (Young, 1994a; Young & Klosko, 1993/1994) as an expansion of Beck's cognitive therapy model (Beck, Rush, Shaw, & Emery, 1979), specifically to address more difficult, chronic life patterns and disorders. This chapter outlines a schema-focused view of satisfaction in intimate relationships. We describe the etiology of relationship satisfaction, discuss the obstacles to obtaining satisfaction, and finally suggest treatment strategies to enhance relationship satisfaction.[1]

CONCEPTUAL MODEL

Core Needs and Domains

The schema-focused model suggests that relationship satisfaction occurs when early core needs and later adult needs are both fulfilled. Core needs begin at birth and continue throughout the lifespan. We describe how these needs can be satisfied in childhood, and how they subsequently affect adult relationship satisfaction. Adult needs begin to emerge in adolescence and also play a prominent role in relationship satisfaction. However, this chapter focuses on core needs, since they are central to the schema-focused model.

Young (1994a) has suggested that core needs can be categorized into several broad domains that appear to be valid across individuals. We have adapted Young's original list of core domains for this chapter, in order to address more specifically the topic of close relationships. The six domains hypothesized to be related to romantic relationships are Basic Safety and Stability; Close Connection to Another; Self-Determination and Self-Expression; Self-Actualization; Acceptance and Self-Esteem; and Realistic Limits and Concern for Others. We outline the core needs associated with each domain, describe how these needs can be fulfilled in childhood, and relate them to adult relationship satisfaction.

The first domain is Basic Safety and Stability. Successful resolution of this domain results in children's expectation that their needs for security, consistency, and predictability will be met. In addition, they experience trust and respect for their boundaries. Finally, these children are not exposed to verbal, physical, or sexual abuse. Parents who provide this environment tend to be even-tempered, reliable, and respectful of their children. Furthermore, they rarely leave their young children alone for long periods.

Children who are raised in this type of environment generally seek stable and reliable partners when they become adults, and they feel that they can count on their partners. Their adult relationships are usually committed and secure. They expect that their partners will not leave them, which produces a sense of security.

The second domain is Close Connection to Another. In this arena, children feel nurtured, loved, understood, and accepted. They receive physical affection, as well as guidance. Parents who are warm, compassionate, involved, and loving will fulfill these needs.

As adults, these individuals usually enter relationships that are loving and warm, often involving a great deal of affection and empathy. These partners are comfortable expressing their feelings toward each other, and they value both physical and emotional intimacy. They derive great joy from being part of a couple, and can both give love to and accept it from their partners, which contributes to their rich relationships.

Third, the domain of Self-Determination and Self-Expression includes the freedom to express and assert individual preferences and feelings in daily situations. Children who are healthy in this domain possess a strong sense of self-determination without excessive control by others. Their needs and feelings are valued by others. They are encouraged to make their own decisions, and a sense of competence is fostered.

In adult relationships, these individuals usually choose partners who respect their ideas and value their input in decision making. They are encouraged to express their own needs in daily situations by partners who are neither selfish nor domineering. In addition, their partners are not intimidated or made uncomfortable by expressions of emotion; thus, these individuals know that they can express their desires and feelings, and their partners will still be supportive.

The fourth domain, Self-Actualization, reflects individuals' freedom to pursue their own interests and natural inclinations autonomously, without undue interference from others. Individuals high on this domain do not feel held back by others, and generally are able to develop and maintain an independent identity. Parents who foster self-actualization in their children are often flexible and easygoing, encouraging growth and independence. These parents maintain appropriate interpersonal boundaries and minimize enmeshment with their children.

In intimate adult relationships, these individuals are able to retain their own identity, and expect that their partners will do so also. The members of such couples have both shared and independent interests, so that the preferences and inclinations of both individuals are taken into account when choices are made. For example, if one partner is offered a job in a different city, the impact of the move on the other individual will weigh heavily in the decision-making process.

Fifth, the domain of Acceptance and Self-Esteem includes the need for praise and unconditional acceptance, along with freedom from punishment. To fulfill these needs, parents are firm but fair. Although rules are enforced, these children feel highly respected and valued.

As adults, these individuals choose partners who take pride in and value them. Their partners are thoughtful, caring, and appreciative; they reassure and bolster confidence when the individuals have self-doubts, and they are the individuals' biggest fans.

The final domain, Realistic Limits and Concern for Others, includes the need to develop empathy for others, and to accept the normal expectations and limitations imposed on all individuals by society. Individuals understand and follow rules of fairness and reciprocity, and they accept responsibility for behaving in a way that enhances others' well-being. To encourage this development, parents teach by modeling appropriate and considerate interpersonal behaviors. They also invoke consequences when their children misbehave, thus setting limits and teaching self-discipline.

This domain is evident in adult relationships when both partners are fair and willing to compromise. These relationships are marked by empathy for and understanding of each person's position, as well as a sense of reciprocity. In addition, partners behave in a way that is considerate and respectful of each other; for example, they are consistently faithful and honest.

The six domains outlined above reflect what we hypothesize to be some of the basic needs of all individuals, in regard to relationship satisfaction. When these core needs are fulfilled, most individuals experience satisfaction from their relationships. However, many factors can interfere with achieving a full degree of satisfaction. We focus primarily on three psychological barriers to intimacy: early maladaptive schemas (EMSs), emotional temperaments, and maladaptive coping styles.

Early Maladaptive Schemas

According to Young's (1994a) model, EMSs are viewed as the core of personality disturbance. These EMSs are broad, pervasive life themes regarding oneself and others, and encompass the primary cognitive and emotional obstacles to satisfying relationships. Schemas[2] have several defining characteristics:

1. They are accepted as truths about oneself and others, regardless of objective evidence to the contrary.
2. They are self-perpetuating, rigidly held, and difficult to change.
3. They are dysfunctional, either to oneself or to others.
4. They are often triggered by environmental events.
5. They are associated with high degrees of affect when they erupt.
6. They block an individual from meeting one or more of the core needs discussed earlier in this chapter.

When children's core needs *are* met, they develop adaptive schemas and are more likely to experience satisfying relationships. Unfortunately, because schemas function primarily outside of awareness, individuals usually do not recognize when they are influencing interpersonal functioning in maladaptive ways.

We hypothesize that EMSs develop in childhood as a response to ongoing negative interactions with significant others, particularly parents and other family members. These negative developmental events interact with a child's temperament to produce a schema.

Eighteen EMSs have been identified thus far; 11 of these are directly relevant to close relationships. Because these schemas are the cognitive and emotive structures that interfere with children's attempts to meet their core needs, they can be grouped into the same six domains described earlier (see Table 14.1). We now discuss how individual schemas are linked to the domains and core needs we have outlined above.

TABLE 14.1. Domains Linked with Early Maladaptive Schemas

Domain: Basic Safety and Stability

1. Abandonment/Instability

The perceived instability or unreliability of those available for support and connection. Involves the sense that significant others will not be able to continue providing emotional support, connection, strength, or practical protection because they are emotionally unstable and unpredictable (e.g., angry outbursts), unreliable, or erratically present; because they will die imminently; or because they will abandon the patient in favor of someone better.

2. Mistrust/Abuse

The expectation that others will hurt, abuse, humiliate, cheat, lie, manipulate, or take advantage. Usually involves the perception that the harm is intentional or the result of unjustified and extreme negligence. May include the sense that one always ends up being cheated relative to others or "getting the short end of the stick."

Domain: Close Connection to Another

3. Emotional Deprivation

Expectation that one's desire for a normal degree of emotional support will not be adequately met by others. The three major forms of deprivation are:

   a. *Deprivation of nurturance:* Absence of attention, affection, warmth, or companionship.

   b. *Deprivation of empathy:* Absence of understanding, listening, self-disclosure, or mutual sharing of feelings from others.

   c. *Deprivation of protection:* Absence of strength, direction, or guidance from others.

Domain: Self-Determination and Self-Expression

4. Subjugation

Excessive surrendering of control over one's behavior, emotional expression, and decisions, because one feels coerced—usually to avoid anger, retaliation, or abandonment. Involves the perception that one's own desires, opinions, and feelings are not valid or important to others. Frequently presents as excessive compliance, combined with hypersensitivity to feeling trapped.

   Almost always involves the chronic suppression of anger toward those perceived to be in control. Usually leads to a build up of anger that is manifested in maladaptive symptoms (e.g., passive–aggressive behavior, uncontrolled outbursts of temper, psychosomatic symptoms, withdrawal of affection, "acting out," substance abuse).

5. Dependence/Incompetence

Belief that one is unable to handle one's everyday responsibilities in a competent manner, without considerable help from others (e.g., take care of oneself, solve daily problems, exercise good judgment, tackle new tasks, make good decisions). Often presents as helplessness.

Domain: Self-Actualization

6. Unrelenting Standards/Hypercriticalness
   The underlying belief that one must strive to meet very high internalized standards of behavior and performance, usually to avoid criticism. Typically results in feelings of pressure or difficulty slowing down, and in hypercriticalness toward oneself and others. Must involve significant impairment in pleasure, relaxation, health, self-esteem, sense of accomplishment, or satisfying relationships.
   Unrelenting standards typically present as (a) *perfectionism*, inordinate attention to detail, and an underestimate of how good one's own performance is relative to the norm; (b) *rigid rules* and "shoulds" in many areas of life, including unrealistically high moral, ethical, cultural, or religious precepts; or (c) preoccupation with *time and efficiency*, so that more can be accomplished.

7. Enmeshment/Undeveloped Self
   Excessive emotional involvement and closeness with one or more significant others (often parents), at the expense of full individuation or normal social development. Often involves the belief that at least one of the enmeshed individuals cannot survive or be happy without the constant support of the other. May also include feelings of being smothered by, or fused with, others, or insufficient individual identity. Often experienced as a feeling of emptiness and floundering, having no direction, or in extreme cases questioning one's existence.

8. Approval Seeking
   Excessive emphasis on gaining approval, recognition, or attention from other people, or fitting in, at the expense of developing a secure and true sense of self. One's sense of esteem is dependent primarily on the reactions of others, rather than one's own internalized values, standards, or natural inclinations. Sometimes includes an overemphasis on status, appearance, social acceptance, money, competition, or achievement—being among the best or most popular—as a means of gaining approval. Frequently results in major life decisions that are inauthentic or unsatisfying; hypersensitivity to rejection; or envy of others who are more popular or successful.

Domain: Acceptance and Self-Esteem

9. Defectiveness/Shame
   The feeling that one is defective, bad, unwanted, inferior, or invalid in important respects, or that one would be unlovable to significant others if exposed. May involve hypersensitivity to criticism, rejection, and blame; self-consciousness, comparisons, and insecurity around others; or a sense of shame regarding one's perceived flaws. These flaws may be *internal* (e.g., selfishness, angry impulses, unacceptable sexual desires) or *external* (e.g., undesirable physical appearance, social awkwardness).

10. Punitiveness
    The tendency to be angry, intolerant, harshly critical, punitive, and impatient with those people (including oneself) who do not meet one's expectations or

(cont.)

TABLE 14.1. (continued)

standards. Usually includes difficulty forgiving mistakes or tolerating limitations in oneself or others, because of a reluctance to consider extenuating circumstances, allow for human imperfection, empathize with feelings, be flexible, or see alternative points of view.

Domain: Realistic Limits and Concern for Others

11. Entitlement
Insistence that one should be able to do or have whatever one wants, regardless of what others consider reasonable or the cost to others; or the excessive tendency to assert one's power, force one's point of view, or control the behavior of others in line with one's own desires—without regard to others' needs for autonomy and self-direction. Often involves excessive demandingness and lack of empathy for others' needs and feelings.

Note. Copyright 1996 by Jeffrey Young, PhD. Unauthorized reproduction without written consent of the author is prohibited. For more information, write Cognitive Therapy Center of New York, 3 East 80th Street, Penthouse, New York, NY 10021.

Schemas Linked to Basic Safety and Stability

Two schemas are closely linked to the domain of Basic Safety and Stability. Abandonment/Instability reflects the view that others will be unstable or unreliable in giving support. Individuals may expect that loved ones will leave or die. This schema may develop if a child is raised by inconsistent parents or in a chaotic environment. It may also emerge if a parent leaves the home or leaves a child alone for long periods.

Adults with this schema are continually afraid that their partners will leave them. They do not have a sense that their relationships are secure, which produces ongoing anxiety. They may seek constant reassurance from partners that they will not be abandoned, or they may perpetuate the schema by choosing unreliable partners. Conversely, in the absence of this schema, healthy individuals choose partners who are dependable and committed. A sense of security is thus maintained.

Mistrust/Abuse includes the expectation that others will hurt, humiliate, or exploit the individual. This harm is believed to be intentional or malicious. This view may develop if children experience abuse, betrayal, manipulation, or dishonesty.

In unhappy adult relationships, individuals may choose partners who are verbally or physically abusive. Others may believe that they cannot trust their partners, perhaps accusing them of infidelity. In the absence of this schema, satisfying relationships occur because individuals tend to select partners who are loyal and respectful. These individuals feel safe and protected when with their partners.

Schema Linked to Close Connection to Another

Emotional Deprivation is the schema most relevant to the domain of Close Connection to Another. Individuals with this schema expect that their need for support will not be adequately met by others. Three types of deprivation are prominent. Deprivation of nurturance involves the lack of attention and warmth. Deprivation of empathy includes an absence of understanding and listening. Deprivation of protection occurs if children do not receive guidance and safety. Typically, individuals with this schema are raised by parents or other caretakers who are emotionally unavailable, withholding, or detached.

Adults with this schema may have an overwhelming need for support, attention, or affection from their partners that is impossible to fulfill, and thus dissatisfaction results. Other individuals may become involved with partners who are cold and withholding, similar to their childhood caretakers. When this schema is not present, individuals feel understood and cared for by their partners. Such partners are attentive and offer input, so each individual feels nurtured.

Schemas Linked to Self-Determination and Self-Expression

The schema of Subjugation involves relinquishing control to others to avoid negative consequences (e.g., anger or rejection). Individuals may subjugate needs by suppressing opinions or preferences, or they may inhibit emotional expression. Individuals with this schema may experience conditional acceptance as children. For example, they may only be valued for the assistance they give with household responsibilities. They are taught to suppress their daily needs in order to avoid retaliation by parents, and they learn that their desires are insignificant. Their parents are probably controlling and domineering.

Individuals with this schema in adult relationships are often dissatisfied because they put their partners' needs and desires first. For example, they may never express an opinion about shared activities, such as vacations or entertainment. They are subsequently disappointed and angry when their partners choose something they do not really want. They may also choose partners who need to dominate and control. Without this schema, partners in healthy relationships are able to express and fulfill their needs. The partners are willing to negotiate and compromise, leading to satisfaction for both.

Dependence/Incompetence involves individuals' belief that they are incapable of adequately handling daily responsibilities. Such individuals may perceive themselves as helpless and requiring much assistance from others. Parents who are overprotective may foster this schema in their children. Through criticism, they may undermine their children's confidence in their own ability to make decisions and function competently. Unsatisfying adult relationships for these individuals may include partners who are overprotective, but make them feel safe. Though they may feel infantilized, they believe that they cannot function without a caretaker. Individuals without this schema select partners who support their strengths and encourage them to strive toward new and challenging goals. The partners reassure each other about their competence, talents, and abilities.

Schemas Linked to Self-Actualization

The schema of Unrelenting Standards/Hypercriticalness reflects extremely rigid and perfectionistic internalized standards, usually to avoid feeling shame. Individuals with this schema may be critical of themselves and others. Typically they are raised by perfectionistic parents who focus on their children's performance and who would not tolerate mistakes. These children were unable to follow their "true selves," because their focus is always on meeting the parents' expectations for achievement.

Adults with this schema may be very demanding of their partners, with unrealistically high expectations. When the partners cannot fulfill these demands, these individuals become angry and disappointed. Others with this schema may choose "trophy" partners who meet their high standards on the surface, but the relationships may be superficial and dissatisfying in terms of intimacy. Some individuals with this schema may choose partners whom they can never satisfy, in a repetition of the relationship they had with their parents; they are too concerned with meeting high standards to develop a true sense of self. In satisfying relationships without this schema, partners accept each other as imperfect, with both assets and weaknesses. By holding a realistic view and reasonable expectations, individuals are more likely to be pleased with their partners and to develop in line with their natural inclinations.

The schema of Enmeshment/Undeveloped Self is also linked to the domain of Self-Actualization. Individuals with this schema are overly involved with their significant others and possess a limited sense of individual identity. This schema may result from parents who are overinvolved with their children, do not respect the children's boundaries or privacy, and thus limit the children's independent development.

Individuals with an Enmeshment/Undeveloped Self schema may select adult partners who are similarly intrusive and do not respect boundaries or encourage independent growth. These individuals may feel that they are extensions of their partners, without their own identity. A common example is a wife who has never worked outside of the home, but instead focuses solely on furthering her husband's career. In a healthy adult relationship without this schema, the couple is interconnected, but each partner maintains some separate interests. Each individual is recognized and appreciated for his or her unique contribution to the relationship, and thus self-actualizes.

Approval Seeking is the final schema associated with Self-Actualization. These individuals focus on receiving recognition or attention from others. Their self-worth is derived from others' opinions of them. As children, these individuals may receive positive attention only if they behave or perform in certain ways.

As adults, they may repeat this pattern by choosing partners who admire them for specific attributes, such as attractiveness or wealth. Thus, they may feel pressure to maintain a certain image or else lose their partners. Others may seek out loved ones who never accept them as they are, although they continually try to please. Individuals with Approval Seeking may become frustrated when they are unable to gain approval or recognition. In healthy relationships without this schema, love is not contingent on performance. Individuals realize that they can make mistakes or have flaws, and their partners will still approve of them. In this environment, partners can pursue their unique interests and talents without worrying unduly about seeking approval.

Schemas Linked to Acceptance and Self-Esteem

The Defectiveness/Shame schema is linked to the domain of Acceptance and Self-Esteem. These individuals believe that they are bad or inferior in core realms. They may view themselves as inherently unlovable. This schema may develop if a child's parents are critical or rejecting.

Unhappy adult relationships for these individuals may involve partners who reinforce their negative self-view. Their partners may be critical or demeaning. Potential partners who treat them well may be rejected, because this experience is so contrary to what they have experienced as children. Adaptive, satisfying relationships for individuals without this schema involve partners who enhance their self-esteem. Such partners are proud of the individuals and contribute to their sense of worth.

A Punitiveness schema is defined by the view that people should be severely punished for their mistakes. Individuals with this schema are intolerant and impatient with themselves and others. Their parents were probably unnecessarily harsh when they made even minor mistakes.

In adult relationships, individuals with a Punitiveness schema are often rejecting or harshly punitive if their partners do almost anything wrong. Others with this schema may choose partners who are rigid and unforgiving like their parents. In healthy adult relationships without this schema, partners are accepting and forgiving of each other's mistakes. They work together to resolve errors by solving problems, instead of making one partner feel ashamed or punished.

Schema Linked to Realistic Limits and Concern for Others

Individuals who are impaired in the domain of Realistic Limits and Concern for Others often have an Entitlement schema. They may believe they are superior and deserving of special privileges, and usually lack empathy and concern for others. Parents who are very indulgent, who actively teach their children to view themselves as superior, or who have trouble setting limits and invoking consequences usually encourage the development of Entitlement.

In adult relationships, individuals with this schema are often inconsiderate and self-focused. They may not understand why their partners are unhappy, but instead just feel hassled or nagged. They may be involved in extramarital relationships, without concern about how this might affect their partners. In satisfying relationships without Entitlement, individuals treat their partners with respect and concern. The well-being of the couple is as important as each individual's happiness, and healthy partners often sacrifice many of their own desires, without resentment, for the good of the relationship.

Emotional Temperaments

Basic temperament can also serve as an obstacle to interpersonal satisfaction. Recently, temperament theorists (see Millon, 1981, for a review) have focused on biological etiologies of personality. These personality styles are long-standing and difficult to change.

The schema-focused model suggests that several specific emotional temperaments can affect close relationships (Young & Gluhoski, 1996). We have presently identified seven temperaments: "emotional," "dysthymic," "anxious," "obsessive," "irritable," "nonreactive," and "cheerful" (see Table 14.2). Temperament may affect the degree, associated affect, and direction (i.e., inward or outward) of behavior in relationships. Each of these temperaments can strongly influence how individuals interact with their partners; unfortunately, individuals have limited control over this aspect of their makeup, except sometimes through psychotropic medication.

Serious relationship dissatisfaction may arise as a result of temperament, particularly when one or both partners have one of the more

TABLE 14.2. Emotional Temperaments

1. *Emotional, reactive:* Emotionally intense, inconsistent, labile, impulsive, highly sensitive.
2. *Dysthymic, discouraged:* Easily discouraged, bouts of low energy and desire, pessimistic, depressive.
3. *Anxious, frightened:* Easily frightened, focuses on "uncontrollable" danger, catastrophizes.
4. *Obsessive, worried:* Obsesses about "controllable" things that could go wrong, decisions, etc. Has difficulty relaxing and putting mind at peace. Overly focused.
5. *Irritable, angry:* Short-tempered, impatient, irascible, Type A.
6. *Flat, nonreactive:* Calm, consistent, unemotional, flat, insensitive.
7. *Cheerful, optimistic:* High-spirited, resilient, rebounds quickly, positive.

Note. Copyright 1996 by Jeffrey Young, PhD. Unauthorized reproduction without written consent of the author is prohibited. For more information, write Cognitive Therapy Center of New York, 3 East 80th Street, Penthouse, New York, NY 10021.

emotionally intense temperaments, or if the partners have markedly different temperaments. For example, individuals who are extremely irritable and impatient may exhibit behavior that leads their partners to reject or leave them. Partners with contrasting styles may come to feel a deep sense of incompatibility. For example, an individual who is flat and nonreactive may be unhappy with a partner who is emotional and labile. Thus, compatibility of temperaments can greatly influence relationship satisfaction.

Schema Processes and Coping Styles

So far in this chapter, we have focused primarily on domains, schemas, and temperaments. All of these are essentially *internal* constructs— components of cognition and emotion. We now focus more on how these internal constructs lead to specific *behaviors* that influence satisfaction in close relationships.

Schema Processes

Schemas are translated into behavior via three general processes: "maintenance," "avoidance," and "compensation." Schema maintenance includes maladaptive behaviors that directly support the EMS. For example, individuals with a Mistrust/Abuse schema often choose dishonest, manipulative, or abusive partners who reinforce their view of others as malevolent. Alternatively, other individuals with this schema may select honest, reliable partners, yet they still behave suspiciously toward them. For example, they may exhibit unrealistic jealousy or make unjustified accusations, consistent with their distorted expectations of mistreatment and betrayal.

Schema avoidance includes mechanisms to avoid activating the schema and its related affect. For example, individuals with an Abandonment/Instability schema may engage in avoidance by not allowing themselves to become intimate in their close relationships; by maintaining distance, they feel they can prevent themselves from being hurt if their partners leave them. Individuals with a Subjugation schema may avoid it by not discussing areas of conflict with their partners, or by hiding their anger to avoid arguments.

Finally, schema compensation involves developing a style that is opposite to the core schema. This may be particularly prevalent in individuals who appear narcissistic. Their grandiosity and entitlement may actually be means of compensating for core feelings of defectiveness or emotional deprivation. For example, narcissists may believe: "No one would love me for my true self; I have no inherent value." They may then try to attract others by focusing on and pointing out aspects of their surface desirability, such as their important jobs or material wealth. They may hope that these attributes will attract partners, not realizing that they usually appear self-absorbed and superficial.

Coping Styles

These three broad schema processes have been refined into 11 specific coping styles (see Table 14.3). These are the actual behaviors that people engage in to cope with their schemas. For example, individuals with a Mistrust/Abuse schema may treat their partners with aggression–hostility when their schema is triggered. The aggression is a tangible, observable result of the individual's attempt to cope or adapt to the maladaptive schema. These coping styles are believed to develop early in life, as a result of both basic temperament and parental modeling. The concept of coping styles has been further refined by Young to address satisfaction in close relationships; the next section presents this adaptation of the coping style concept for intimate relationships.

Spectrums and Poles

In examining close relationships, Young proposes five spectrums of behavior: Connection, Power, Feeling, Mutuality, and Valuing. A "spectrum" is a dimension of behavior that partners engage in moment to moment as they relate to each other. We believe that the success of

TABLE 14.3. Maladaptive Coping Styles

1. *Aggression–hostility:* Vents anger directly and excessively: defies, abuses, blames, attacks, or criticizes.

2. *Manipulation–exploitation:* Meets own needs through *covert* manipulation, seduction, dishonesty, or conning.

3. *Dominance, excessive self-assertion:* Controls others through *direct* means to accomplish goals, with little regard for needs or feelings of others.

4. *Recognition seeking, status seeking:* Overcompensates through impressing, high achievement, status, attention seeking, etc.

5. *Distraction, stimulation seeking:* Seeks excitement or distraction, often through risk taking, action, or novelty.

6. *Dependence, approval seeking:* Reliant on others, seeks affiliation, passive, dependent, submissive, clinging, avoids conflict, people-pleasing.

7. *Excessive self-reliance:* Exaggerated focus on independence, rather than depending on others. (Note: Is reasonably comfortable around people and is not socially isolated.)

8. *Compulsivity, overcontrol:* Maintains strict order, tight self-control, or high level of predictability through compulsive order and planning, or excessive adherence to routine or ritual.

9. *Psychological withdrawal:* Copes through addiction, dissociation, denial, fantasy, or other internal forms of psychological escape.

10. *Passive–aggressiveness:* Appears overtly compliant while venting anger or punishing others covertly through procrastination, pouting, "backstabbing," lateness, complaining, rebellion, nonperformance, etc.

11. *Social withdrawal, situational avoidance:* Avoids life situations that might trigger discomfort or negative outcomes; and/or experiences social contact as aversive and copes through social isolation.

a romantic relationship depends to a considerable degree on how well partners resolve conflicts along each of these five spectrums.

Conflicts arise when partners move to the extreme points at either end of a spectrum. For example, the extreme points along the Connection spectrum are Smother and Isolate. Young calls these extreme points on a spectrum "poles" (or "coping stances"). Poles are the extremes of maladaptive behavior that partners move toward when their schemas are triggered (see Table 14.4.). Thus poles are the specific coping styles that partners exhibit in close relationships; they represent individuals' maladaptive attempts to get their core needs met.

TABLE 14.4. Spectrums and Poles

SPECTRUM	Pole	↔	Pole
CONNECTION	Smother	↔	Isolate
POWER	Submit	↔	Dominate
FEELING	Emotionalize	↔	Intellectualize
MUTUALITY	Self-Sacrifice	↔	Self-Serve
VALUING	Idealize	↔	Devalue

Note. Copyright 1996 by Jeffrey Young, PhD. Unauthorized reproduction without written consent of the author is prohibited. For more information, write Cognitive Therapy Center of New York, 3 East 80th Street, Penthouse, New York, NY 10021.

Dissatisfaction in close relationships often develops when a dispute or life event activates one partner's early core schema. This individual then (without awareness) moves toward a pole (an extreme coping stance) on one of the five spectrums of behavior. Subsequently, this maladaptive, extreme behavior activates a schema in the other partner, who then also moves toward a pole on either the same or a different spectrum. Consequently, each partner is stuck at an extreme pole, creating a cycle of chronic dissatisfaction.

We use the case of David and Melissa to illustrate our model. David has a Mistrust/Abuse schema, which resulted from growing up with an abusive father. Melissa has a Dependence/Incompetence schema, as a consequence of her parents' coddling and overprotecting her. One quality of Melissa's that draws David to her is her air of vulnerability. This helps him trust her.

David and Melissa have been dating for 2 years. Now Melissa's parents are pressuring her to get married. As she feels her parents' support for her situation lessening, Melissa begins to feel frightened. She worries about ending up with no one to take care of her. Her Dependence schema is triggered. She goes to the Dominate pole: She yells at David, cries and demands that they get married, and behaves punitively when he resists. This triggers David's Mistrust schema, and he withdraws from her. He moves toward the Isolate pole. This further frightens Melissa, retriggering her Dependence schema and pushing her to an even more extreme position at the Dominate pole; this further drives David away, until the quality of the relationship is significantly eroded over time. Figure 14.1 illustrates this sequence.

We now describe the five spectrums and elaborate on their associated life poles.

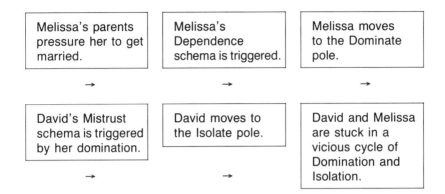

FIGURE 14.1. Illustrative diagram of conflict cycle. Copyright 1996 by Jeffrey Young, PhD. Unauthorized reproduction without written consent of the author is prohibited. For more information, write Cognitive Therapy Center of New York, 3 East 80th Street, Penthouse, New York, NY 10021.

Connection

On the Connection spectrum, partners either attach and move toward intimacy, or move away from intimacy by withdrawing and detaching. In healthy relationships, partners maintain a balance between attachment and autonomy. Problems arise when an extreme style is utilized. Smother and Isolate are the two poles associated with this spectrum. Individuals who feel deprived may compensate for this feeling by seeking too much of an attachment with their partners. Partners may feel overwhelmed and retreat. Conversely, individuals may withdraw first from their loved ones and become detached. Both of these behaviors are maladaptive and lead to dissatisfaction.

Power

The Power spectrum is associated with issues of control. Finding balance on this spectrum is one of the greatest challenges couples face. At one extreme, an individual may let the partner control the situation by relinquishing all power. The other extreme consists of one partner's dominating and bullying the other. The poles on this spectrum are Submit and Dominate. Individuals who believe that their safety or control is threatened may react by becoming domineering and bossy. Others may become increasingly passive or overly compliant. Both extreme styles usually result in unhappiness.

Feeling

The spectrum of Feeling is characterized by differences in emotional expression. Most often, women emotionalize while men intellectualize, although sometimes the reverse is the case. Women often go to their male partners seeking comfort and sympathy for a problem. Men may move into a problem-solving mode and try to generate solutions. The women then feel misunderstood and patronized. The men may become frustrated because their input is disregarded.

This spectrum thus includes the poles of Emotionalize and Intellectualize. Some individuals may become too emotionally expressive, weeping or complaining excessively. Individuals at the other extreme are rigid problem solvers who often lack empathy. The result is frequently that the conflict moving the partners toward dysfunctional poles is not resolved and the dispute is intensified.

Mutuality

On the Mutuality spectrum, the goal is a balance between give and take. However, problematic relationships may be characterized by one partner who gives too much, and another who is selfish and disregards the other's needs. The sacrificing partner may eventually burn out; anger builds and compassion fades. Self-sacrifice and Self-serve are the poles on this spectrum. Individuals who relinquish their own needs and desires, and thus put their partners first, are self-sacrificing. Those who are selfish and demanding demonstrate the other pole, self-serving. Both styles, if extreme, may produce dissatisfaction.

Valuing

Healthy goals on the Valuing spectrum include respecting and valuing the partner, but within a realistic light. Problems arise when stances involving either too much adoration or a very critical approach develop. The poles on this spectrum are Idealize and Devalue. A Defectiveness/ Shame schema is often associated with this spectrum. Individuals who themselves feel defective may compensate for this schema by criticizing and devaluing their partners. Others may maintain their negative self-view by unrealistically idealizing their partners. They view their partners as having extreme positive value that they cannot achieve themselves. Thus, these individuals hold extreme views of their loved ones that are unrealistic and cannot be fulfilled.

SCHEMA-FOCUSED TREATMENT

We now describe how to intervene with couples to enhance their relationship satisfaction. We briefly review the general treatment model, and then outline four stages of schema-focused therapy for couples: the initial sessions, assessment and education, individual change, and couple work. We assume that the therapist is working with both partners, as couple works is most effective in enhancing close relationships. However, our model of couple work often involves individual sessions with each partner, as well as couple sessions.

Overview of Schema-Focused Therapy

Schema-focused therapy (Young, 1994a) is divided into two components: assessment and change. The assessment component emphasizes identifying and activating those EMSs that are particularly salient for each client. This is accomplished through several mechanisms: (1) a life review, which identifies patterns and links current problems with their early origins; (2) educating clients about schemas, through such sources as Reinventing Your Life (Young & Klosko, 1993/1994); (3) reviewing the client's scores on schema inventories; (4) activating schemas through imagery, dialogues, and other experiential techniques; (5) noting patterns in the therapeutic relationship; and (6) identifying long-term maladaptive behavior patterns and coping styles.

The change component of schema-focused therapy involves modifying the most relevant and problematic schemas and coping styles. This component of treatment includes integrating four types of interventions: (1) cognitive strategies, such as disputing the validity of the schemas, reframing negative events, and carrying out dialogues between the negative schemas and the healthier perspective; (2) experiential techniques, to achieve emotional change, including imagery and role playing; (3) the therapeutic relationship, in which the therapist may serve a limited reparenting role, or may interpret and confront the influence of schemas in the therapy relationship; and (4) breaking of behavioral patterns which involves changing the negative self-defeating behaviors activated by schemas, including couple work and modification of coping styles.

Early Sessions: Establishing Problems and Patterns

In couple work, the early sessions focus on assessing the reasons for the couple's dissatisfaction and the areas of dispute. In the first two or three sessions, the therapist meets together with both partners to establish each person's view of what would increase satisfaction. Each partner explains, as specifically as possible, what the other person does to contribute to his or her dissatisfaction. To facilitate understanding of the situation, the therapist may ask such questions as "What do you want that you're not receiving from your partner?", "What does your partner do that frustrates you?", or "What expectations are not being met?"

The therapist then tries to obtain and analyze one or two prototypical problematic interactions between the partners, by having them reenact these in the session. A "prototypical problem" refers to an ongoing theme or pattern in disputes. For example, some couples may have ongoing fights about money, while others typically argue about sex or affection. The therapist then asks both partners to identify their thoughts and feelings during the reenactments. At this stage, the therapist makes some tentative hypotheses about the poles and schemas that each partner manifests; these hypotheses may or may not be shared with the clients at this phase.

We will describe one couple, Mark and Julia, throughout this part of the chapter to illustrate schema-focused treatment. They sought therapy because Julia viewed Mark as cold and aloof. In session, she described a recent fight in which she had had a bad day at work and wanted his support. He asked whether they could discuss it later, as he was relaxing then. In reenacting the fight, Julia reported that she thought, "I'm not important to him. I feel alone." Her subsequent emotions were sadness and loneliness. Mark stated that he thought, "She's so demanding and needy. I just need some time to myself now." He felt nagged and annoyed. The therapist began to hypothesize that Julia had an Emotional Deprivation schema and that Mark held a Subjugation schema. However, she did not yet share this view with the couple, as she wanted to gather more information.

During these early sessions, each partner is also asked to fill out for homework various questionnaires that are part of schema-focused therapy, including the Multimodal Life History Inventory (Lazarus & Lazarus, 1991), the Young Schema Questionnaire, second edition (Young & Brown, 1994), the Young Parenting Inventory (Young, 1994b), the Young–Rygh Avoidance Inventory (Young & Rygh, 1994), and the Young Compensation Inventory (Young, 1995a). These questionnaires are reviewed later with the couple, as we explain below.

Assessment and Education

The next few sessions are conducted either individually or with the couple together, depending on the level of trust and preferences of each partner. Usually partners will alternate sessions if they are held individually. During these sessions, the therapist reviews the assessment materials with each client, describing each client's high-scoring schemas and coping styles (i.e., poles).

Each of the questionnaires has a different function. The Multimodal Life History Inventory (Lazarus & Lazarus, 1991) includes a broad range of questions to assess family history, current symptoms, self-views, fears, images, cognitions, physical sensations, expectations of therapy, and psychosocial functioning. The Young Schema Questionnaire (Young & Brown, 1994; Schmidt, Joiner, Young, & Telch, 1995) enables the therapist to pinpoint which specific schemas are salient for each partner. Two other inventories assess coping styles. The Young–Rygh Avoidance Inventory (Young & Rygh, 1994) uncovers avoidant behaviors that partners may employ. The Young Compensation Inventory (Young, 1995a) examines coping behaviors that involve overcompensation (e.g., excessive recognition seeking or rebelliousness) and that may result from maladaptive schemas.

The rationale for reviewing the questionnaires is to teach clients about their particular schemas, and about how these schemas influence their behavior, relationships, and emotions. Often it is beneficial to review each individual's results in the presence of the partner; this approach facilitates greater understanding of and empathy for the other partner. It is emphasized that understanding schemas and their associated coping processes is the first step toward change, but that insight alone will not usually increase satisfaction significantly.

Clients are also encouraged to begin reading *Reinventing Your Life* at this point as an adjunct to the sessions. This book explains the schema-focused model in a manner that is easy for clients to absorb. Each schema is described, along with its origins, sustaining mechanisms, and tools for change. Partners are assigned the chapters relevant to their schemas. The therapist points out that this assignment will enable them to understand and apply the model faster, and thus may lead to satisfaction earlier.

The next stage of assessment consists of partners' engaging in early childhood imagery involving their mothers and fathers. In this exercise, clients are asked to close their eyes and evoke a childhood image of themselves with one of their parents. Clients are encouraged to describe the scene in detail, noting their emotions and cognitions. They are also encouraged to carry on a dialogue with the parent in the image, expressing their needs and feelings to the parent. This exercise is then repeated with the other parent. The purpose of this exercise is to identify themes developed early in life that are linked to schemas. For example, when Mark described a scene with his father, he recalled a time when he was excited about winning a softball trophy and was eager to show his award to his father. However, when he happily burst into the house, his father yelled at him for being so noisy. His father was angry because Mark's excitement had disrupted his nap. Mark knew that his father's needs came first and did not bother to show him the trophy. He felt that his own emotions had to be held back, and, although he was now angry at his father, he did not express it. This image revealed Mark's Subjugation schema.

After both partners have completed these tasks, the therapist reviews their results on the Young Parenting Inventory (Young, 1994b). On this inventory, they rate each of their parents separately on items associated with each of the maladaptive schemas. Sample items include "My mother lied to me, deceived me, or betrayed me" and "My father overprotected me." This inventory, along with the imagery, further enables the therapist and the couple to understand how particular schemas developed and how they are linked to current problems.

As a final stage of assessment, couples rate each other on each of the 10 poles, on a scale from 0 to 10. This exercise enables the therapist to see how each of the partners typically copes with problem areas. It also highlights which spectrums are particularly problematic for the couple. For example, Mark and Julia had problems primarily on the Connection and Power spectrums. She viewed their problem as one of disconnection. When her Emotional Deprivation schema was activated, she moved toward the Smother pole on the Connection Spectrum. Julia thus dealt with conflict by smothering Mark with demands for closeness. However, this behavior activated Mark's Subjugation schema. He viewed the problem as a power struggle. Subsequently, he reacted through retreating as a coping stance—that is, moving toward the Isolate pole. Both partners continued to feel dissatisfied.

After all of this information is compiled, the therapist has an extensive understanding of the presenting problem, relevant schemas, and coping styles. Feedback is then given to the couple. The presenting problems and prototypical interactions are linked to each partner's maladaptive schemas, childhood origins, and poles. The partners begin to understand how early experiences have led to the development of certain schemas and poles. They recognize that their current problems and typical ways of interacting with each other are the culmination of long-term patterns. This feedback is usually enlightening and validating for couples. Clients generally emerge from these sessions with an enhanced understanding of themselves and their partners; this sets the stage for the change process to begin.

For instance, Julia saw that Mark had never learned to be comfortable with intimacy because of his cold, domineering parents. She recognized that her demands only caused him to feel burdened and then to avoid her. Mark learned more about the impact of Julia's parents' divorce: Although she was smothered by her mother, she had little contact with her father. These two extreme experiences contributed to her problems with connection. He learned to see that when she made requests of him, it was because she wanted a connection to him, not because she was trying to control him.

Change Phase I: Individual Cognitive and Experiential Work

Schema-focused couple therapy incorporates two phases of change: individual work and couple work. In this section we discuss the individual component; the couple work is outlined below, in the discussion of Phase II. The individual schema work may be done in couple sessions, individual sessions, or both.

The individual phase uses schema-focused strategies similar to those utilized for clients who come to therapy alone (not as part of a couple). There is a focus in this phase on cognitive and experiential techniques for changing schemas. Cognitive tools include teaching the client to examine schemas rationally and seek evidence supporting or refuting the negative views. The negative thoughts and alternative responses are written out in the Schema Diary (Young, 1993). Schema Flashcards (Young, 1995b) are also developed, which involve writing out statements challenging the maladaptive schemas. The client then reads these cards whenever these schemas are activated, to lessen their intensity. Schema dialogues are another valuable technique. The client practices developing a "healthy voice" to argue back against the "schema voice." This strengthens a new, positive view and diminishes the maladaptive schema.

Julia made extensive use of schema dialogues. In session, she had the "schema voice" begin by discussing how she thought that her needs for affection, understanding, and guidance would never be met by others. She then switched chairs and had the "healthy voice" respond by pointing out how her needs could be met if she asked others in a more appropriate, less overwhelming style. The "healthy voice" reassured her that others could be available to her if she did not smother them. Julia later reported that this exercise helped her see how her intense demands pushed others away and only left her feeling more deprived.

Other experiential strategies, such as those found in gestalt therapy, are also employed. These techniques may include imagery, role playing, dialogues, and venting of affect. For example, Mark was instructed to create an image in which he expressed his anger toward his father for being so controlling and angry. He was hesitant at first, but as the image unfolded, he became quite emotional. The purpose of using such tools is to further modify the maladaptive schemas into healthier, more functional views by empowering clients to assert their rights. In Mark's case, he learned that he had the ability to stand up to his father and express himself. He realized that he did not have to feel subjugated, because he had the tools to be assertive.

A focus on the therapeutic relationship may also be utilized. The therapist may provide personal observations about each client in relation to the therapist, to point out negative styles and enhance change. Links among maladaptive in-session interactions, maladaptive schemas, and coping styles are discussed. The goal here is to teach clients about their impact on others when their schemas are activated. For example, at the end of Mark and Julia's sessions, Julia frequently lingered and asked the therapist many questions. The therapist began to feel controlled and answered in a curt manner. In a subsequent session, the therapist pointed out this interaction. She explained how Julia's Emotional Deprivation schema triggered her smothering demands, which in turn led the therapist to isolate, as Mark often did.

Change Phase II: Couple Work

In Phase II, most of the work is done with both partners together in session. The focus now is on specific partner interactions, blending cognitive, experiential, and behavioral exercises. In this phase, partners utilize their Schema Diaries, dialogues, and Schema Flashcards from Phase I to modify their interactions. For example, when Mark was late returning from work one day, Julia thought, "He doesn't love me." She was upset because her Emotional Deprivation schema had erupted, and she began to retaliate by crying and insisting that Mark hold her and comfort her. Her coping style again was to smother, which led him to isolate, which further intensified her Emotional Deprivation schema. However, she was now able to see that her reaction was schema-driven. Realistically, she knew that he did love her. When she was able to view the situation this way, she calmed down and apologized.

The focus in this phase shifts more to the behavioral coping styles (poles) both partners move toward when their schemas are triggered. Partners help each other by empathizing with each other's schemas, and then using a helpful coping style to enable each other to heal the schemas, instead of moving toward a maladaptive pole. In addition, the prototypical interactions identified in the initial sessions are replayed in healthier ways, with both partners attending to and modifying their schemas and coping behaviors. Finally, homework is assigned to enable the partners to practice the new interaction styles.

For example, as noted earlier, Julia's Emotional Deprivation schema led her to develop a clinging, dependent coping style. Her predominant pole was Smother. The therapist recognized that Mark had a Subjugation schema for which he compensated by moving toward the Isolate pole. The relationship was problematic because she wanted more closeness and he appeared to want more distance. They gradually learned more moderate styles of interacting. Julia began to challenge her beliefs that Mark did not love her, and subsequently was able to give him more space. He then felt less overwhelmed and wanted more time with her. They also completed homework assignments that focused on giving and receiving more moderate signs of affection, which eventually became more intimate. This enabled Mark to be less aloof as he gradually increased his attention to Julia.

Alternative coping behaviors are also rehearsed in session to substitute for negative poles. For example, because they had problems along the Connection spectrum, Mark was instructed to hold Julia's hand as she described her sense of loneliness. This small gesture made her feel much more connected, and also showed him that he did not have to make elaborate gestures to satisfy her.

Each of the spectrums and associated poles discussed earlier in this chapter can be modified with similar techniques. The goal is to teach couples less extreme ways of coping and interacting. On the Connection spectrum, problems are the result of a smothering or isolating style. Smothering individuals are taught to seek intimacy without overwhelming their partners. They observe their thoughts, feelings, and behaviors each time they have the urge to smother. They then use techniques such as Schema Flashcards or Schema Diaries to ease the intensity of their schemas. Isolating partners are shown how to provide support so their significant others see that they care. They are taught mirroring techniques and empathic, active listening skills.

Submit and Dominate are the poles of the Power spectrum. Couples with problems in this area are taught how to compromise and solve problems. The partners learn negotiation skills, such as the importance of making specific requests and avoiding criticism of each other. Learning how to be appropriately assertive, rather than too passive or domineering, is usually valuable for individuals at both extremes of this spectrum. Individuals at the Dominate pole see that their requests will be met without resorting to an aggressive style.

Emotionalize and Intellectualize are the extreme poles associated with the Feeling spectrum. Individuals with an emotional style can learn how to manage their reactions through rational thinking or relaxation strategies. Eventually, they are able to express their feelings without overreacting. Overly logical partners can begin attending to emotions and developing perspective-taking skills. They practice identifying and expressing feelings, focusing on bodily sensations, and mirroring their partners' feelings.

On the Mutuality spectrum, the poles are Self-Sacrifice or Self-Serve. Self-sacrificing individuals learn to focus on the disadvantages of their style, as well as the benefits of expressing their needs. They may be encouraged to write out these advantages and disadvantages, and to look at this card in situations when they feel inclined to sacrifice. Self-serving partners learn how to respect others more and focus on what is good for both individuals. In decision making, they learn to ask themselves, "Is this choice good for both of us, or just for me?"

The Valuing spectrum includes the Idealize and Devalue poles. Clients who idealize learn to view significant others in a more realistic light. By viewing partners realistically, idealizing individuals develop a more accurate view of their partners and their relationships. Devaluing individuals are taught noncritical ways of communicating. They learn not to put down their partners, and are instructed to focus on their partners' positive attributes.

We want to emphasize that partners usually have problems along more than one spectrum. Therapists should not be discouraged by this, since progress can occur in multiple areas simultaneously. Modifying schemas and coping styles can have far-reaching results.

SUMMARY AND CONCLUSIONS

This chapter has applied Young's schema-focused therapy to relationship satisfaction. The schema-focused model suggests that individuals have core needs that begin at birth. If these needs are not fulfilled, children develop EMSs. These schemas lead to dysfunctional partner selections, overreactions, and maladaptive coping styles, which lead in turn to relationship dissatisfaction.

As outlined above, these schemas and coping styles can be altered through schema-focused therapy. Initially, the therapist assesses and activates the schemas and coping styles operating in each partner. Subsequently, change procedures are implemented to enhance relationship satisfaction.

The altering of maladaptive schemas and poles is the primary mechanism of change, both in individual and in couple work. Utilizing a broad repertoire of techniques—including cognitive, experiential, interpersonal, and behavioral tools—the clinician can produce significant schema-level change. Subsequently, partners experience enhanced satisfaction in their close relationships.

NOTES

1. Throughout this chapter, we use the term "relationship satisfaction" to refer to close, intimate relationships with a romantic component.
2. The term "schema" is used throughout the rest of this chapter interchangeably with "early maladaptive schema" (EMS).

REFERENCES

Beck, A. T., Rush, A. J., Shaw, B. F., & Emery, G. (1979). *Cognitive therapy of depression*. New York: Guilford Press.

Lazarus, A., & Lazarus, C. (1991). *Multimodal Life History Inventory*. Champaign, IL: Research Press.

Millon, T. (1981). *Disorders of personality: DSM-III, Axis II*. New York: Wiley.

Schmidt, N. B., Joiner, T. E., Young, J. E., & Telch, M. J. (1995). The Schema Questionnaire: Investigation of psychometric properties and the hierarchical structure of a measure of maladaptive schemas. *Cognitive Therapy and Research, 19*, 295-321.

Young, J. E. (1993). *Schema diary*. (Available from the Cognitive Therapy Center of New York, 3 East 80th Street, Penthouse, New York, NY 10021)

Young, J. E. (1994a). *Cognitive therapy for personality disorders: A schema-focused approach* (rev. ed.). Sarasota, FL: Professional Resource Press.

Young, J. E. (1994b). *Young Parenting Inventory*. (Available from the Cognitive Therapy Center of New York, 3 East 80th Street, Penthouse, New York, NY 10021)

Young, J. E. (1995a). *Young Compensation Inventory*. (Available from the Cognitive Therapy Center of New York, 3 East 80th Street, Penthouse, New York, NY 10021)

Young, J. E. (1995b). *Schema flashcards*. (Available from the Cognitive Therapy Center of New York, 3 East 80th Street, Penthouse, New York, NY 10021)

Young, J. E., & Brown, G. (1994). Young Schema Questionnaire (2nd ed.). In J. E. Young, *Cognitive therapy for personality disorders: A schema-focused approach* (rev. ed.). Sarasota, FL: Professional Resource Press.

Young, J. E., & Gluhoski, V. L. (1996). Schema-focused diagnosis for personality disorders. In F. W. Kaslow (Ed.), *Handbook of relational diagnosis and dysfunctional family patterns* (pp. 300–321). New York: Wiley.

Young, J. E., & Klosko, J. S. (1994). *Reinventing your life*. New York: Plume. (Original work published 1993)

Young, J. E., & Rygh, J. (1994). *Young–Rygh Avoidance Inventory*. (Available from the Cognitive Therapy Center of New York, 3 East 80th Street, Penthouse, New York, NY 10021)

PART 5

CONCLUSION

CHAPTER 15

———◆◆———

Satisfaction in Close Relationships: Challenges for the 21st Century

MARK A. WHISMAN

> On entering into family life he saw at every
> step that it was not at all what he had
> imagined. At every step he felt as a man might
> feel who, after admiring the smooth, cheerful
> motion of a boat on the water, actually gets
> into the boat himself. He saw that apart from
> having to sit steadily in the boat without
> rocking, he also had to keep in mind, without
> forgetting for a moment where he was going,
> that there was water beneath his feet, that he
> had to row, that his unaccustomed hands hurt,
> and that it was easy only when you looked at
> it, but that doing it, though it made you very
> happy, was very hard.
> —LEO TOLSTOY, *Anna Karenina*

Understanding "satisfaction" in close relationships would appear, at first blush, to be an easy task. After all, most individuals have been in one or more intimate relationships. However, upon closer examination, one feels like the character in *Anna Karenina*: One quickly sees that a myriad of factors contribute to satisfaction, and that maintaining the satisfaction in close relationships, like maintaining stability of a boat in water, requires skillful coordination of these factors. For, like the character

385

in this novel, one quickly finds out that satisfaction in close relationships is not a static, unmoving "thing," but rather a fluid, changing "process." Similarly, basic and applied research on satisfaction are ever-changing fields, as suggested by the breadth of the contributions in this volume.

Studies of close relationships have proliferated since the 1930s, when the first book on psychological factors in satisfaction in marriage was published by Terman and his associates (Terman, Buttenweiser, Ferguson, Johnson, & Wilson, 1938). As a rough indicator of the amount of research conducted on satisfaction in close relationships, a computer search of the Psychological Literature (PsycLIT) data base—which contains information from 1967 to the present from the fields of psychology and related social and behavioral sciences—identified over 2,500 entries that included the terms "satisfaction" and "marriage" or "marital."

This volume brings together several of the most recent and enduring themes regarding satisfaction in close relationships. In this chapter, I highlight some common elements discussed by the contributors to this volume, and discuss some issues to be considered in the next generation of research on satisfaction in close relationships. It is not my goal to provide a comprehensive integration of all the perspectives discussed, but to highlight some points of convergence among the various perspectives and to introduce a model for their organization. In the final section of this chapter, I highlight some implications and applications of the chapters for the maintenance of satisfaction in close relationships.

SATISFACTION IN CLOSE RELATIONSHIPS: CONCEPTUAL AND METHODOLOGICAL CONSIDERATIONS

Before I address the correlates and maintenance of satisfaction in close relationships, I believe it is important to consider the methods involved in studying satisfaction. In this section, the common measures and participants involved in studying satisfaction in close relationships are briefly reviewed, and suggestions for future research are offered.

What Is the "Satisfaction" That Is Being Evaluated?

First, let us review how "satisfaction" in close relationships is typically quantified in scientific investigations. Although there are numerous measures for assessing satisfaction, and these differ in length and content (as reviewed by Sabatelli, 1988), most measures are paper-and-pencil (i.e., self-report) instruments that ask individuals to provide subjective evaluations of their relationships. A typical item on these scales is something similar to "How satisfied are you with your relationship?" Thus, although there may be some differences among self-report questionnaires in the number and kinds of questions included, measures of relationship satisfaction are highly correlated; this is cited as evidence of the validity of these measures (Sabatelli, 1988).

More recently, however, investigators have challenged whether commonly used self-report questionnaires are pure measures of "satisfaction" (i.e., happiness). As reviewed in greater detail elsewhere (e.g., Fincham & Bradbury, 1987; Norton, 1983), the assessment of satisfaction through questionnaires is often confounded by the inclusion of items other than satisfaction items (e.g., items measuring frequency of sexual relations, and items regarding how often partners disagree about a variety of topics). For example, Eddy, Heyman, and Weiss (1991) reported that although the factor structure of one commonly used measure—the Dyadic Adjustment Scale (Spanier, 1976)—suggests that the items are highly interrelated and compose one higher-order factor, the items referring directly to "satisfaction" accounted for only 25% of the variance in the total score. Because of the inclusion of these other items, investigators (e.g., Fincham & Bradbury, 1987; Norton, 1983) have proposed that the construct being measured by such scales may best be viewed as "adjustment" (or "quality"), rather than as "satisfaction."

The issue, however, is more than an academic debate regarding the appropriate label for these measures. Of greater concern is the risk of overlap (or confounding) of closely related if not identical concepts. That is, if the dependent variable (i.e., the "satisfaction" measure) includes items similar if not identical to those included in the independent variables (i.e., measures of the correlates of satisfaction), then there may be a thinly veiled tautology in obtaining an association between "satisfaction" and other variables. To address this problem, researchers (e.g., Fincham & Bradbury, 1987; Norton, 1983) have argued for instruments that do not confound the measurement of satisfaction with other relational events.

Besides challenging the validity of self-report measures of "satisfaction," researchers have recently questioned the equivalence of existing measures. That is, using a common label to describe various measures as instruments for assessing "satisfaction" may obscure differences that exist among measures. For example, we (Whisman & Jacobson, 1992) reported that two measures of satisfaction that are commonly used in evaluating the effectiveness of marital therapy yielded different estimates of the effectiveness of therapy. These results suggest that existing measures are not "created equal" and should not be viewed as interchangeable.

Besides these issues regarding the validity and equivalence of self-report measures of satisfaction, a methodological problem stems from the exclusive reliance on self-report measures in evaluating the quality of close relationships. Because many correlates of satisfaction are also measured by self-report, the association between satisfaction and the correlates of satisfaction may be artificially inflated because of "shared-method variance." That is, individuals' responses to paper-and-pencil self-report measures are influenced by a range of idiosyncratic response biases. For example, those who use extreme scores on one self-report measure are likely to use extreme scores on other measures, whereas those who choose socially desirable response alternatives on one self-report measure are likely to do so on other measures. Thus, if both satisfaction and correlates of satisfaction are assessed by means of self-report, the relation between these measures will be artificially inflated, because the identical response biases will be picked up by both measures.

Although most self-report measures of relationship satisfaction primarily treat satisfaction as a unitary construct, Fincham, Beach, and Kemp-Fincham (Chapter 11) propose that relationship quality consists of both positive and negative elements; the simultaneous existence of satisfaction and dissatisfaction in close relationships is also discussed by Erbert and Duck (Chapter 8). Furthermore, Fincham and colleagues present findings suggesting that positive and negative evaluations of relationship quality are differentially related to relationship behavior and attributions. Although conceptualizing relationship quality as independently consisting of positive and negative evaluations may have important theoretical implications, additional research is needed to establish whether these two aspects of relationship quality are truly independent. In particular, such research should employ multiple assessments (using different formats) of positive and negative evaluations, to ensure that their seeming independence is not the result of biases stemming from random and nonrandom response error—a problem observed in purportedly independent positive and negative aspects of mood (Green, Goldman, & Salovey, 1993).

The following suggestions are offered for future research on satisfaction in close relationships to address the preceding issues. First, investigators should carefully consider the potential overlap in content in their measures of "satisfaction" and the correlates of satisfaction. This may require selecting as dependent variables measures that assess only relationship satisfaction. Alternatively, the degree of overlap can be reduced by removing items from one scale that are confounded with another scale. However, it should be noted that dropping items may alter the psychometric characteristics of a scale (i.e., its reliability and validity); therefore, the psychometric properties of the revised scale should be evaluated. Finally, use of multiple measures of satisfaction that differ in response format may provide a more valid measure of satisfaction in close relationships than any one measure can provide.

Second, greater attention should be paid to using multimethod assessments in studies of close relationships. For example, if satisfaction is to be measured by self-report, then the correlates of satisfaction could be measured by other methods (e.g., observation of actual behavior). Such a practice is common in behavioral studies of communication in close relationships, but has been rarely used in evaluating other models. Obtaining corroborative information about the correlates of satisfaction from other people in an individual's social network (e.g., ratings provided by another family member or friend) would also address the problem of shared-method variance. Alternatively, if the correlates of satisfaction (e.g., love) are to be measured via self-report, then satisfaction could be measured by other means. Although assessment of relationship "satisfaction," which entails a subjective evaluation of the relationship, may require the use of self-report instruments, the assessment of relational "quality" can be evaluated by using other assessment methods. For example, interview-based rating scales of relationship quality could be developed that would supplement the use of self-report measures. There already exist clinician rating scales for evaluating family functioning (e.g., Miller, Kabacoff, Epstein, Bishop, & Keitner, 1994), and the fourth edition of the *Diagnostic and Statistical Manual of Mental Disorders* (American Psychiatric Association, 1994) includes a proposed rating scale—the Global Assessment of Relational Functioning—to be used as "an overall judgment of the functioning of a family or other ongoing relationship" (p. 758). Use of these measures, or the development and use of similar measures of satisfaction other than self-report instruments, would increase confidence in the validity of the observed associations between satisfaction and the correlates of satisfaction in close relationships.

Who Are the Typical Participants of Research on "Close Relationships"?

Second, let us review who is typically evaluated in research on "close relationships." Most studies of intimate relationships include either legally married couples or, less frequently, dating couples. Therefore, the degree to which many findings from these studies generalize to other kinds of romantic relationships (e.g., cohabiting couples, same-sex couples) or to other close relationships (e.g., parental relationships) remains to be evaluated. Moreover, in studying satisfaction in married couples, investigators often use "samples of convenience." For example, researchers often recruit couples through newspaper advertisements, fliers, and other media announcements. Although convenient, this sampling procedure may result in the recruitment of couples that are not representative of the population of interest. For example, couple members who respond to media announcements may be higher in extraversion or neuroticism than people who do not respond. Nonsystematic recruitment may therefore result in a biased sample (i.e., couples with an exaggerated prevalence of certain risk factors that are confounded with the members' probability of volunteering). Moreover, couples recruited in this fashion are often quite satisfied with their relationships. Such a procedure may result in a restricted range of satisfaction, thereby attenuating the magnitude of the relation between satisfaction and the correlates of satisfaction.

A related problem with recruitment in studies on satisfaction in close relationships concerns underrepresentation of individuals from ethnic minority groups. For example, U.S. census data for 1990 suggest that the racial composition of marital couples living in the United States is 84% white (not of Hispanic origin), 7% black, 7% Hispanic; and 2% Asian or Pacific Islander (U.S. Bureau of the Census, 1992). Examination of the participants in most studies on close relationships in the United States, however, suggests that the racial composition of such studies does not reflect this distribution; similar comments can be made regarding studies conducted in other countries. The degree to which studies based on predominantly white, middle-class couples will generalize to other racially or ethnically diverse samples is unknown and should not be assumed. Thus, there is a great need to recruit representative samples in future studies on close relationships.

What then, can be done to improve recruitment practices in research on satisfaction in close relationships? Krokoff (1987) discussed a three-stage procedure for recruiting representative samples for research on intimate relationships, which involved (1) random telephone surveys, (2) direct mailings, and (3) informational meetings in the home. Particularly informative were findings that cooperation was high at each recruitment stage, and that the resulting sample was more representative of the U.S. general population than prior studies. Alternatively, recruiting couples through marital registers may also result in a more representative sample, given that such registers include all couples in a given area. This procedure, however, may result in highly satisfied couples (as most couples are quite satisfied during the very early stages of marriage); it has the added limitation of recruiting only legally married couples, and therefore is inappropriate for research on dating couples, cohabiting couples, and same-sex couples. Although such procedures may require more time and resources than recruiting samples of convenience, investing in similar recruitment procedures may improve the generalizability of findings regarding the correlates of satisfaction in close relationships.

Summary and Recommendations

Satisfaction in close relationships has been measured in prior studies primarily with self-report measures that often include items assessing correlates of satisfaction. Future research should place greater emphasis on using multimethod assessments of satisfaction and on eliminating items from self-report measures that are confounded with correlates of satisfaction. Furthermore, many prior studies have used samples of convenience to evaluate satisfaction in close relationships. Greater attention to recruiting representative samples (in terms of race, socioeconomic status, satisfaction, and the like) is needed in future studies.

A UNIFYING MODEL OF THE CORRELATES OF SATISFACTION IN CLOSE RELATIONSHIPS

There is a vast literature on various characteristics proposed over the years by scientists in their search for the correlates of satisfaction in close relationships. Generally speaking, these fall primarily into one of two categories. One category consists of characteristics that describe something about one or both partners (i.e., intrapersonal characteristics), whereas the other category consists of characteristics that describe the relationship between partners (i.e., interpersonal characteristics). There has been comparatively less research on a third category— environmental characteristics—that may also influence relationship satisfaction.

Figure 15.1 depicts a model based on these three categories, which I have developed to organize and integrate the various characteristics discussed as correlates of satisfaction in close relationships (including those discussed in this volume). The bidirectional arrows between relationship satisfaction and each of the determinants of satisfaction categories illustrate the theoretical position that satisfaction and its determinants can reciprocally influence one another. For example, a satisfying intimate relationship can affect a person's basic trust in others (which is an aspect of the intrapersonal characteristic of attachment), and people in satisfied relationships may become more similar over time (which is an aspect of the interpersonal characteristic of homogamy). In addition, the bidirectional arrows among the three categories of satisfaction correlates represent the theoretical position that characteristics

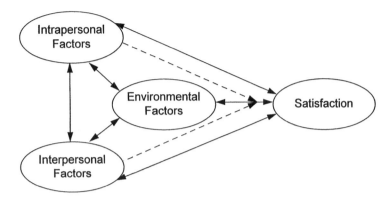

FIGURE 15.1. A heuristic model designed to illustrate the potential integration of the intrapersonal, interpersonal, and environmental influences on satisfaction in close relationships.

in each category are likely to have a reciprocal influence not only on other characteristics within the same category, but on characteristics in the other categories. Therefore, it is acknowledged that the organization of correlates of satisfaction into these three categories is rather arbitrary and does not suggest that the categories are independent or mutually exclusive. As such, the three categories can have an indirect (i.e., mediated) effect on satisfaction. For example, an individual's personality (an intrapersonal characteristic) can influence the individual's communication with his or her partner (an interpersonal characteristic), which in turn can affect each partner's satisfaction. Finally, as discussed in greater detail below, the dotted arrows represent the theoretical position that the intrapersonal and interpersonal categories *moderate* the relation between environmental influences and satisfaction (i.e., intrapersonal and interpersonal characteristics affect the strength and/or direction of the relation between environmental characteristics and relationship satisfaction). In the sections that follow, this model and the three categories of correlates of satisfaction in close relationship are reviewed, and directions for future research are suggested.

Intrapersonal Influences on Satisfaction in Close Relationships

As discussed in many chapters in this volume, considerable attention has been given to evaluating the association between relationship satisfaction and intrapersonal characteristics (i.e., those that reside within the individual). What follows is a partial (i.e., illustrative) listing of some

intrapersonal characteristics identified as important correlates of satisfaction in close relationships.

First, investigators have studied the role of personality in relationship outcomes. That is, researchers have been interested in detecting
whether certain personality characteristics are related to relationship
satisfaction. One personality characteristic that has been linked to satisfaction is "neuroticism" (e.g., Kelly & Conley, 1987), which includes
such behavior or characteristics as worry, anxiety, and emotional reactivity. The chapter by Shackelford and Buss (Chapter 1) adds to the
literature on personality correlates of satisfaction. Specifically, in reviewing research based on the five-factor model of personality, they conclude that "men and women married to agreeable, conscientious,
emotionally stable, and open spouses are happier with their marriages"
(p. 22). Moreover, they review relational behavior and attitudes associated with personality characteristics, thereby offering suggestions about
the mechanisms by which personality may influence satisfaction.

Second, researchers have been interested in how cognitions influence relationship satisfaction. The importance of cognitive processes in adapting to life's circumstances has long been recognized. For
example, Epictetus, a philosopher in the 1st century A.D., wrote, "Men
are disturbed not by things, but by the view which they take of them";
Shakespeare wrote in *Hamlet* that "there is nothing either good or bad
but thinking makes it so." Regarding the scientific study of relationships, Baucom, Epstein, Sayers, and Sher (1989) have proposed five important cognitive variables involved in relationship functioning: selective
attention, attributions, expectancies, assumptions, and standards. Young
and Gluhoski (Chapter 14) add to this literature in discussing core needs
and early maladaptive schemas, which they believe are important to
relationship satisfaction. A particularly interesting aspect of this cognitive model is that these authors propose schema processes and coping styles to explain how schemas are sustained over time. These schema
processes and coping styles may in turn offer points of convergence between intrapersonal and interpersonal (i.e., communication) models of
relationship satisfaction. In addition, whereas most research conducted on cognitive components of relationships has focused on cognitive
contents and products (e.g., beliefs, attributions), the theory and research
discussed by Fincham and colleagues (Chapter 11) are among the first
to examine the role of cognitive *operations* (i.e., means by which relational information is processed). That is, whereas other studies have
primarily focused on *what* people think about their own relationships
and relationships in general, the work discussed by Fincham and colleagues focuses on *how* people think about their relationships. Specifically, the idea that correlates of satisfaction may be more strongly related

to relationship satisfaction for individuals whose happiness with their relationship is more easily "accessible" (i.e., happiness is more highly associated with their representations of their partners in memory) is an important concept that warrants continued systematic investigation.

Third, emotional or affective components of relationship satisfaction have been the focus of many empirical studies. One primary emotion addressed in both theoretical and empirical writings is love. There are many theories of love, as reviewed in the chapters by Barnes and Sternberg (Chapter 4) and Hendrick and Hendrick (Chapter 3). However, the research conducted by Barnes and Sternberg suggests that types of love can be hierarchically organized; these authors conclude, "Theories of love do not differ so much in their validity as they do in their respective emphases on different levels of the overall phenomenon of love" (p. 97). Interestingly, both chapters conclude that although there may be different types of love, two types of love seem particularly salient and important to relationship satisfaction: a "hot" or passionate type of love, and a "warm" or companionate type of love. The fact that both chapters converge on the importance of these two types of love underscores the potential importance of both types in relationship functioning.

Fourth, investigators have examined the influence of attachment styles on relationship satisfaction. Although attachment has long been studied in the context of parent–child relationships, its importance in adult relationships has only more recently been investigated. However, support for the importance of attachment in adult relationships, including romantic relationships, is quickly accumulating, as suggested by the literature reviewed by Koski and Shaver (Chapter 2). Furthermore, whereas many models of relationships (particularly those based on behavioral theory) have not specified the origins of the intrapersonal influences on satisfaction, Koski and Shaver review theoretical and empirical literature suggesting that attachment theory offers a developmental model of how attachment may develop and be maintained across the lifespan.

Interpersonal Influences on Satisfaction in Close Relationships

A second category that scientists have evaluated in their search for the correlates of relationship satisfaction consists of interpersonal characteristics. Indeed, one definition of "satisfaction"—fulfillment of a need or desire—underscores the importance of considering dyadic (i.e., interpersonal) influences on relationship satisfaction, in that a partner and/or a relationship with a partner fulfills an individual's need or want. Interpersonal characteristics can in turn be divided into relationship characteristics (e.g., communication) and between-partner similarity in intrapersonal characteristics (e.g., partner homogamy).

Communication

One of the best-documented findings in the field of close relationships is that communication is a primary determinant of relational satisfaction and outcome (Gottman, 1994). Furthermore, communication problems are the problems most commonly reported by couples seeking couple therapy in the 1990s (Whisman, Dixon, & Johnson, in press). It should come as no surprise, therefore, that studies using self-report measures of communication have consistently reported a relation between positive communication and satisfaction in close relationships. The research conducted by Feeney, Noller, and Ward (Chapter 7) adds to this literature in identifying specific aspects of positive communication associated with relationship satisfaction.

Communication in intimate relationships has also been studied through observing couples' interactions. Early research in the association between communication and relationship satisfaction primarily evaluated the frequency of occurrence of *specific* behavior or affects. For example, as reviewed by Gottman (1994), compared to couples who are satisfied with their relationship, the communication of unsatisfied couples is associated with "(a) enhanced levels of negative interaction and affect; (b) low levels of agreement compared to disagreement; (c) lower levels of humor and laughter, and less reciprocated laughter; (d) fewer assents, agreements, approval, and compliance; and (e) more disagreement, criticism, and put downs" (p. 65). In sum, early research suggested that the interactions of satisfied couples were more positive and less negative than the interactions of couples that were not satisfied with their relationships.

Besides base rates of specific behavior, investigators have examined the *sequences* or patterns of communication associated with satisfaction and stability in close relationships. Several interesting findings have emerged from this literature. One early pattern identified as an important correlate of relationship satisfaction was "negative reciprocity" (Gottman, 1979). This term refers to the probability that the members of a couple will stay in a negative affective state once they enter it. As might be expected, compared to their satisfied counterparts, individuals who are unsatisfied with their relationships tend to be more likely to reciprocate negative affect in their interaction with their partners.

A second pattern of communication that has generated considerable interest in satisfaction in close relationships is one in which one partner demands, complains, and criticizes, while the other partner withdraws with defensiveness and passive inaction. Various labels have been given to this pattern, such as the "demand–withdraw" pattern (Christensen, 1988), and there is an accumulating body of literature supporting an inverse relation between this interaction pattern and satisfaction in close relationships in both cross-sectional (Heavey, Layne, & Christensen, 1993) and longitudinal (Heavey, Christensen, & Malamuth, 1995) research.

Most recently, Gottman (1994) has identified a third pattern of communication that is associated with declines in satisfaction and relationship dissolution. According to Gottman, the important interaction sequence is one in which "complaining and criticizing leads to contempt, which leads to defensiveness, which leads to listener withdrawal from interaction (stonewalling)" (p. 110). Gottman refers to these behaviors as "The Four Horsemen of the Apocalypse" to underscore the corrosive nature of this interaction sequence.

In summary, prior research has shown that the communication of satisfied couples differs from the interaction of unsatisfied couples, both in terms of specific behaviors and in terms of sequences or patterns of interaction.

Homogamy

A second interpersonal characteristic that has been associated with satisfaction in close relationships is "homogamy," which is the pairing of like with like (i.e., partner similarity). The importance of similarities between partners in influencing satisfaction has long been recognized in both professional and popular conceptualizations of relationships. However, do "birds of a feather flock together" or do "opposites attract"? There is a considerable body of literature (for a review, see White & Hatcher, 1984) that suggests that greater partner similarity is associated with greater relationship satisfaction. The association between partner consensus and satisfaction reported by Feeney and colleagues (Chapter 7) is consistent with this research. Although prior research suggests that homogamy may be related to satisfaction, there has been relatively little theoretical discussion of how dissimilarity leads to relationship unhappiness. Christensen and Walczynski's (Chapter 10) model of how dissimilarity and change in satisfaction are mediated through conflict provides a theoretical advance in our understanding of this process.

One difference between partners in close relationships that has generated considerable interest in recent years has been the interest in gender differences in relationships. Although research suggests that correlates of satisfaction are generally similar for women and men (for a review, see Karney & Bradbury, 1995), gender differences have been observed for some correlates of satisfaction. For example, Koski and Shaver (Chapter 2) review evidence for gender differences in the influence of attachment on satisfaction. Furthermore, the popularity of self-help books on gender differences in relationships suggests that couples resonate to discussions of differences between women and men in relationships, particularly as these apply to differences in styles of communication. Empirical studies have identified gender differences in some, but not all, aspects of communication. For example, Clements, Cordova, Markman, and Laurenceau (Chapter 13) review findings suggesting (1) that the construct of satisfaction may be unidimensional for men but multidimensional for women; and (2) that men tend to withdraw from conflict more than women. Explanations for this gender difference in communication are discussed by Notarius, Lashley, and Sullivan (Chapter 9). The findings that gender differences in communication seem to "ring true" for couples involved in relationships, and that preliminary research provides evidence for some gender differences, suggest that gender differences in relationship satisfaction and its correlates may be an important topic for continued systematic investigation.

Moreover, there may be other partner characteristics, as yet unexamined, for which homogamy may be important for relationship satisfaction. For example, Hojjat (Chapter 5) introduces the view that partner similarity in "philosophy of life" influences the degree of relationship satisfaction. Thus, whereas prior research suggests that similarity may play an important role in satisfaction, research on other variables— including the variables discussed in this volume—is needed for a fuller understanding of the nature of the relation between homogamy and satisfaction in close relationships.

Environmental Influences on Satisfaction in Close Relationships

In their search for the correlates of relationship satisfaction, researchers have often emphasized the importance of intrapersonal and interpersonal correlates of satisfaction, and have seemingly deemphasized the role of environmental influences on relationship functioning. In this section, the importance of stressful life circumstances and other environmental influences on satisfaction in close relationships is discussed.

Stressful Life Circumstances

There has been comparatively little research on the impact of stressful life circumstances on satisfaction in close relationships, relative to the sizeable body of research on interpersonal and intrapersonal correlates of satisfaction. Yet decreases in relationship satisfaction may be attributable in large part to the occurrence of stressful life circumstances.

Several types of stressful life circumstances may have an impact on satisfaction in relationships. First, satisfaction may be influenced by "life events," which are traditionally defined as objective experiences that are sufficiently disruptive or threatening as to require a substantial readjustment by the individual. Such events may include a death, loss of a job, and the like. Second, relationship satisfaction may be influenced by "chronic life stressors," which are traditionally viewed as ongoing problematic conditions and difficulties. Examples of such stressors include environmental stress (e.g., crowding, noise, air pollution), economic stress (e.g., unemployment, inability to pay bills), and living situations (e.g., urban vs. rural residence, type of neighborhood). Finally, satisfaction may be influenced by "microstressors," which are defined as frustrating demands or minor stressors that affect an individual's everyday life. Microstressors include such things as traffic problems, concerns about weight and/or appearance, and having too many things to do.

Besides their direct influence on relationship satisfaction, stressful life circumstances may interact with intrapersonal or interpersonal characteristics in determining satisfaction. One of the most common models for explaining emotional and behavioral problems is the "diathesis–stress" (or "vulnerability–stress") model. In this model, it is proposed that people have certain diatheses or vulnerabilities that make them more or less vulnerable to the impact of stress. Some characteristics contribute to adaptive processes that protect a person from the negative effects of stress, whereas other characteristics may increase the negative effects of stress. Vulnerabilities therefore contribute to an individual's behaving, feeling, and thinking in specific and characteristic ways when he or she is confronted with stressful life circumstances. Thus, emotional and behavioral problems are more likely to develop when a person both has a vulnerability and is under stress. In similar fashion, people may have a vulnerability to develop relational problems (i.e., declines in satisfaction), but this tendency may not become a reality until certain environmental events occur that trigger the vulnerability.

For example, consider how different couples might respond to the birth of a child. When the members of a couple desire to have children, and have prepared for their child, the transition to parenthood may have little impact on their satisfaction with their relationship. However, transition to parenthood may be more difficult for a couple in which one or both partners do not want to have children, or for a couple in which one person is burdened with most of the child rearing because of a lack of support from the other partner or a lack of desire on the other's part to be the primary caretaker. In each case, the same event is presumed to have very different outcomes, depending upon the characteristics of each partner and of the couple. As this example illustrates, dissatisfaction should be greatest when the vulnerability and the stressful condition are both present. When not challenged by exogenous stressful life circumstances, therefore, a vulnerability may remain latent and exhibit little association with relationship satisfaction.

Although other theoretical models have discussed the potential role of stressful life events (e.g., Karney & Bradbury, 1995), other theorists have generally not specified the nature of the relation between such events and satisfaction, or have primarily suggested a main effect for life circumstances. In comparison, based on the empirical support garnered in research on emotional and behavioral problems, I propose that stressful life circumstances influence satisfaction primarily through their interaction with intrapersonal and interpersonal vulnerabilities. Furthermore, the influence of stressful life circumstances may be particularly important for some correlates of satisfaction. For example, as briefly discussed by Koski and Shaver (Chapter 2), the attachment system is hypothesized to be activated only under certain conditions, whereas at other times it is "quiescent." In comparison, however, most studies that have evaluated the importance of attachment styles on relationship satisfaction have not included environmental conditions in their assessments. Consequently, because investigators have not routinely included measures of stressful life circumstances in their research, empirical support for the importance of correlates of satisfaction may be attenuated in existing studies, if the relation between these variables and satisfaction varies as a function of the occurrence of stressful life circumstances.

Other Environmental Factors

Berscheid and Lopes (Chapter 6) discuss how various environmental forces serve to "compel or repel interaction [between partners]" (p. 143). These environmental factors have often been neglected by relationship researchers, who have instead focused on intrapersonal and interpersonal factors. However, a particularly interesting aspect of the model discussed by Berscheid and Lopes is not only that both endogenous and exogenous forces influence the probability of interaction, but that partners exert an influence on the environmental forces governing the probability of continued interaction. Identifying and evaluating the role of these often overlooked factors may help increase our understanding of longitudinal and societal changes in relationship satisfaction and dissolution.

Summary and Recommendations

The correlates of satisfaction evaluated in prior studies fall generally into one of two categories: intrapersonal (i.e., individual) characteristics and interpersonal (i.e., relationship) characteristics. Less attention has been given to a third category—environmental characteristics— that may influence satisfaction, both as a main effect and in interaction with intrapersonal and interpersonal characteristics. Although the findings discussed above are informative, several methodological issues in existing studies limit the conclusions that can be drawn. In the paragraphs that follow, these limitations are discussed, and suggestions are offered for improving the study of relationship satisfaction.

First, in evaluating the literature on the correlates of satisfaction, it should be noted that many of these correlates have been measured with paper-and-pencil (i.e., self-report) measures. Implicit in the use of these measures is the belief that partners' reports represent accurate portrayals of the assessed variables. However, this implicit assumption may be invalid. Weiss (1980) has proposed that responses to self-report measures in research on close relationships are largely influenced by partners' global evaluations of the relationship—a response style that he has labeled "sentiment override." That is, when people are happy with their partners, they endorse almost any positive item about their relationships, their partners, and themselves; when they are unhappy, they endorse almost any negative item. Thus, partners' responses to self-report measures of correlates of satisfaction may be largely influenced by their global evaluations of their relationships as a whole. Because the veridicality of partners' reports may be suspect as a result of sentiment override, there is a greater need for multimethod assessments of the correlates of satisfaction.

Second, it should be noted that most studies of satisfaction in relationships examine the role of a single correlate of satisfaction in isolation from other variables that are important to relationship functioning—a practice criticized by others (e.g., Newcomb & Bentler, 1981). Examining variables in isolation does not provide information regarding how various correlates are related to and influence one another. As discussed by Erbert and Duck (Chapter 8), making connections among factors is necessary for an understanding of how the contradictions and competing demands that individuals encounter are related to satisfaction. Examining correlates of satisfaction in isolation, therefore, does not address how the influence of one correlate may depend on its context (i.e., the presence or absence of other correlates). Moreover, examining correlates of satisfaction in isolation from other correlates does not provide evidence that each variable is uniquely related to satisfaction. That is, if correlates of satisfaction are highly related, then the variance accounted for by one variable may be shared by another variable (i.e., the first variable may not be uniquely related to satisfaction). For example, noting the similarities between attachment theory and social cognition theory (i.e., both theories offer cognitive conceptual frameworks for understanding close relationships), we (Whisman & Allan, 1996) evaluated the incremental validity of these two theories in accounting for relationship satisfaction in dating couples. Our results suggested that measures derived from the two theories, although modestly associated, each accounted for unique variance in couples' satisfaction. Thus, there is a need for future research to include multiple correlates of satisfaction in one study, in order to evaluate (1) the association among hypothesized correlates of satisfaction, and (2) the unique association between each variable and relationship satisfaction. Integrative research such as this is needed to develop and refine theoretical models of satisfaction in close relationships.

Third, an (implicit) assumption in most studies of satisfaction in close relationships is that the correlates of satisfaction are similar across couples. It is quite likely, however, that the reasons for the degree of satisfaction with a relationship may differ for different kinds of people. Accordingly, there may be different kinds or types of satisfied and unsatisfied couples, and these may differ in important ways. There have been attempts to develop typologies of intimate relationships in past research (e.g., Fitzpatrick, 1988; Gottman, 1993), and the chapter by Fincham and colleagues (Chapter 11) introduces a fourfold couple typology based on patterns of positive and negative evaluations of the relationship. In recent years, there has been increasing interest in the attachment categorization system, as reviewed by Koski and Shaver (Chapter 2). In comparison, however, most studies on the correlates of satisfaction have not addressed the potential heterogeneity among couples. Consequently, the importance of specific correlates of satisfaction may have been underestimated, if such correlates apply only to a subset of individuals. Besides differing among subtypes, the correlates of satisfaction may vary for couples at different times in their lives. For example, recent research suggests that the correlates of satisfaction may differ for older and younger couples (e.g., Carstensen, Gottman, & Levenson, 1995; Levenson, Carstensen, & Gottman, 1994). As such, there is a greater need for studies evaluating whether types or stages of close relationships differ in terms of (1) correlates of satisfaction, (2) relationship satisfaction over time, and (3) other relationship outcomes (e.g., relationship stability, outcome to couple therapy).

Finally, many studies on relationship satisfaction have evaluated the correlates of satisfaction via cross-sectional designs, in which both

satisfaction and the correlates of satisfaction are measured concurrently. In discussing the results obtained from cross-sectional studies, authors
often implicitly or explicitly suggest that these factors cause or maintain relationship satisfaction. For example, these correlates are discussed
as "predictors" or "determinants" of satisfaction in close relationships.
Statistical association (i.e., correlation), however, is only one of two
essential criteria for establishing causality. The other criterion—temporal
precedence—can only be evaluated by using longitudinal designs.
Without longitudinal research, we cannot know whether a variable is
a cause, a concomitant, or a consequence of the degree of relationship
satisfaction. Furthermore, recent studies suggest that the characteristics associated with concurrent satisfaction may not be the same characteristics associated with longitudinal changes in satisfaction (e.g.,
Gottman & Krokoff, 1989), and that changes in satisfaction attributed
to life cycle changes may be greater in cross-sectional studies than in
longitudinal studies (Vaillant & Vaillant, 1993). Although a thorough
discussion of longitudinal research is beyond the scope of this chapter,
readers interested in the major theoretical perspectives, empirical findings, and methodological issues involved in longitudinal changes in relationship (i.e., marital) satisfaction and marital status are referred to a
recent review by Karney and Bradbury (1995). Furthermore, as discussed
by Erbert and Duck (Chapter 8), repeated assessments of both satisfaction and the correlates of satisfaction are needed for a full understanding of the nature of change in close relationships.

THE MAINTENANCE OF SATISFACTION
IN CLOSE RELATIONSHIPS

In any long-term relationship between two individuals, it is inevitable
that one partner will engage in behavior that the other person finds
unsatisfactory, and that there will be disagreements between the partners. There is growing agreement that how people react to negative
partner behavior and between-partner disagreement is critical in deciding
how likely they are to maintain their satisfaction in their relationships
(e.g., Gottman, 1994). Thus, the ability to handle conflict constructively may be one of the keys, if not the major key, to long-term satisfaction in close relationships. A thorough review of methods for
improving conflict management through improving communication is
beyond the scope of this chapter. Notarius et al. (Chapter 9) have provided many helpful suggestions, particularly in regard to anger management. Because many well-intentioned partners try to make changes in
their relationships, but get discouraged and give up when widespread

changes do not immediately occur, readers may find Notarius and colleagues' discussion of reasons why it is difficult to make changes in one's relationship particularly interesting and motivating.

In this section, chapters in this volume that address the maintenance and treatment of satisfaction are reviewed, and the implications and applications of the preceding sections for the maintenance of satisfaction are discussed. Specifically, implications for maintaining satisfaction that follow from recognition of the three categories of correlates of satisfaction are outlined. The basic premise behind the following discussion is that if "dysfunctional marital interaction consists of inflexibility and a constriction of alternatives" (Gottman, 1994, p. 37), then the maintenance of satisfaction requires flexibility, openness, and creativity. This is hardly a unique perspective; others have also discussed methods for promoting flexibility (e.g., Cordova & Jacobson, Chapter 12), and an identified therapeutic component shared by all forms of therapy is providing individuals with "potentially helpful alternate ways of looking at themselves and their problems" (Frank, 1985, p. 65). Furthermore, in keeping with the model presented by Erbert and Duck (Chapter 8), the following suggestions are not offered as an "ideal" or "generalized" way of handling differences that people "should" follow as one would follow a recipe in a cookbook. Instead, the following suggestions are offered as *examples* of ways of fostering creativity, spontaneity, and flexibility in handling the inevitable difficulties and differences that arise between partners in close relationships. Throughout the sections that follow, I stress the importance of one's *appraisal* of one's partner, oneself, and one's life situation in maintaining satisfaction in close relationships.

Recognizing Alternate Explanations and Perspectives for a Partner's Behavior

One long-standing theme in psychology is that people are "naive psychologists" who attempt to explain the behavior of other people (Heider, 1958). Interestingly, it has been found that people make different explanations or "attributions" about their own behavior than they do about someone else's behavior—a difference referred to as the "actor–observer discrepancy" (Nisbett, Caputo, Legant, & Marecek, 1973). Specifically, an individual who performs an action (the "actor") commonly attributes the action to the situation, whereas another person who sees the same action (the "observer") is more likely to attribute it to the actor's internal characteristics.

As applied to close relationships, the actor–observer discrepancy suggests that individuals are likely to make different attributions for their own behavior than for their partners' behavior. For example, readers might ask themselves this question: "When my partner does something that bothers me, do I think that my partner is the cause of the behavior?" Or, more importantly, "If I were to engage in the same behavior, would I think that I was the cause of the behavior?" Readers who answer "yes" to the first question and "no" to the second question are among the many people who engage in actor–observer discrepancies in their attributions for interpersonal behavior.

Furthermore, the kinds of attributions people make for their partners' undesirable behavior varies as a function of their satisfaction with their relationships. A consistent finding in research on close relationships is that, compared to people in satisfied relationships, people who are unsatisfied with their relationships are more likely to believe that their partners' negative behavior is caused by their partners (for a review of this literature, see Bradbury & Fincham, 1990). The implication of this line of research is that developing alternative explanations for a partner's negative behavior should increase an individual's own satisfaction with the partner and the relationship.

How can awareness of attributions help to maintain satisfaction in close relationships? First, a person can look for alternate explanations for a partner's upsetting behavior—for example, a person may ask "Is there another reason for why my partner did X?" In searching for alternate explanations for the partner's behavior, the person might think of the kinds of explanations he or she would provide if he or she were acting like the partner. In addition, awareness of the reciprocal relation between environmental and intrapersonal characteristics might encourage the person to think about environmental and situational explanations for the partner's behavior (e.g., "My partner is doing X because he [she] has been under stress at work").

Besides forming an explanation for "why" other people act the way they do, people often pass judgment on the behavior of others. That is, a person may be upset with a partner not only because he or she did something that bothered the person, but also because implicit in the person's perspective is the belief that the partner "should do something about it" (i.e., the partner should be able to change). Indeed, a sizeable body of research (as reviewed by Bradbury & Fincham, 1990) suggests that people who are unsatisfied with their relationships are more likely to blame their partners and believe that the partner's negative behavior is intentional and selfishly motivated. As reviewed earlier, however, some characteristics that influence people's behavior are characteristics that are not readily amenable to change. For example, research suggests that there is considerable stability in personality characteristics in adulthood (as reviewed by Costa & McCrae, 1986). Furthermore, there is some evidence that relationship outcomes are genetically based (i.e., inherited). For example, in a study of over 1,500 same-sex twin pairs, McGue and Lykken (1992) reported that concordance for divorce was significantly higher for monozygotic (i.e., identical) than for dizygotic (i.e., fraternal) twins, thus suggesting a strong influence of genetic factors on divorce. Although no one is suggesting the existence of a "divorce gene," these findings suggest that there is a genetic influence on correlates of relationship satisfaction, such as personality characteristics. Recognizing that a partner's behavior may result in part from factors outside his or her control (e.g., genetics or early parental and familial relationships, as discussed by Young and Gluhoski, Chapter 14) may influence a person's emotional and behavioral reaction to the partner. Thus, not passing judgment on the partner's behavior (i.e., not blaming and holding him or her responsible for something that bothers the person) may serve to improve the person's relationship satisfaction, in part by encouraging greater tolerance and acceptance.

A recent development in couple therapy has been an emphasis on promoting "acceptance" between partners. This approach to treatment is described in greater detail in the chapters by Cordova and Jacobson (Chapter 12) and Christensen and Walczynski (Chapter 10). Under this treatment modality, partners in a relationship are encouraged to accept the inevitable differences that exist between them, instead of trying to change such differences. Preliminary research suggests that this approach to therapy improves satisfaction in couples, and that this improvement is mediated by greater acceptance. Thus, although these findings are in need of replication, they suggest that promoting acceptance holds promise for improving outcome in couple therapy. Although Cordova and Jacobson (Chapter 12) offer some guidelines, a major challenge facing clinicians promoting greater acceptance in relationships as a therapeutic intervention, however, is in teaching couples (and therapists!) which problems and behavior are amenable to change, and which are to be accepted.

Recognizing One's Own Intrapersonal Influences on Satisfaction

When people are having problems in their relationships, they most often look to their partners as the sources of the problems. The previous discussion of correlates of relationship satisfaction, however, would suggest that satisfaction is determined in part by one's *own* intrapersonal characteristics. That is, an individual may become upset with a partner because of something that the partner did (or didn't do), or because something that happened to the individual or the partner struck a chord with the individual's own intrapersonal characteristics (i.e., his or her own vulnerabilities).

The implication of this idea is that before blaming the partner or getting irritated, upset, or angry with him or her, the person might want to take a moment and see whether his or her reaction really stems from something about himself or herself. For example, a person may ask, "Am I hurt because my partner commented on my weight, or am I hurt because my weight is a vulnerable topic for me?" or "Was what my partner said or did really that insensitive, or is it that I viewed my partner's comment or behavior negatively because I have recently been feeling irritable?" Recognizing that the reaction arises in part from something about himself or herself may help reduce the person's negative emotional response (i.e., decrease reactivity to the partner's negative behavior), and may lessen the impact of the partner's behavior on the person's relationship satisfaction.

Recognizing the Role of Environmental Influences in Satisfaction

As reviewed in the section on correlates of satisfaction in close relationships, environmental factors such as stressful life circumstances can influence relationship satisfaction. Recognizing these environmental influences may have important implications for the maintenance of satisfaction.

One implication of recognizing the role of environmental influences concerns the kinds of explanations or attributions people make for declines in their relationship satisfaction. As previously reviewed, partners in unhappy relationships often attribute the cause of their problems to their partners (e.g., something about the partners' personalities). They are therefore more likely to blame their partners and to be angry with them. However, the current model suggests that the causes of many relationship problems may reside outside each partner and outside the relationship. For example, financial problems (e.g., unemployment) may make a person more reactive to perceived provocations from a partner. Similarly, relational problems with someone other than one's partner (e.g., problems with family members or friends) may increase the likelihood of feeling rejected by one's partner. Consequently, a person may ask, "Am I really feeling upset because of something my partner did, or is it because of something that is happening outside our relationship?" Identifying the presence of external factors may help to reduce the tendency to blame the partner, thereby increasing relationship satisfaction.

A second implication of recognizing environmental correlates of relationship satisfaction concerns problem solving about an issue. For example, stressful life circumstances often become divisive wedges that force partners apart because they take opposite positions regarding a problem. Furthermore, as discussed by Christensen and Walczynski (Chapter 10), partners often get into conflicts because of the attributions that each partner is making regarding the problem. However, viewing a problem as an external "it" may help partners become more problem-focused, and may thus draw them together as they work on a solution of how to solve the problem.

A third implication of recognizing environmental correlates of relationship satisfaction is related to helping heighten couples' awareness of high-risk situations for relationship problems before such problems occur. That is, keeping a watchful eye on environmental influences may help partners predict when they or their relationship may be vulnerable, and therefore when to take precautions to protect their relationship. To use an analogy, when there are warning signs of impending environmental changes in the weather (e.g., warning signs of a blizzard, tornado, or hurricane), people take precautions to protect themselves and their possessions (e.g., they install snow tires, they board up their windows). In similar fashion, by recognizing the warning signs of impending environmental influences on a relationship (e.g., increase in stress, major life transitions), partners can learn to take precautions to protect their relationship (e.g., doing something special for each other, being especially considerate of each other).

Summary and Recommendations

How couples handle conflict may be the single best predictor of success in close relationships (e.g., Gottman, 1994). Learning and improving methods for handling conflict, therefore, may be among the most important aspects of maintaining long-term satisfaction. Awareness of the multiple correlates of satisfaction (e.g., intrapersonal, interpersonal, and environmental), in particular, may influence a person's *appraisal* of his or her partner and their separate and mutual problems, and thus may contribute to constructive management of the inevitable conflicts that develop between two people involved in a close relationship. Such awareness may help couples to develop greater flexibility in solving problems that can be solved, and greater acceptance of problems that cannot be solved. Learning methods for maintaining relationship satisfaction may be difficult at first, just as learning any other skill may be, and there may be setbacks in which a person falls into old patterns. However, with practice, people can become more flexible, creative, and open in the ways in which they cope with the inevitable disagreements that arise between partners, and thus they can do more to maintain their satisfaction in their close relationships.

CONCLUSION

Since publication of the first book on psychological factors in happiness in marriage nearly 60 years ago (Terman et al., 1938), there has been a proliferation of theoretical and empirical articles addressing the assessment, understanding, and maintenance of satisfaction in close relationships. To paraphrase the quotation from *Anna Karenina* at the beginning of this chapter, upon entering into either the science of close relationships or an actual close relationship, one recognizes that understanding and maintaining relationship satisfaction look easy only from a distance. However, confronting the challenges inherent in the ever-changing processes addressed in this chapter and in this volume, although difficult, can be a "satisfying" (i.e., fulfilling) journey—both for the scientists who investigate satisfaction in close relationships and for the partners who seek to maintain relationship satisfaction. The closing comments written by Terman and colleagues (1938) are as relevant today as they were nearly 60 years ago:

> With every generation, new causes of marital [and relational] unhappiness become operative, and some of the earlier causes lose their effects. These changes in mores may be relatively slow, or they may come about with almost cataclysmic speed; in any case they call for endless modification of diagnostic and research procedures and for plasticity of interpretation on the part of all who use them. (p. 378)

REFERENCES

American Psychiatric Association. (1994). *Diagnostic and statistical manual of mental disorders* (4th ed.). Washington, DC: Author.

Baucom, D. H., Epstein, N., Sayers, S., & Sher, T. G. (1989). The role of cognitions in marital relationships: Definitional, methodological, and conceptual issues. *Journal of Consulting and Clinical Psychology, 57,* 31–38.

Bradbury, T. N., & Fincham, F. D. (1990). Attributions in marriage: Review and critique. *Psychological Bulletin, 107,* 3–33.

Carstensen, L. L., Gottman, J. M., & Levenson, R. W. (1995). Emotional behavior in long-term marriage. *Psychology and Aging, 10,* 140–149.

Christensen, A. (1988). Dysfunctional interaction patterns in couples. In P. Noller & M. A. Fitzpatrick (Eds.), *Monographs in social psychology of language: No. 1. Perspectives on marital interaction* (pp. 31–52). Clevedon, England: Multilingual Matters.

Costa, P. T., & McCrae, R. R. (1986). Personality stability and its implications for clinical psychology. *Clinical Psychology Review, 6,* 407–423.

Eddy, J. M., Heyman, R. E., & Weiss, R. L. (1991). An empirical evaluation of the Dyadic Adjustment Scale: Exploring the differences between marital "satisfaction" and "adjustment." *Behavioral Assessment, 13,* 199–220.

Fincham, F. D., & Bradbury, T. N. (1987). The assessment of marital quality: A reevaluation. *Journal of Marriage and the Family, 49,* 797–809.

Fitzpatrick, M. A. (1988). *Between husbands and wives: Communication in marriage.* Newbury Park, CA: Sage.

Frank, J. D. (1985). Therapeutic components shared by all psychotherapies. In M. J. Mahoney & A. Freeman (Eds.), *Cognition and psychotherapy* (pp. 49–79). New York: Plenum Press.

Gottman, J. M. (1979). *Marital interaction: Experimental investigations.* New York: Academic Press.

Gottman, J. M. (1993). The roles of conflict engagement, escalation, and avoidance in marital interaction: A longitudinal view of five types of couples. *Journal of Consulting and Clinical Psychology, 61,* 6–15.

Gottman, J. M. (1994). *What predicts divorce? The relationship between marital processes and marital outcomes.* Hillsdale, NJ: Erlbaum.

Gottman, J. M., & Krokoff, L. J. (1989). Marital interaction and satisfaction: A longitudinal view. *Journal of Consulting and Clinical Psychology, 57,* 47–52.

Green, D. P., Goldman, S. L., & Salovey, P. (1993). Measurement error masks bipolarity in affect ratings. *Journal of Personality and Social Psychology, 64,* 1029–1041.

Heavey, C. L., Christensen, A., & Malamuth, N. M. (1995). The longitudinal impact of demand and withdrawal during marital conflict. *Journal of Consulting and Clinical Psychology, 63,* 797–801.

Heavey, C. L., Layne, C., & Christensen, A. (1993). Gender and conflict structure in marital interaction: A replication and extension. *Journal of Consulting and Clinical Psychology, 61,* 16–27.

Heider, F. (1958). *The psychology of interpersonal relations.* New York: Wiley.

Karney, B. R., & Bradbury, T. N. (1995). The longitudinal course of marital quality and stability: A review of theory, method, and research. *Psychological Bulletin, 118,* 3–34.

Kelly, E. L., & Conley, J. J. (1987). Personality and compatibility: A prospective analysis of marital stability and marital satisfaction. *Journal of Personality and Social Psychology, 52,* 27–40.

Krokoff, L. J. (1987). Recruiting representative samples for marital interaction research. *Journal of Social and Personal Relationships, 4,* 317–328.

Levenson, R. W., Carstensen, L. L., & Gottman, J. M. (1994). Influence of age and gender on affect, physiology, and their interrelations: A study of long-term marriages. *Journal of Personality and Social Psychology, 67,* 56–68.

McGue, M., & Lykken, D. T. (1992). Genetic influence on risk of divorce. *Psychological Science, 3,* 368–373.

Miller, I. W., Kabacoff, R. I., Epstein, N. B., Bishop, D. S., & Keitner, G. I. (1994). The development of a clinical rating scale for the McMaster Model of Family Functioning. *Family Process, 33,* 53–69.

Newcomb, M. D., & Bentler, P. M. (1981). Marital breakdown. In S. Duck & R. Gilmour (Eds.), *Personal relationships 3: Personal relationships in disorder* (pp. 57–94). New York: Academic Press.

Nisbett, R. E., Caputo, C., Legant, P., & Marecek, J. (1973). Behavior as seen by the actor and as seen by the observer. *Journal of Personality and Social Psychology, 27*, 154–164.

Norton, R. (1983). Measuring marital quality: A critical look at the dependent variable. *Journal of Marriage and the Family, 45*, 141–151.

Sabatelli, R. M. (1988). Measurement issues in marital research: A review and critique of contemporary survey instruments. *Journal of Marriage and the Family, 50*, 891–915.

Spanier, G. B. (1976). Measuring dyadic adjustment: New scales for assessing the quality of marriage and similar dyads. *Journal of Marriage and the Family, 38*, 15–28.

Terman, L. M., Buttenweiser, P., Ferguson, L. W., Johnson, W. B., & Wilson, D. P. (1938). *Psychological factors in marital happiness.* New York: McGraw-Hill.

U. S. Bureau of the Census. (1992). *1990 census of population: General population characteristics: United States.* Washington, DC: U.S. Government Printing Office.

Vaillant, C. O., & Vaillant, G. E. (1993). Is the U-curve of marital satisfaction an illusion? A 40-year study of marriage. *Journal of Marriage and the Family, 55*, 230–239.

Weiss, R. L. (1980). Strategic behavioral marital therapy: Toward a model for assessment and intervention. In J. P. Vincent (Ed.), *Advances in family intervention, assessment and theory* (Vol. 1, pp. 229–271). Greenwich, CT: JAI Press.

Whisman, M. A., & Allan, L. E. (1996). Attachment and social cognition theories of romantic relationships: Convergent or complementary perspectives? *Journal of Social and Personal Relationships, 13*, 263–278.

Whisman, M. A., Dixon, A. E., & Johnson, B. (in press). Therapists' perspectives of client problems and treatment issues in couple therapy. *Journal of Family Psychology.*

Whisman, M. A., & Jacobson, N. S. (1992). Change in marital adjustment following marital therapy: A comparison of two outcome measures. *Psychological Assessment, 4*, 219–223.

White, S., & Hatcher, C. (1984). Couple complementarity and similarity: A review of the literature. *American Journal of Family Therapy, 12*, 15–25.

Author Index

Acitelli, L. K., 115, 116, 195, 204, 337
Addis, M. E., 264
Adler, N. L., 57, 201
Adler, Z., 307
Agostinelli, J., 208
Ainsworth, M. D. S., 27, 30, 31, 34, 35, 48
Albersheim, L. J., 34
Albrecht, S. L., 130, 197
Algeier, E. R., 17
Allan, L. E., 401
Allen, A., 115
Alpern, L., 33
Altman, I., 137, 192, 193, 194, 197, 205
American Psychiatric Association, 317, 389
Amato, P. R., 102
Amolozo, T. O., 142, 190, 339
Anderson, S., 164
Anderson, S. A., 339
Andrews, B., 307
Andrews, D. W., 190, 195
Antonucci, T. C., 44, 337
Applegate, B., 58
Argyle, M., 163, 165, 183
Arias, I., 115, 121
Aristotle, 97
Aron, A., 69, 79, 86, 87, 138, 338
Aron, A. P., 79
Aron, E. N., 79, 138
Aseltine, R. H., 307

Asher, S. J., 102
Attridge, M., 60, 148, 152, 155
Augustine, 84
Aved, B. M., 307
Ax, A. F., 222

Babcock, J. C., 266
Badura, B., 307
Bailey, J., 289
Bakhtin, M. M., 191, 192, 193, 194, 202, 206
Banmen, J., 278
Barnard, K. E., 32
Barnas, M. V., 46
Barnes, M. L., 62, 79–101, 137
Barnett, D., 31
Barnett, P. A., 336
Bartholomew, K., 36, 38, 41, 43
Barry, W. A., 253
Bassili, J. N., 290
Baucomb, D. H., 118, 120, 293, 297, 309, 348, 393
Baxter, L. A., 191, 192, 193, 194, 201, 202, 204, 205, 207–208, 209
Beach, R. H., 115, 121
Beach, S. R. H., 275–304, 307, 308, 388
Beall, A. E., 61, 86, 87
Beck, A. T., 356
Beeghly, M., 32
Beeghly-Smith, M., 32
Behrens, B. C., 348

Bellack, A. S., 277
Belsky, J., 30, 32, 261
Benesch, K. F., 108, 109
Bengston, V. L., 163, 164, 183, 285
Benim, M. H., 208
Benoit, D., 41
Benson, H., 245
Bentler, P. M., 12, 82, 115, 400
Berger, P., 115, 116, 117
Berlin, L. J., 32, 33
Bernard, J., 185
Bernstein, M., 87
Berscheid, E., 60, 61, 79, 84, 97, 115,
    129–159, 274
Best, P., 115, 118
Betzig, L., 7, 8, 18
Biblarz, T. J., 209
Bienvenu, M. J., 278
Bifulco, A., 307
Billings, A. G., 307
Billig, M., 192
Biringen, Z., 42
Birtchnell, J., 307
Bishop, D. S., 389
Blades, J., 102
Blair, G. E., 208, 209
Blair, S. L., 201
Blais, M. R., 149
Blascovich, J., 291
Blaylock, B., 115
Blehar, M. C., 30
Blood, R. O., 2, 164
Bloom, B. L., 102
Blumberg, S. L., 47, 342, 348
Blustein, D. L., 38
Boles, A. J., 353
Bonnell, D., 185
Booth, A., 142, 149, 156, 190, 286,
    339
Booth, C. L., 32
Bowlby, J., 26, 27, 28, 29, 46, 48, 109,
    228
Bradburn, N. M., 163, 285, 286
Bradbury, T. N., 119, 120, 121, 130,
    148, 153, 190, 195, 201, 202, 203,
    249, 250, 257, 260. 261, 278, 281,
    282, 287, 294, 337, 338, 396, 399,
    402, 404
Bradshaw, D., 28, 79–80
Braunwald, K., 31
Brengelmann, J. C., 309
Brennan, K. A., 28, 39, 41

Bretherton, I., 32, 42
Brett, J., 208
Bridge, L., 307
Brinton, C., 41
Broderick, C. B., 252
Broderick, J. E., 201
Brodsky, A., 80
Bromet, E. J., 307
Brown, B. B., 137, 192, 194
Brown, D., 7, 8, 23
Brown, G. W., 307, 374, 375
Buck, R., 61
Buehlman, K. T., 118–119
Bugaighis, M. A., 78, 303
Bumpass, L., 102, 129
Burgess, E. W., 12, 336
Burleson, B. R., 65
Burman, B., 275
Burnett, C. K., 307
Buss, D. M., 7–25, 60, 61, 80, 137,
    226, 393
Buttenweiser, P., 102, 386
Buunk, B. P., 202, 250
Byrne, D., 80, 115

Cacioppo, J. T., 224
Callan, V. J., 43, 185
Campbell, B., 60, 134–135, 146–147,
    150
Cannon, C., 339
Cannon, K., 164
Cannon, W. B., 222
Caputo, C., 403
Carlson, E., 33
Carlson, V., 31
Carnelley, K. B., 40
Carroll, J. B., 80
Carstensen, L. L., 44, 45, 114
Carter, L., 220
Cassidy, J., 29, 32, 33, 230
Cate, R. M., 201, 202
Catlin, G., 109–110
Cattell, R. B., 80
Chaiken, S., 283
Chevron, E., 308
Choo, P., 68
Christian, J. L., 307
Christensen, A., 158, 202, 205,
    249–274, 309, 313, 342, 344, 396,
    405, 407
Cicchetti, D., 31, 32
Cicirelli, V. G., 45

Clark, C. L., 28, 35
Clark, L. A., 285, 300
Clements, M. L., 155, 197, 250,
335–355, 341, 348, 397
Clore, G. L., 80
Cohn, D. A., 42
Cole, C., 183
Cole, H. E., 37
Collins, N. L., 28, 39, 41
Conley, J. J., 12, 137, 249, 260, 390
Connell, M. M., 307
Contreras, R., 65, 69
Conville, R. L., 193
Conway, B. E., 87
Copeland, J. M., 78, 303
Cordova, A. D., 335–355
Cordova, J. V., 307–334, 397, 403,
405
Cornforth, M., 192, 194
Cornwall, M., 170
Corsini, R. J., 115
Cortese, A., 78
Cosmides, L., 7
Costa, P. T., 404
Cottrell, L. S., 336
Cowan, C. P., 42, 340
Cowan, P. A., 42, 353
Coysh, W. S., 353
Craddock, A. E., 115, 116
Cramer, L., 149
Cronkite, R. C., 307
Crosby, J. F., 281
Cross, D. G., 282
Crouter, A., 340
Cummings, E. M., 46, 243
Curtis Boles, H., 353

Dahlstrom, W. G., 291
Daly, M., 7, 8, 9, 10, 14, 15, 18, 19
Davies, P. T., 243
Davis, K. B., 336
Davis, K. E., 28, 39, 41, 65, 67, 79,
85
Dawson, D. A., 102
de Werth, C., 14, 19
Deimling, G., 46
DeLillo, D. A., 206
Denton, W. H., 65
Deutsch, M., 201
Dindia, K., 208
Dion, K. K., 2, 81
Dion, K. L., 2, 81

Dixon, A. E., 395
Dobasch, R. E., 14
Dobasch, R. P., 14, 19
Dobson, K., 308
Doherty, R. W., 68
Dougher, M. J., 308, 309
Douvan, E., 116, 275, 336
Dozier, M., 37
Duby, G., 160
Duck, S. W., 79, 190–216, 388, 400,
402, 403
Dugan, E., 45
Duncan, S. W., 307
Dunn, R. L., 338, 348
Duran, R. L., 206
Dutton, D. G., 79

Eagly, A. H., 283
Eckland, B. K., 11
Eddy, J. M., 300, 387
Edmunds, V. H., 185
Edwards, J. N., 286
Egeland, B., 31, 32
Eidelson, R. J., 118, 119
Eisenstadt, D., 289
Ekman, P., 222
Elder, G. H., Jr., 11
Elicker, J., 33, 49
Ellis, A., 120
Emerson, C., 191
Emery, G., 356
Englund, M., 33
Epstein, E., 7, 8, 23
Epstein, N. B., 110, 118, 119, 297,
389, 393
Epstein, S., 104, 105, 109–110, 111
Erbert, L. A., 190–216, 388, 400, 402,
403
Erickson, M. R., 32
Ernst, J. M., 301
Esterly, E., 118

Farber, E., 31
Fazio, R. H., 149, 290–291, 300
Feeney, J. A., 40, 41, 43, 160–189,
234, 395, 396
Fehr, B., 62, 73, 86
Feldman, H., 164, 285
Felmlee, D. H., 73
Ferenz-Gillies, R., 37
Ferguson, L. W., 102, 386
Fernandes, L. O., 120, 278

Ferreira, A. J., 115
Ferster, C. B., 318, 327
Festinger, L., 142
Field, D., 185
Fincham, F. D., 119, 120, 121, 149,
  190, 195, 201, 202, 203, 204, 227,
  250, 257, 260, 275–304, 337, 338,
  387, 388, 393, 401, 404
Fine, M. A., 58
Finkel, J. S., 164
Fisher, H. E., 7
Fitzpatrick, J. H., 201–202
Fitzpatrick, M. A., 115, 118, 198, 200,
  206, 401
Fleming, A. S., 340
Fleming, W. S., 37
Fletcher, G. J. O., 39, 143, 149
Floyd, F. J., 197, 348
Foley, S. H., 308
Follette, V. M., 309
Follette, W. C., 265
Fowers, B. J., 58, 209, 281, 337
Frank, J. D., 403
Frazier, P. A., 118
Freedman, J., 129
Frenkel, O. J., 31
Freud, S., 81, 108
Friesen, W. V., 222
Fruzzetti, N. E., 308
Furnham, A., 163, 165, 183

Gamble, W., 37
Gangestad, S. W., 147
Gano-Phillips, S., 292
Garnier, P. C., 292
Garret, E., 353
George, C., 34
Ghiselin, M. T., 15
Gilford, R., 163, 164, 183, 285
Gilligan, C., 339
Gilner, F., 81
Ginat, J., 194
Ginsberg, G. P., 204
Glenn, N. D., 11, 57–58, 129, 148,
  190, 195, 276
Glucksberg, S., 115
Gluhoski, V. L., 356–381, 393, 405
Goldberg, L., 12
Goldberg, S., 31
Goldman, S. L., 388
Goldsamt, L. A., 261
Goldsmith, D., 192

Gonso, J., 346
Gosse, R., 102
Gotlib, J. H., 275, 336
Gottman, J. M., 45, 47, 48, 102, 114,
  115, 118–119, 190, 195, 196, 197,
  198, 199, 200, 201, 202, 203, 206,
  219, 235, 236, 245, 251, 279, 343,
  346, 348, 395, 396, 401, 402, 403,
  407
Grajek, S., 80, 81, 85, 87, 91
Gray, J., 206
Graziano, W., 139
Green, D. P., 388
Greenberg, L. S., 49
Greenberg, M. T., 32
Griffin, D. W., 283
Grossman, K. E., 33
Groth, G., 7
Guldner, G. T., 58
Gurman, A. S., 309
Guthrie, D. M., 171
Guttman, R., 7, 8, 23

Hackbert, L., 312
Hackel, L. S., 340
Hahlweg, K., 264, 309, 338, 339, 348
Halverson, C. F., 65
Hamilton, G. V., 336
Hammock, G., 62
Hammond, J. R., 39
Hansen, F. J., 164
Harel, Z., 46
Harlow, H., 79
Harris, T., 307
Hartigan, J., 91
Harvey, J. H., 158, 274
Hass, R. G., 289, 296
Hatch, R. C., 78, 303
Hatcher, C., 115, 396
Hatfield, E., 41, 60, 61, 67, 68, 74, 79,
  83, 97
Haven, C., 44
Hayes, S. C., 309, 312
Hazan, C., 28, 35, 36, 37, 41, 43, 48,
  62, 67, 79, 85, 230, 231, 233–234
Heaton, T. B., 130, 197
Heavey, C. L., 202, 205, 251, 259,
  342, 347, 396
Hecht, M. L., 69, 71
Hegel, G. W. F., 191–192, 193
Heider, F., 117, 145, 403

Heming, G., 353
Hendrick, C., 56–78, 85, 201, 394
Hendrick, S. S., 56–78, 85, 201, 394
Henkemeyer, L., 338
Henton, J. M., 202
Heron, N., 149
Hesse, E., 31, 34
Heyman, R. E., 250, 261, 277, 279, 300, 387
Hindy, C. G., 41
Hocker, L. J., 201
Hoffman, J. A., 309
Hojjat, M., 102–126, 397
Holman, T. B., 208
Holmes, J. G., 149
Holquist, M., 191
Holtzworth-Munroe, A., 265, 309
Holzinger, K. J., 80
Homans, G., 139
Honeycutt, J. M., 195
Hong, G. K., 109
Hops, H., 256
Horn, J. L., 80
Horowitz, L. M., 36, 38, 41
Horwitz, A. V., 307
Houseknecht, S. K., 340
Houts, R. M., 260
Howes, P. W., 307, 338
Huba, G. J., 82
Humphreys, K., 120, 279
Huston, T. L., 158, 194, 196, 203, 260, 338, 340, 341
Hutt, M., 37

Ibrahim, F. A., 104, 105, 116
Ilfield, F. W., Jr., 316
Inman-Amos, J., 65, 66
Isabella, R. A., 30, 31
Izard, C. E., 222

Jacobson, N. S., 253, 258, 262, 264, 265, 266, 271, 281, 296, 300, 307–334, 336, 387, 403, 405
Jacquart, M., 208
Jamieson, K., 348
Janoff-Bulman, R., 104
Jarvis, I. L., 261
Jaspers, J. M., 227
Johnson, B., 386, 395
Johnson, D. J., 147
Johnson, D. R., 142, 148, 190, 195, 286, 339

Johnson, M. P., 133–134, 137, 138, 140, 144, 152
Johnson, S. M., 149
Johnson, W. B., 102
Joiner, T. E., 375
Jones, M. E., 118, 119
Jordan, P. L., 347
Julien, D., 337

Kahn, H., 104, 105, 116
Kahn, R. L., 44
Kalma, A. P., 14, 19
Kamo, Y., 69
Kaplan, K. J., 285, 286
Kaplan, N., 29, 33, 34, 230
Karney, B. R., 121, 130, 148, 153, 201, 249, 250, 251, 260, 261, 338, 396, 399, 402
Katz, I., 115, 289, 296
Katz, L. F., 118–119
Keith, B., 102
Keitner, G. I., 389
Kelley, H. H., 86, 130–131, 132–133, 135, 136, 138, 140
Kellner, H., 115, 116, 117
Kelly, E. L., 12, 137, 249, 260, 390
Kelly, G. A., 104, 109, 201, 207, 211, 257, 258
Kelsy, R. M., 301
Kemp-Fincham, S. I., 275–304, 388
Kenney, M. E., 38
Kenny, D. A., 115, 116
Kenrick, D. T., 7
Kerkstra, A., 250
Kessler, R. C., 307
Ketton, J. L., 87
Kinninmonth, L. A., 143
Kirkpatrick, L. A., 39, 41, 48
Kitayama, S., 2, 109
Klosko, J. S., 356
Kluckhohn, C., 105–106, 107, 111
Kluckhohn, F. R., 104, 105–106, 108, 110, 116
Kniskern, D. P., 309
Koback, R. R., 37, 38, 43, 49
Koch, W. R., 226
Kohlenberg, R. J., 312
Koltko-Rivera, M. E., 125
Koski, L. R., 26–55, 62, 394, 397, 399
Kraft-Hanak, S., 342
Krauss, R., 115

Krokoff, L. J., 102, 114, 196, 199, 201, 203, 235, 390, 402
Kroonenberg, P. M., 31
Kulka, R. A., 275, 336
Kurdek, L. A., 137, 155, 202, 340

LaFraniere, P. J., 32
Lang, F. R., 44
Lang, M., 340
Langis, J., 209
Larkey, L. K., 69
Larsen, H. L., 162
Larsen, R. J., 9
Larson, J. H., 63, 202
Larus, J. M., 348
Lashley, S. L., 219–248, 397
Latty-Man, H., 65, 85
Laurenceau, J.-P., 335–355, 397
Layne, C., 202, 342, 396
Lazarus, A., 374, 375
Lazarus, C., 374, 375
Lazarus, R. S., 222–223, 227
Lee, G. R., 129
Lee, J. A., 62, 70, 74, 80, 85, 97
Legant, P., 403
Lemke, L. K., 202
Lemryre, L., 307
Leonard, K. E., 43, 121
Lerma, M., 147
Lerner, H., 220
Lerner, R. M., 162, 164, 171
Levenson, R. W., 45, 114, 195, 197, 198, 199, 201, 222, 279, 401
Levinger, G., 1–4, 133, 137, 139, 140, 274
Levitskaya, A., 78
Levy, M. B., 28, 41
Lewin, K., 133
Lewis, R. A., 63, 160, 161–162, 163, 165–167, 168–169, 172–173, 175, 177, 181–183, 186–187, 278, 337
Lindahl, K., 155, 250, 251
Linfield, K., 286, 287, 288, 300
Lipkus, I., 43
Lively, E. L., 276
Lloyd, S. A., 201, 202
Locke, H. J., 155, 198, 276, 336
Long, E. C., 190, 195
Lopes, J., 129–159
Lowenthal, M. F., 44
Luckey, E. B., 164
Lussier, Y., 209

Lye, D. N., 208, 209
Lykken, D. T., 405
Lyons-Ruth, K., 33

MacDermid, S. M., 338
MacDougall, E., 277
Main, M., 29, 30, 31, 32, 33, 34, 230
Malamuth, M. M., 251, 396
Marecek, J., 403
Margolin, G., 235, 250, 251, 253, 258, 262, 275, 309
Marini, M., 163
Marini, M. M., 286
Markman, H. J., 47, 48, 152–153, 155, 203, 219, 226, 231, 235, 236, 245, 250, 251, 264, 307, 335–355, 397
Marks, S. R., 200
Markus, H. R., 2, 109, 292, 293
Marsella, A. J., 108, 109
Marston, P. J., 69
Martin, J. D., 201
Martin, T., 102, 129
Maslow, A. H., 83–84
Mathes, E. W., 81
Mathieu, M., 208
McAdams, D. P., 97
McAllister, I., 114, 115
McCabe, S. B., 275
McCall, G. J., 200, 206
McClintock, E., 158, 274
McCrae, R. R., 404
McCubbin, H. I., 162
McDonald, K., 226
McGoldrick, M., 116
McGue, M., 405
McGuire, W., 107
McHale, S. M., 338, 340
McKay, J., 220
McKay, M., 102, 220
McNew, S., 32
Medvin, N., 62
Meens, J. M., 78
Meens, L. D., 303
Mellen, S. L., 61
Mendell, N. R., 307
Merrick, S. K., 34
Middleton, C. F., 65
Miller, I. W., 389
Miller, W. R., 323
Millon, T., 366
Minirth, F., 220
Monroe, S. M., 307

Monsma, B. R., 208
Montgomery, B., 191, 192, 193, 194, 196, 201, 205, 208, 209
Moos, R. H., 307
Morisset, H., 32
Morris, C., 60
Morson, G. S., 191
Moss, M. S., 45
Moss, S. Z., 45
Mullins, L. C., 45
Murstein, B. I., 73, 81, 84, 139–140
Muxen, M. J., 162

Nelligan, J. S., 41
Nelson, G. M., 307
Nevels, R., 201
Newcomb, M. D., 12, 115, 400
Newcomb, T. M., 117
Nisbett, R. E., 403
Nock, S. L., 148
Noller, P., 41, 43, 160–189, 171, 185, 190, 395
Norman, W. T., 12
Norton, R., 163, 167, 276, 281, 282, 292, 387
Notarius, C. I., 47, 48, 219–248, 342, 343, 346, 347, 397, 402–403
Nygren, A., 96, 97
Nye, F. I., 277

Obiorah, F. C., 78, 303
Ochs, E., 202
O'Leary, K. D., 201, 280, 285, 307, 308, 317
O'Leary, L. D., 201
Olson, D. H., 58, 162, 164, 171
Omoto, A. M., 97
Orden, S. R., 163, 285, 286
Osborne, L. N., 292
Osgood, C. E., 281

Paff-Bergen, L. A., 78, 303
Pagel, M., 265, 309
Palladino-Schultheiss, D., 38
Paris, B. L., 164
Parker, K. C. H., 41
Parkes, C. M., 104
Pasch, L., 261
Patterson, G. R., 256
Patton, D., 336
Paulhus, D. L., 82
Paykel, E. S., 307

Pearson, J., 42
Peele, S., 80
Pensky, E., 261
Peplau, L. A., 158, 274
Peterson, D. R., 158, 274
Petty, R. E., 224
Pfaff, H., 307
Philliber, W. W., 209
Pietromonaco, P. R., 40
Pinsof, W. M., 309
Pistole, M. C., 39, 41, 202
Plato, 97
Pollina, L., 46
Pomerantz, B., 58
Ponterotto, J. G., 108, 109
Potapova, E., 78
Potter-Efrom, R., 220
Powell, J. S., 80
Powell, M. C., 291
Preto, N., 116
Prezioso, M. S., 38
Prusank, D. T., 206

Rapson, R., 60, 68, 74
Rausch, H. L., 2
Rawlins, W. K., 194, 200
Read, S. J., 28, 39, 41
Reik, T., 82, 84
Reis, H. T., 137, 138
Rempel, J. K., 149
Renick, M. J., 197, 348
Repecholi, B., 33
Repetti, R. L., 261
Revenstorf, D., 309
Rhodes, N., 337
Rholes, W. S., 41
Richardson, D. R., 62, 64
Ridgeway, D., 32, 42
Riso, L. P., 307
Rizzo, N., 289
Robertson, J., 29
Rodin, M. J., 286
Rogers, P. D., 102, 220
Rokeach, M., 104
Rollins, B. C., 164, 285, 339
Rosch, E., 86
Roskos-Ewoldsen, D. R., 291
Rotheram, M. J., 209
Rotter, J., 108
Rounsaville, B. J., 308
Rovine, M., 30
Rubin, T. J., 220

Rubin, Z., 79, 81, 97
Ruble, D. N., 340
Ruckdeschel, K., 49
Rusbult, C. E., 43, 132, 140, 147
Rush, A. J., 356
Russell, C. S., 185, 339
Russell, J. A., 86
Russell, R. J. H., 58
Rychlak, J. F., 193
Rygh, J., 374, 375

Sabatelli, R. M., 58, 195, 198, 386–387
Sabourin, S., 149, 209
Sacher, J. A., 58
Sadella, E. K., 7
Salomon, K. L., 301
Salovey, P., 388
Saltzburg, J. A., 261
Salusky, S., 308
Sanders, M. R., 348
Satir, V., 234
Sayers, S. L., 115, 277, 393
Sceery, A., 38
Schaap, C., 250, 251
Schaefer, E. S., 307
Scharfe, E., 41, 43
Schindler, L., 309
Schmaling, K. B., 265, 308, 309
Schmidt, N. B., 375
Schmitt, D. P., 7, 8, 9, 10, 23
Schott, T., 307
Schuum, W. R., 58, 164, 281, 339
Schuster, T. L., 307
Schwabel, A. L., 348
Schwartz, D. J., 41
Schwartz, G. E., 222
Scott, C. K., 203, 294
Seccombe, K., 129
Seligman, C., 149
Seligman, M. E., 323
Semmelroth, J., 9
Senchak, K., 129
Shackelford, T. K., 7–25, 60, 393
Sharpley, C. F., 282
Shaver, P. R., 26–55, 62, 67, 79, 85, 138, 230, 231, 233–234, 394, 397, 399
Shaw, B. F., 356
Shehan, C. L., 129
Shenk, J. L., 258, 261

Sher, T. G., 115, 348, 393
Sholomaskas, D., 308
Shotter, J., 204
Shulman, S., 33
Siavelis, R. L., 202
Silver, D. H., 42
Silverberg, S. B., 209
Silvern, L., 342
Simmel, G., 200, 201, 206
Simpson, J. A., 39, 40, 41, 60, 147, 152, 155
Singer, J. A., 222
Singer, I., 60, 96
Skinner, B. F., 265
Slough, N. M., 32
Slovik, L. F., 43
Slugoski, B. R., 204
Smith, D. A., 201, 285
Smith, G. T., 202, 208
Smith, J., 44, 292, 293
Smollen, D., 138
Snell, W. E., 226
Snyder, D. K., 58, 121, 175, 208, 271, 277, 280
Snyder, M., 97
Soble, A., 96, 97
Sokoloski, D. M., 66, 69
Solomon, J., 31, 33
Spanier, G. B., 63, 160, 161–162, 164, 165–167, 169, 171, 172–173, 175, 177, 181–183, 186–187, 276, 278, 281–282, 336, 337, 387
Spearman, C., 80, 81
Sperling, M. B., 79
Spieker, S. J., 32
Sprecher, S., 60, 67, 69, 79, 87
Sroufe, A. L., 32, 33
Sroufe, L. A., 27
Srull, T. K., 292
Stangor, C., 340
Stanley, J., 47
Stanley, S. M., 152–153, 197, 342, 344, 345, 346, 348
Stanton, A. L., 118, 119
Steinberg, L., 209
Steiner, S. C., 307
Sternberg, R. J., 61, 62, 67, 79–101, 394
Stone, L., 1
Storaasli, R. D., 307, 338, 348
Strodtbeck, F. L., 104, 105–106, 108, 110, 116

Stuart, R. B., 262, 263
Suci, E. J., 281
Sue, D., 106, 107–108, 109
Sue, D. W., 104, 106, 107–108, 109
Suitor, J. J., 208
Sullivan, B. O., 83, 121
Sullivan, D. J., 219–248, 397
Sullivan, K. T., 12, 201, 338
Swensen, C. H., 58, 81
Symons, D., 11

Tannen, D., 171, 185
Tannenbaum, P. H., 281
Taylor, D. G., 30
Taylor, P. A., 11
Telch, M. J., 375
Tellegren, A., 285, 300
Tennov, D., 82
Terman, L. M., 102, 336, 386, 408
Tesser, A., 82
Thibaut, J. W., 130–131, 140
Thomas, D. L., 170
Thompson, J. S., 121
Thompson, K., 68
Thompson, M. M., 283, 285, 289
Thompson, T., 115
Thomson, G., 88
Thurstone, L. L., 80
Ting-Toomey, S., 202
Todd, M. J., 65, 67, 79
Tomaka, J., 301
Tooby, J., 7
Treboux, D., 34
Trivers, R., 14, 19
Troll, L., 44
Trost, J. E., 276
Trost, M. R., 7
Troy, M., 32, 33
Truax, P., 271
Trull, T. J., 208
Tucker, P., 69, 338

Udry, J. R., 11, 137
U.S. Bureau of the Census, 390

Vaillant, C. O., 164, 339, 402
Vaillant, G. E., 164, 339, 401
Vallerand, R. J., 149
van den Boom, D. C., 42
van Ijzendoorn, M. H., 31, 41
Vandenberg, S., 7, 8, 23
Vangelisti, A. L., 194, 196, 203, 338, 341

VanLear, C. A., 205
Vannoy, D., 209
VanYperen, N. W., 202
Verette, J., 43
Vernon, P. E., 80
Veroff, J., 116, 275
Vinsel, A., 192
Vivian, D., 201
Vogel, N. A., 278
Volosinov, V. N., 192
von Eye, A., 30

Walczynski, P. T., 249–274, 396
Wall, S., 30
Wallace, K. M., 155, 198, 336
Wallen, P., 12
Waller, N. G., 42
Wallin, P., 102, 336
Walster, E., 61, 67, 83, 123
Walster, E. H., 79, 97
Walster, G. W., 61, 67, 83
Waltz, M., 307
Wampler, K. S., 65
Wampold, B. E., 235
Ward, C., 160–189, 395
Waring, E. M., 336
Waters, E., 27, 30, 34, 49
Watson, D., 285, 287, 300
Weaver, C. N., 129
Weghorst, S. J., 9, 10
Weinberger, D. A., 222
Weiner, N., 209
Weishaus, S., 185
Weiss, R. L., 250, 261, 291, 307, 387,
    400, 405, 407
Weissman, M. M., 307, 308
Wells, P. A., 58, 185
Werner, C. M., 137, 192, 194, 201,
    202
West, L., 204
Westbay, L., 86, 87
Westen, D., 9
Wetzler, S., 220
Whelan, M., 337
Whisman, M. A., 300, 307, 385–410
White, H. R., 307
White, J. M., 117
White, L. K., 130, 134, 149, 156, 276,
    286
White, S., 396
White, S. G., 115, 116
White, S. W., 102

Whitney, G. A., 43
Wiederman, M. W., 17
Wilmot, W. W., 193, 201
Williams, C. J., 290–291
Wilson, D. P., 102, 386
Wilson, E. O., 7, 8, 9, 16
Wilson, M. A., 10, 14, 18, 19, 162
Winch, R. F., 253
Winter, W. D., 115
Wolfe, D. M., 164
Woll, S. B., 62, 64
Wood, J. T., 196, 197, 200, 201, 207
Wood, J. V., 261

Wood, W., 337
Wyer, R. S., 292

Yelsma, P., 202
Yogev, S., 202
Young, J. E., 356–381, 405
Yum, J. O., 108, 109

Zanna, M. P., 149, 283
Zavalloni, M., 103
Zimbardo, P. G., 108
Zimmer, T. A., 148
Zuo, J., 198

Subject Index

Abandonment, fear of, 360, 362
Abusive relationships, 360, 362
Acceptance, emotional, 266-270,
   309-331, 365-366, 405, 407
  components of, 310-313
  techniques, 313-316
  unconditional, 358
Adaptive challenges, 8-10, 229, 319
Adjustment, marital, 57, 65, 170, 277
  vs. satisfaction, 195
Adolescence, 240-243, 357
  relationship styles in, 34, 36, 37
Adult Attachment Interview (AAI),
  34-35, 36, 37, 41, 42
  predictive capability of, 42
Affect-regulating emotions/defenses, 28,
  29
Affection, 57, 72, 173, 357
Agape, 62, 64, 75, 85, 97
  and Eros, 96-97
  as satisfaction predictor, 66
Age
  and longitudinal vs. cross-sectional
    reports, 164-165
  and mate value, 11
Agreeableness, 12-13, 15, 22
Alcohol abuse, 13, 20, 21
Ambivalence; see Anxious-ambivalent
  feelings
Anger, 4, 219-246
  behavioral expressions of, 223-224
  components of, 221-224, 225

definition of, 220, 221
examples of, 224-225, 230-231,
  237-238, 240-244
handling, 220, 235-238, 241-243,
  245-246
vs. hurt, 225, 239; see also Self-
  esteem
sources of, 18-19, 228-230, 245
riggers of, 226-228
Anxious-ambivalent feelings, 30-31,
  32-33, 85, 229
in adolescents, 37
in adult relationships, 35, 40-41,
  283-284, 288-289, 296, 362
and communication, 43
and social loneliness, 33, 38
in women, 39
Approval seeking, 361, 365
Asian society, 2, 69, 108, 109
Assumptions, 118, 393
Attachment; see also Parent-child attachment relationships
adult styles in, 34-36, 38-39, 85,
  231, 357-366, 394
categories, 30-36
developmental changes in, 29, 33,
  49, 230, 240
and emotion regulation, 28, 40
in infancy, 27-28, 29-31, 228-229
in marital relationships, 43,
  232-234, 283-284
in old age, 44-46

Attachment (*continued*)
  romantic, 35, 39, 394
  theory, 26–28, 29, 46, 47–49, 228,
    394
  transgenerational, 41
Attitude, 277, 281, 285, 289,
  290–294, 393
Attraction forces, 133
Attractiveness, physical, 10–11, 162,
  176, 180, 182, 183
Attribution process, 120–121,
  203–204, 249, 257, 260, 393,
  403–404
Autonomy vs. connectedness, 192,
  200, 207, 208, 209
Avoidance behavior, 201, 323–324, 375
Avoidant feelings, 30, 31, 32, 34, 85,
  201
  in marriage, 283–284, 288–289
  in young adults, 37–38, 39
  in romantic relationships, 35, 40, 41

Barrier forces, 133, 134, 140, 141
Behavior exchange, 262–263, 272, 313
Behavioral systems, 27, 107, 229
Behavioral therapy, 253, 262–271; *see
  also* Couple therapy
  clinical trials, 264, 271
  strategies, 262–264, 266–270
  traditional vs. integrative, 271, 272
Being vs. doing, 106, 107, 108–109
Beliefs, 103, 104, 111, 113, 200, 222;
  see also Philosophy of life
  dysfunctional, 119–120, 240
Bipolar adjective scales, 281, 286
Bipolar personality attributes, 12
Blame, 311, 314, 322, 329, 404, 406

Caregiving, 236–237
Caritas, 84
Centripetal–centrifugal forces,
  191–192, 202
Change process, 192–193, 202–205,
  289
  and acceptance, 266, 272, 308–313,
    330–331
  and behavioral therapy, 309–310
  and identity, 204
  and incompatibility, 254–255
  negotiated, 329–331
  and rigid repertoire, 318–319
  in schema-focused therapy, 377–380

Children
  and attachment encounters, 229–230
  cognitive/communication skills in, 32
  and core domains, 357–366
  effects of on marriage, 171–172,
    174, 180–181, 185–186, 261,
    340–341, 398–399
  and Strange Situation classifications,
    32–33, 34–35
Chronotope, 194
Cluster analysis, 91, 92, 93, 95
Coercion theory, 256
Cognition–behavior relations,
  290–298
  in marital therapy, 297–298, 348
Cognitive–experiential self-theory,
  110; *see also* Schema-focused
  therapy
Commitment, 65, 86, 131–133, 138,
  155n1, 350
  and investment model, 131–132
    personal-dedication, 351
  in premarital stage, 347
  and security, 148
  subjective experience of, 133
  and triangular theory of love, 62, 83,
    87
Communication, 43–44, 49, 117–118,
  184, 185, 187, 204
  and attribution, 112, 121
  avoiding, 48
  in long-term marriages, 45, 46
  and marital quality, 161, 162, 167,
    168, 171, 176–178, 180, 182,
    250, 395
  nonverbal, 43, 162, 349
  parent–child, 47
  patterns, 395–396
  sexual, 72
  training, 262, 263–264, 272, 313,
    348–350
Companionate love, 61–62, 66–68,
  83, 394
  in cross-cultural study, 69
  in hierarchical model, 91, 94, 96, 97
  maintaining, 72–73
Comparison level alternatives,
  130–132, 137
Compatibility
  loss of, 254–259
  in marriages without children, 180
Complementarity of needs, 253

Conflict, 205, 209
  areas for young couples, 342
  factors influencing, 260–262
  management, 219, 233, 342–343, 346, 352, 402, 407
  and polarization, 369
  as positive, 201, 236–238, 270, 326
  and relationship breakup, 249–272
  resolution, 47, 238, 243, 244, 261
  structure vs. process in, 251–252
  in therapy, 298
Congeniality, as factor in hierarchical model, 89, 90
Connection spectrum, 368, 369–371, 376, 377
Conscientiousness, 12, 13, 22
  and female infidelity, 14, 22
Consensus, 169, 170, 171–172, 180, 181, 185, 186
Contempt, 48, 114, 221, 396
Contradiction, 191, 196–202, 209–210, 211
  essential features of, 194
  in ideal vs. real, 202
  internal vs. external, 207, 209
  responses to, 207–208
  symbolic vs. materialistic, 193
Coping styles, 393
  assessment of, 375
  maladaptive, 369–371, 378–379
  practicing, 378–380
Core needs/domains, 356–366; *see also* Early maladaptive schemas
Couple therapy, behavioral, 262–271, 297, 348; *see also* Schema-focused therapy
  vs. cognitive therapy, 308
  and depression, 307, 329
  examples of, 319–322, 323–326, 327–328
  integrative, 266–272, 309, 312–318, 326, 329
Couple types, 198–199, 206, 401
Criticism, 48, 114, 361, 364, 396
Cupiditas, 84

Dating relationships
  and attachment style, 39–41
  predicting satisfaction in, 65
Deactivation strategy, 37, 38
Decision making, 344

Defensiveness, 48, 114, 225, 235, 242, 314
  and guilt feelings, 321
  and withdrawal, 267, 269, 396
Deficiency theory, 82, 83–84
Demand–withdraw pattern, 252, 259, 315, 396
Denver Family Development Study, 338
Dependence, 360, 363–364
Depression, 4, 307, 317
  repertoires in, 318–329
  resignation as, 310, 313
  symptoms of, 317–318
  therapy for, 316–331
Detachment, emotional, 229–230, 232
  unified, 268–269, 313, 314–315, 325, 326
Dialectical theory, 191–211
Dialogue, 193, 204–205
Disorganized/disoriented feelings, 30, 31, 33, 34
Divorce, 23, 49, 102
  predictors of, 119, 344–347, 405
  rates, 2, 7, 102, 160
  and societal conditions, 134
Dyadic Adjustment Scale (DAS), 58, 276, 277–283, 300, 387
  factors, 282

Early maladaptive schemas (EMSs), 359–380, 393
  assessment of, 373, 374–377
  and behavior, 367–368
  and coping styles, 368–372, 373, 378–380
  education about, 375, 379–380
  and overcompensation, 375
Emotional gratification, 161, 162, 167, 253
  deprivation of, 360, 363
Emotional manipulation, 17, 22
Emotional stability/instability, 12, 13, 22, 357, 360; *see also* Moodiness
  and infidelity, 19
  and physical abuse, 13, 15, 19
Empathic joining, 266–268, 313–314, 326, 358
  and hard vs. soft emotions, 314, 320–321
Endogenous forces, 142, 143–144, 147, 150, 154
Enmeshment, 358, 364–365

Entitlement, 362, 366
Environment, 139, 143–155, 156n4,
  392, 397–400, 406
  awareness of, 143, 144–145, 155
  change in, 319–320
  closed vs. open, 139–140
  exogenous vs. endogenous, 143–145,
    399
  exploring, 27, 29, 30, 227, 327–328
  manipulation of, 144, 145, 147,
    151–152, 155
  measuring, 152–153, 155; *see also*
    Quality–environment grid
  multifaceted, 194
Eros, 62, 63, 74, 75, 85, 96–97
  Agape in, 75, 96–97
  as satisfaction predictor, 64, 65–66,
    69, 74, 75
  strategies for maintaining, 71–72
  universality of, 68, 70, 74
Erosion theory, 342–352
  and conflict, 342–343
  and prevention strategies, 347–351
Escalation, 345, 346
Ethnic groups, 65, 68, 69, 390
Evaluation vs. descriptive assessment,
  163–164
Evolutionary psychology, 3, 7–23
  adaptive challenges in, 8–10
  and love, 60–61, 67–68, 71
  and mate guarding, 22
  and personality factors, 13–14
  and reproduction, 8–9, 18–19
Exogenous forces, 141–142, 143, 150,
  152
Experiential strategies, 377
Expressive speaking skills, 263
Extramarital relationships, 2

Facial expression, in anger, 222,
  235
Factor analysis, 89, 90–92
Field theory, 133
Flexibility, 316, 319, 403, 407
Friendship; *see* Companionate love,
  Peer relationships, Storge
Fulfillment, as factor in hierarchical
  model, 91
  and satisfaction index, 92, 93,
    95–96
Functional opposites, 201; *see also*
  Contradictions

Gender differences
  and communication, 171, 180, 185,
    396–397
  in conflict management, 342, 346,
    397
  in love styles, 62, 64, 65, 66
  in marital satisfaction, 337–339
  in relationship beliefs, 118, 122
Generalization, vs. individuality,
  206–207
Global Assessment of Relational
  Functioning, 389
Guilt, feelings of, 321

Happiness, 129, 156n5, 160, 194, 195,
  206; *see also* Satisfaction
  evaluation of, 210
Homogamy, 253, 392, 395, 396–397
Human nature, evaluation of, 105,
  107–108
Husbands
  complaints about wives, 13, 19, 23
  and mate value discrepancy, 12, 20,
    21
  and mental illness, 337
  and perceptions of marital satisfac-
    tion, 338–339
  and predictors of marital satisfaction,
    20, 22, 177–178
  and withdrawal, 345

Ideal relationship, 197–202
Identity, 202, 204, 222–223, 358, 364
Imagery, 373, 375–376, 377–378
Importance of Dyadic Interaction
  Scale, 166, 167, 169–171,
    174–178, 183–187
Individual differences, 63, 107
Individualism–collectivism, cultural,
  68, 106, 109
Infancy
  bonding in, 27
  exploratory behavior in, 27, 29, 30, 229
  and internal working models, 28
  and Strange Situation classification,
    30–31
Information processing, 290–294, 297,
  393–394
  automatic vs. controlled, 297, 300n4
Intelligence, theories of, 80, 81
Interdependence theory, 130–132,
  133, 137

Intermarriage, 116
Internal working models, 28, 40,
    46–47, 48, 229, 230
Intimacy, 67, 83, 87, 97, 142, 330, 350
    barriers to, 359–368
    and education level, 179
    as factor in hierarchical model,
        89–90, 91
    in ideal relationship, 197, 199
    in marriages without children, 172,
        180–181, 186
    in Quality Marriage Index, 168, 170,
        176, 180, 181–182, 183
    and satisfaction index, 92, 96
Invalidation, 345, 346
Involuntary relationships, 130, 140

Jealousy, 20, 21, 311–312
    provoking, 17

Kansas Marital Satisfaction Scale, 281,
    282

Learned helplessness, 323, 360
Life review, 373
Limerance, 82
Lineal systems, 106, 109
Locus of control, 108
Loss/separation experiences, 28, 29, 32,
    34, 35
    in college students, 37–38
Love, 56, 58–75, 79, 142
    components of, 83–84
    across cultures, 68
    definitions of, 81–82, 83, 96–97
    finding/keeping, 70–74
    hierarchical model of, 80, 87–96, 97
    kinds of, 59, 61–62, 83
    passionate (see also Eros) vs. compan-
        ionate, 61–62, 66–68, 83, 91,
        96, 97, 394
    psychometric studies of, 67, 81, 86–96
    and reality constraints, 82
    and sex, 81
    as story, 85–86
    styles, 59, 62–75, 85, 394
    theories of, 59–63, 79–87, 96–97
    and transition periods, 69
Love Attitudes Scale, 62, 66, 67, 69, 70
Ludus, 62, 64, 85
    as satisfaction predictor, 6, 66,
        70–71, 74–75

Mania, 62, 64, 85
    and culture, 68
    as satisfaction predictor, 64, 66, 75
Marital Adjustment Test (MAT),
    155n3, 276, 277, 279, 281–283,
    287–288, 292–294
Marital Communication Inventory, 278
Marital quality, 3, 130, 275–300; see
    also Satisfaction, Stability
    and attitude accessibility, 290–294,
        295, 297, 299, 300n4
    dimensions of, 162, 165–169,
        282–283, 297, 299
    and educational level, 170, 179
    and gender, 170–171, 179
    indexes of, 57, 163–164, 165–187,
        277–296
    over the lifespan, 162, 164–165,
        166, 171, 185
    model of, 161–162
    predictors of, 161, 162, 249, 277
    and religiosity, 170, 179
    two-dimensional approach to,
        282–289, 294–295
Marital Satisfaction Inventory (MSI),
    175, 178–179, 184, 271, 280, 282
Marital therapy; see Couple therapy,
    Psychotherapy
Marriage, 160; see also Marital quality,
    Spousal interaction
    and adaptation, 10
    breakup; see Conflict, Divorce
    cognitive factors in, 115, 118, 120
    in contemporary Western society, 2, 276
    danger signals in, 345–346
    evaluative judgments of, 281–283,
        291, 296, 299
    expectations of, 8, 393
    hedonic purpose of, 276
    negotiated, 1, 342
    in old age, 45, 46, 56–57
    positive vs. negative behaviors in,
        47–48
    predictive factors in, 12–15, 20–21,
        22, 249
    and reproduction, 9
    rewards of, 162, 165
    satisfaction in; see Satisfaction
    and societal change, 338
    statistics, 8, 129
    successful, 58, 130, 185, 195,
        197–202, 352

Marriage (*continued*)
  types of, 48, 198–199
  vows, 131, 142, 249
Mate-guarding tactics, 8, 16–19, 20,
    21, 22
Mate selection, 63, 70, 252–254
Mate value, 8, 10–12, 16, 21
  cross-correlation of, 11
  discrepancy in, 12
Memory; *see* Information processing
Monitoring, 2, 135, 343, 351
Moodiness, 19, 23
Multifactorial theory, of love, 83–84,
    96
Multimodal Life History Inventory,
    374, 375
Multiple-cluster theory, of love,
    84–85, 96
Mutual Need, as factor in hierarchical
    model, 89, 90, 91, 94
  and satisfaction index, 92, 96
Mutual Understanding, as factor in
    hierarchical model, 91
  and satisfaction index, 92, 96

Native Americans, 108, 109
Nature, relationship to, 105, 107, 108,
    109
Negative emotions, 220–221, 233,
    342–343
  reciprocity of, 395, 406
  regulating, 343
Neuroticism, 249, 250, 260, 393

Oblique rotation, 89
Openness/intellect, 12, 13
Oppositions, 201–202; *see also*
    Contradictions

Pair bonding, 61, 67
Parent–child attachment relationships,
    26–28, 29–34, 41–42, 43, 47,
    110, 357; *see also* Core
    needs/domains
  and aging parents, 45, 46
  and anger, 228–234, 239–240
  assessment of, 376
  communication in, 47
  negative interactions in, 359–366
  on quality–environment grid, 152
Passionate Love Scale, 67
Peer relationships, 38

Perceptual congruity, 117
Personality
  five-factor model of, 12–15
  and incompatibility, 260
Philosophy of life (POL), 103–122
  compatibility in, 103, 397
  Eastern, 108, 109
  formation of, 109–110
  joint, 117
  processes in, 106–107
  and relationship satisfaction, 104,
    106, 112–114, 115–118, 122,
    397
  reshaping of, 110–112, 113
  terms for, 104
Physical abuse, 14–15, 18–19, 22, 23
Physical arousal reactions, 222, 224
Physical size, 14, 19
Polarization, 257–259, 267, 309, 314,
    369–370, 379–380
Positive and Negative Affect Schedule,
    287
Positive regard, 161, 162, 167
Posttraumatic stress disorder (PTSD),
    110
Power spectrum, 371, 376
Pragma, 62, 64, 75, 85
Praxis, 193, 205–208
Prevention and Relationship Enhance-
    ment Program (PREP), 345,
    348–351
  booster sessions in, 349
  clergy-administered, 348
Problem-solving skills training, 262,
    264, 269, 272, 313, 349–350, 407
Psychotherapy, 49, 387; *see also* Couple
    therapy
  behavioral; *see* Behavioral therapy
  environmental, 145
  schema-focused, 4, 356, 373–380
  and therapeutic relationship, 378
Punitiveness, 361–362, 365–366

Quality, 195; *see also* Marital
    quality
Quality Marriage Index (QMI),
    167–168, 170, 199, 281, 292
Quality of Dyadic Interaction Scale,
    166, 167, 168–170, 171–181,
    183–187
Quality–environment (Q-E) grid,
    146–153, 154–155

Receptive listening skills, 263–264
Reconstituted families, 2
Reinforcement
  erosion, 253–254
  intermittent, 256
  mutual, 252–254, 260
  negative, 311–312
Reinventing Your Life, 373, 375
Relationship Assessment Scale, 58, 59, 64
Relationship Attribution Measure, 287
Relationship bank account (RBA), 342, 343, 349
Relationship Rating Form, 65, 67
Reproduction, 8–9, 11, 18–19, 61
  and mate guarding, 15
  and mate value, 11
Resource provisioning, 17–18, 21, 22
Respect, 169, 170, 176, 182, 358, 359
  in marriages without children, 172, 180, 186
Role fit, 161, 162, 167, 183
Role play, 270, 373, 379

Satisfaction, 28–29, 57, 58, 184–185, 190, 194–196, 210, 336–337; *see also* Marital quality
  and attribution process, 120–121, 203, 257, 260, 287–288, 393, 403–404
  correlates, 287, 380, 391–408
  costs/benefits, 10, 131–133, 146, 154
  dialectical perspective on, 191–211
  and dissatisfaction, 196–197, 199, 201, 205, 207; *see also* Conflict
  elements of, 3, 208–209
  and emotional schemes, 362–366
  environmental factors in, 143–152, 397–400, 406
  erosion theory of, 342–352
  gender differences in; *see* Gender differences
  and lifespan attachment, 26–49, 339, 401
  and love styles, 63–75
  maintaining, 70–74, 195, 201, 234, 330, 351, 402–408; *see also* Stability
  and mate-guarding tactics, 16–19
  measurement of; *see* Satisfaction measurement

  and perceptions of similarity, 65, 103, 116–118, 121, 137, 184, 396
  and personality attributes, 12–15, 39, 136–137, 249, 260, 393, 393–394
  and philosophy of life, 103–122
  predictors of, 20–21, 39, 42, 44, 47, 64–66, 96, 272, 407
  and relationship stability; *see* Stability
  and stressful events; *see* Stress
Satisfaction measurement, 58, 92–96, 190–191, 194, 210, 336, 386–389
  longitudinal vs. cross-sectional, 164–165, 186, 202, 203, 260, 402
  multimethod, 389, 391, 400–401
  sampling procedures in, 389–391
  by self-report questionnaire, 59, 91, 92, 136, 156n4, 165, 210, 277–278, 386–387, 400
  shared-method variance in, 388, 389
Schema-focused therapy, 4, 356, 373–380; *see also* Early maladaptive schemas
  components of, 373
  examples, 370–371, 374, 375–377
  individual work in, 377
  prototypical problems in, 374, 378
  techniques, 377–379
Scripts, 230, 231
Security, feelings of, 40, 46, 85
  in adolescents, 37
  in adults, 34, 35, 36, 357
  in infants and young children, 27–28, 30, 31, 32, 230, 357
  in men, 39
  need to enhance, 49
  in romantic relationships, 39–40, 41
  and verbal expression, 32, 43, 44
Self-actualization, 358, 361, 364–365
Self-care skills, 314, 316, 328–329
Self-esteem, 64, 228, 230, 233, 239–240
  and defectiveness/shame schema, 361, 365
  fostering, 40, 223, 234, 358
  threats to, 48, 222, 223, 226, 235, 239, 361–362
Self-expression, 357–358, 360, 363

Sentiment override hypothesis, 291–292, 400
Sexual fidelity/infidelity
  female, 8, 9, 14, 18, 19
  and jealousy, 17
  male, 10, 14
  and moodiness, 19, 23
  and physical abuse, 18
Sexuality, 72, 234
  as factor in hierarchical model, 89, 90, 91
  and satisfaction index, 92, 96
Similarity, 115–118, 121, 137, 162, 184, 396
  and mutual reinforcement, 260
  perceived vs. actual, 116–117
  in philosophy of life, 103, 397
Sincerity, as factor in hierarchical model, 89, 90, 91
  and satisfaction index, 92, 96
Social exchange theories, 130–135, 142, 152–154, 198, 201, 348
Social networks, 44–46, 161, 331, 389
Social skills, 33
Speaker–listener technique, 349–350
Spousal interaction, 160–186, 201
  curvilinear pattern in, 164, 166, 171, 180, 185–186
  cyclical, 205
  and dialogue, 204–205
  positive vs. negative, 199–202
  and presence of children, 171–172, 180–181, 186
  problem solving in, 207
  rewards, 162, 165, 168, 175–178, 186–187
Stability, in relationships, 203
  compelling/repelling forces in, 140, 141–143, 146, 148–152, 154, 155
  environmental influence on, 135, 139–141, 143–155
  and identity, 204
  and interaction patterns, 136, 138, 141–154; see also Spousal interaction
  predicting, 143, 145, 149, 152, 154
  and satisfaction, 142, 154, 156n4, 198, 203
  theories of, 130–135, 153–154
  threats to, 199
  and voluntariness, 139–140

Standards, 118, 393
  generalized, 206
Sternberg Triangular Theory of Love Scale, 67
Stimulus–value–role theory, 139–140
Stonewalling, 48, 114, 396
Storge, 62, 64, 74, 85
  Agape in, 75
  and age group, 69
  and culture, 68
  maintaining, 72–73
  as satisfaction predictor, 64, 66, 69, 74, 75
Strange Situation, 30–31, 34–35, 41, 42
Stress, 261–262, 397–399, 406–407
  and vulnerability, 398
Structural commitment, 133–134
Surgency, 12

Temperament, 42, 366–367
Time, focus on, 105–106, 107, 108, 112, 122
Togetherness, 197, 198, 199, 200
Tolerance building, 269, 311–312, 313, 315–316, 321–322, 326
Totality, 193–194, 208–210
  and context, 209
Transition periods, 69, 261–262, 340, 347, 398
Triangular theory, of love, 83, 87, 97
Trust, 142, 230, 391
  and commitment, 350
  as factor in hierarchical model, 91
  and satisfaction index, 92, 96
  and vulnerability, 311, 360, 362
Twin studies, 405

Unifactorial theory, of love, 81–82, 96

Value orientation, 105–106, 107, 111, 116
Vilification, 257

Withdrawal, 267, 269, 323, 342, 345
  mutual, 328
Wives
  ambivalent, 288
  complaints about husbands, 12–13, 15, 19
  and mate value discrepancy, 12
  and mental illness, 337

Wives (*continued*)
  and perception of marital satisfaction,
    338–339
  and predictors of marital satisfaction,
    21, 22, 177–178
  and resource investment, 17–18, 22

Young Compensation Inventory, 374,
  375
Young Parenting Inventory, 374, 376
Young Schema Questionnaire, 374, 375
Young–Rygh Avoidance Inventory,
  374, 375